S0-CEE-368

MEDICAL COMPLICATIONS OF MALIGNANCY

MEDICAL COMPLICATIONS OF MALIGNANCY

Edited by

Frank E. Smith, M.D.

Associate Professor
Departments of Pharmacology and Medicine
Associate Director
Clinical Cancer Training Program
Baylor College of Medicine
Houston, Texas

Montague Lane, M.D.

Departments of Pharmacology and Medicine
Clinical Cancer Training Program
Baylor College of Medicine
Houston, Texas

RC262
M425
1984

A WILEY MEDICAL PUBLICATION
JOHN WILEY & SONS
New York · Chichester · Brisbane · Toronto · Singapore

Copyright © 1984 by John Wiley & Sons, Inc.

All rights reserved. Published simultaneously in Canada.

Reproduction or translation of any part of this
work beyond that permitted by Sections 107 or 108
of the 1976 United States Copyright Act without the
permission of the copyright owner is unlawful. Requests
for permission or further information should be addressed
to the Permissions Department, John Wiley & Sons, Inc.

Library of Congress Cataloging in Publication Data:

Main entry under title:
  Medical complications of malignancy.

  (A Wiley medical publication)
  Includes index.
  1. Cancer—Complications and sequelae.   I. Smith,
Frank E. (Frank Edward), 1936-   II. Lane, Montague.
III. Series. [DNLM: 1. Neoplasms—Complications. QZ 200
M4886]
RC262.M425   1984   616.99'4   83-26099
ISBN 0-471-04362-1

Printed in the United States of America

10 9 8 7 6 5 4 3 2 1

To our wives, Karen Smith and Carol Higley Lane, and also to Emily, Muriel, and Bill.

Contributors

Clarence P. Alfrey, Jr., M.D.
Professor of Medicine
Department of Medicine
Baylor College of Medicine
Houston, Texas

James Callen, M.D.
Clinical Associate Professor of Dermatology
University of Louisville School of Medicine
Louisville, Kentucky

Joseph Jankovic, M.D.
Associate Professor
Department of Neurology
Baylor College of Medicine
Houston, Texas

Montague Lane, M.D.
Professor
Head, Division of Clinical Oncology and Section of Medical Oncology
Departments of Pharmacology and Medicine
Clinical Cancer Training Program
Baylor College of Medicine
Houston, Texas

Edward C. Lynch, M.D.
Professor of Medicine
Department of Medicine
Baylor College of Medicine
Houston, Texas

Garrett Rushing Lynch, M.D.
Assistant Professor of Medicine
Section of Oncology
Department of Medicine
Baylor College of Medicine
Houston, Texas

Andrew Rudolph, M.D.
Associate Professor
Department of Dermatology
Baylor College of Medicine
Houston, Texas

Frank E. Smith, M.D.
Associate Professor
Departments of Pharmacology and Medicine
Associate Director
Clinical Cancer Training Program
Baylor College of Medicine
Houston, Texas

Martin R. White, M.D.
Clinical Instructor of Medicine
Department of Medicine
Baylor College of Medicine
Houston, Texas

Paul W. Zelnick, M.D.
Fellow in Hematology
Department of Medicine
Baylor College of Medicine
Houston, Texas

Mary Anne Zubler, M.D.
Professor of Medicine
Department of Medicine
Baylor College of Medicine
Houston, Texas

Preface

Medical events occurring during the course of malignant processes are frequent causes of morbidity or lethal outcome. The recognition of treatable complications of neoplastic diseases can result in highly significant degrees of local control, overall objective palliation, extension of survival in individual patients, as well as enabling definitive therapy of the underlying illness. It is also important to identify those problems for which current treatment approaches are not always satisfactory, so that patients and their families can be informed about medical implications, effects on prognosis, and appropriate elements of supportive care. In addition, the oncologist is frequently called upon to distinguish cancer from noncancer related disease and to advise treatment based upon the conclusions. An appreciation of differential diagnosis and variation in the natural course of specific neoplasms enables the practitioner to separate critical medical questions, making therapeutic intervention possible. The descriptions of complications of malignancy discussed in the following chapters will aid physicians participating in the care of patients with cancer by addressing these often difficult issues.

The organization of chapters is by body system, since this is how the clinician analyzes patient problems. The assumption is made that critical information of pathology, natural course of individual tumor processes, tumor surgery, radiation, chemotherapy, and general therapeutics is readily available in many other oncologic writings and is, therefore, not reduplicated here. The major emphasis of this publication concerns clinical events that may occur as a consequence of malignancy, recognition of these events, and the appropriate general principles of treatment as well as differential diagnosis. In this sense, *Medical Complications of Malignancy* can complement many other sources of information in oncology.

F.E.S.
M.L.

Contents

MEDICAL COMPLICATIONS
OF MALIGNANCY

1
Cardiovascular Complications of Malignancy

Frank E. Smith

Vascular compromise, particularly cardiac dysfunction, often proceeds unrecognized during life in patients with malignancy (1,2). Thurber's retrospective pathology study documents the frequency of problems in the cardiovascular system and points out that many severe clinical situations may go unidentified. In this patient population, 55 of 189 (29%) had significant impairment of cardiac function in life as a direct result of cardiac metastases. In only 8 patients (15%) with metastatic cardiac disease were pericardial lesions considered noncontributory to cause of death, although the tumors interfered with cardiac function. The difficulties of identification of metastatic heart disease can be examined from another point of view as outlined in the report of Goldman and Pearson (3). This study from Toronto General Hospital describes only 15 cases of malignant pericardial effusion seen over a 20-year period. In 4 of 15 patients the diagnosis was only suspected before death. Since 20% or more of cancer victims coming to autopsy may harbor cardiac metastases (1–9), the disparity between pathologic and clinical realization must be wide indeed. Unquestionably, negative bias of the physician when confronted with cardiac difficulties in a patient with widely disseminated neoplasm contributes considerably to inadequate identification of cardiac metastases during life.

CARDIAC METASTATIC MALIGNANCY

The heart may be involved with metastatic malignancy in most types of disseminated neoplasm. In many studies, approximately one-half of the patients with cardiac metastases have an underlying diagnosis of carcinoma of the lung or breast (1,2,4,8,9). Other malignancies frequently associated with cardiac involvement are lymphomas, melanoma, and leukemia. In the last mentioned, as many as 55% will have leukemic cardiac infiltration at postmortem (6,10).

The pericardium and myocardium are most frequently involved, presumably by direct extension, hematogenous dissemination, or lymphatic metastases. Of all solid tumors involving the heart, the most frequent offender is malignant melanoma (11). Since this tumor is much less common in overall incidence than carcinoma of the breast or lung, the awareness of the neoplasm's predilection for cardiac metastases is perhaps less widespread among clinicians. This carcinoma is one of the few epithelial malignancies in which tumor cells may be seen in peripheral blood in a clinical setting of far advanced disease. Hematogenous deposition of cancer cells in multiple organ sites, including the heart, are frequent observations at postmortem.

In many situations cardiac involvement is frequently due to lymphatic metastases and direct extension from mediastinal tumor. Rarely, cardiac tumor may be the presenting problem to the physician in patients not suspected of harboring malignancy. In our experience pericardial fluid cytology is positive in most pathologic examinations when the offending tumor is a carcinoma or sarcoma (18). Similar experiences have been reported by other authors (12,13). Pericardial biopsy may be necessary when Hodgkin's disease or other lymphomas are causatory. Since lymphomas are histologically pleomorphic, microscopic identification may require a biopsy for recognition of histiocytes, lymphocytes, fibrosis, or Reed-Sternberg cells in their architectural relationship to one another. Exfoliative cytology in pericardial fluid is, therefore, quite inaccurate in patients with lymphoma, paralleling general experience of cytologic examination of ascites, pleural effusion, or cerebrospinal fluid in these patients.

If local anatomic metastases are present, specific events, including heart block, may occur (14–16). In this setting bradycardia and syncope have led to the diagnosis of underlying lung carcinoma, myeloma, lymphoma, leukemia, or mesothelioma.

Leukemic infiltration of cardiac muscle is a common postmortem finding and may be seen in as many as half of the patients. During life, generalized cardiomegaly radiographically, usually without concomitant pericardial effusion, may cause heart failure responsive to radiation therapy (17).

Endocardial metastases are extremely rare, and individual cases are reportable events. This uncommon site of metastasis has been attributed to the relative avascularity of the endocardium.

In most patients a previous diagnosis of carcinoma has been made. Symptoms of fatigue, weight loss, shortness of breath, cough, and chest pain or peripheral edema may be seen. In contrast to many disease states, malignant pericardial effusion is much less frequently associated with classic findings during the physical examination at presentation (18). Thus, pericardial rub, muffled heart sounds, increased jugular venous distension, Ewart's sign, and pulsus paradoxus are present in a minority of patients at initial evaluation. This may be accounted for by the fact that the amount of pericardial fluid present in patients with effusion ranges from several hundred to 1500 cc. The average amount of pericardial fluid aspirated is approximately 850 cc in patients undergoing pericardiocentesis (18). The accumulation of fluid is, therefore, usually subacute or chronic, and, when this develops in the face of known and advanced malignancy, clinical identification can be difficult. The most commonly observed radiographic finding of malignant pericardial effusion is coincident pleural effusion (Fig. 1-1) (18). The presence of pleural effusion may further distract the clinician away from the heart as the responsible pathophysiologic mechanism causing intra-

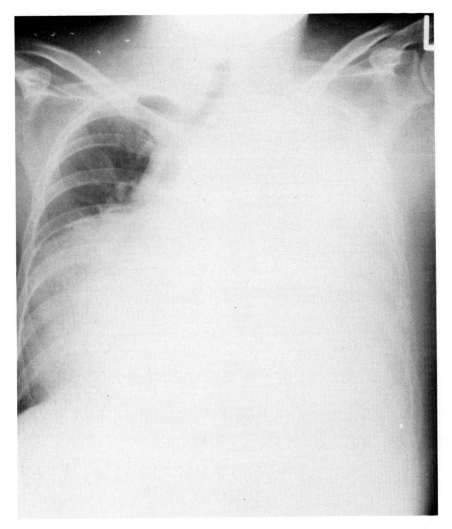

Figure 1-1. Malignant thymoma causing massive left and right pleural effusion, pericardial tamponade, and mediastinal encasement.

thoracic fluid accumulation. Thoracentesis fluid is consistently negative for tumor, and attention must be progressively directed toward a cardiac origin of pleural fluid accumulation. When pleural fluid is positive for malignant cells, pulmonary parenchymal lesions, mediastinal shedding, or pleural implants exist singly or combined. Pleural fluid cytology is positive for malignant cells in approximately two-thirds of patients with carcinoma who have metastases to the above mentioned sites. Reliability of cytology increases to approximately five of six patients when breast or ovarian cancer result in pleural studding of tumor (12).

X-ray findings showing a "water-bottle heart" without significant pleural fluid may also be observed (Fig. 1-2).

Diagnostic measures in patients with suspected malignant pericardial effusion

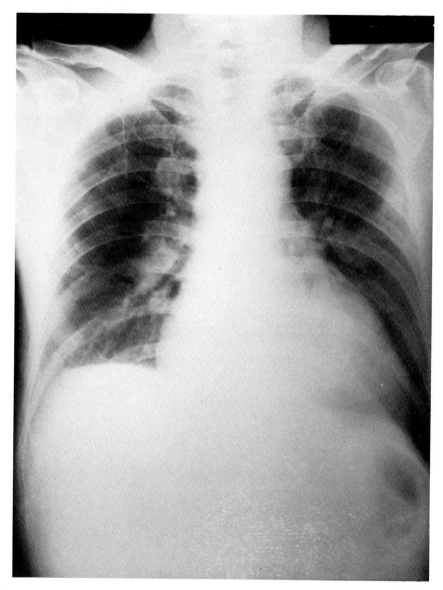

Figure 1-2. Adenocarcinoma of the right lung with pericaridal tamponade at initial clinical presentation.

may include (*1*) echocardiography, (*2*) cardiac angiography, (*3*) radioisotopes, (*4*) pericardiocentesis, and (*5*) computed tomographic scanning.

Cardiac ultrasound examination is the most used and least expensive noninvasive diagnostic technique in the recognition of pericardial effusion. The procedure has been in use since the mid-1960s, being introduced at that time by Feigenbaum (19). False-negative studies are not infrequent, particularly if pleural effusion coexists.

Angiographic studies may show an abnormal separation of intracardiac contrast medium from the pericardial border. The area between the pool of dye within the heart cavities and the outer border of the heart represents fluid in the pericardial space (Fig. 1-3).

Radioisotopic studies may also show a separation of the intracardiac pool of isotopically labelled blood from the cardiac border if visualized on a superimposed chest x-ray film. The hepatic radioactivity is normally confluent with the

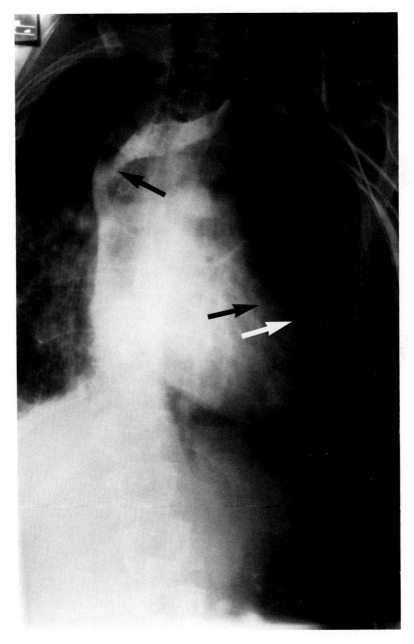

Figure 1-3. Cardiac angiography in metastatic breast carcinoma. Arrows indicate partial superior vena cava obstruction, the edge of the intracardiac pool of dye, and the outer cardiac silhouette.

cardiac pool of isotopes. These two areas of radioactivity are separated when intervening pericardial fluid is present (24).

Pericardiocentesis with injection of 50–75 cc of air or carbon dioxide precisely identifies effusion (Figs. 1-4 and 1-5). As mentioned previously, cytologic examination of pericardial fluid at the time of pericardiocentesis is most frequently positive when carcinomas or sarcomas are the causative tumors.

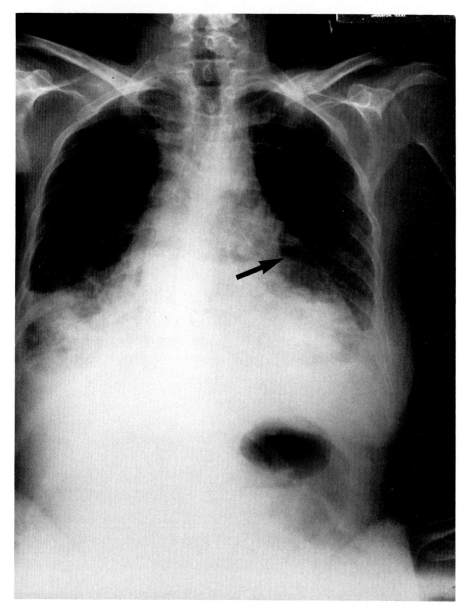

Figure 1-4. Intrapericardial injection of air following pericardiocentesis showing a thin pericardium with masses located in the pericardial sac (arrow). A drainage catheter was left in place for one week without incident.

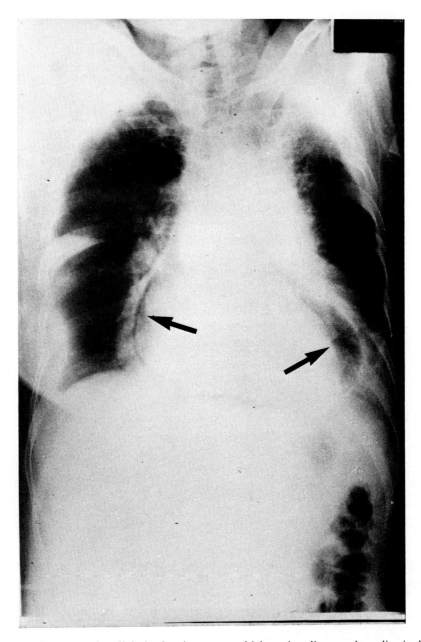

Figure 1-5. Intrapericardial air showing a very thick pericardium and mediastinal encasement. The bulk of intrathoracic disease portends poor prognosis in carcinoma, although lymphoma may respond well.

Each time a pericardiocentesis is attempted, concomitant electrocardiographic monitoring should be performed in order to identify evidence of muscle injury should the needle penetrate the myocardium. Unfortunately, electrocardiographic examinations are in themselves not diagnostic of malignant cardiac involvement (25). All types of rhythm disturbances, voltage abnormalities, and ST segment aberrations have been seen. If pericardial effusion is present, it is fortunate if sinus tachycardia, low voltage, and ST segment elevation are also present.

Computed thoracic tomography (CT) can be an important diagnostic aid in the recognition of pericardial effusion, particularly when concomitant pleural effusion exists (Fig. 1-6). This technique is more accurate than cardiac ultrasound. Pericardial effusion may be seen independently of accompanying pleural fluid. Computed scanning can also demonstrate differences in composition of pericardial fluid. Loculated pericardial effusion and intrapericardial masses may be missed on electrocardiographic examination in as many as 10% of patients. The thickness of the pericardium is easily demonstrated with CT scanning. In this situation echocardiography is extremely limited. CT scans may also identify mediastinal encasement, fat, or blood clots in the pericardium. Finally, scanning may reveal pertinent anatomic information that can be used for potential pericardiocentesis or thoracic surgery (19–23,26–29).

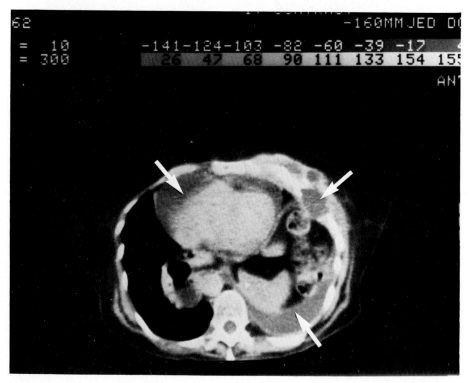

Figure 1-6. Thoracic scan demonstrating pericardial effusion and rib metastases (upper arrows) and pleural effusion in the left pleural space (lower arrow). The underlying disease is breast carcinoma.

Treatment of metastatic cardiac neoplasms can frequently result in successful, even long-term, palliation. Measures employed include (*1*) appropriate systemic therapy for the underlying disease; (*2*) radiation to the heart itself or mediastinal and cardiac irradiation; (*3*) pericardiocentesis with instillation of alkylating or sclerosing agents; and (*4*) establishment of a pericardial window.

Our longest survivor was a patient with breast cancer and cardiac tamponade. Five years elapsed between tamponade and death from widely metastatic disease (Figs. 1-7 and 1-8). Acute phase treatment employed an alkylating agent (thio-

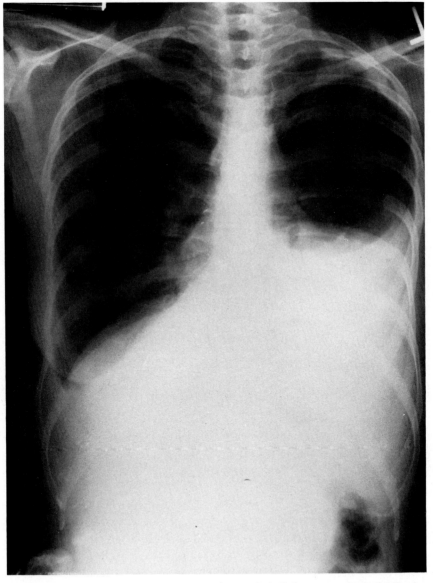

Figure 1-7. Metastatic breast carcinoma causing pericardial tamponade and left pleural effusion. Echocardiogram was negative because of the overlapping effusions.

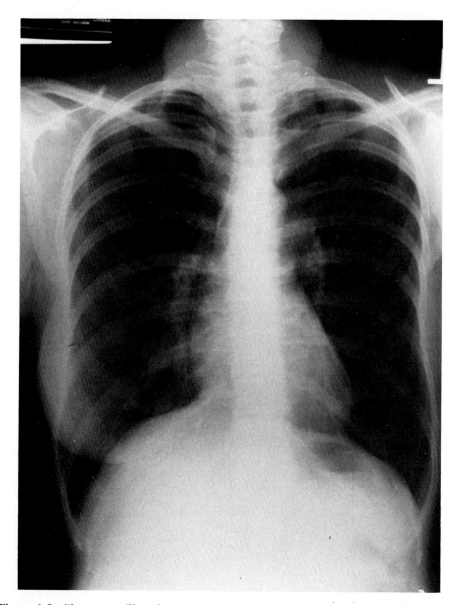

Figure 1-8. Chest x-ray film of patient in Figure 1-7, five years later. In the intervening time local radiotherapy and chemotherapy was supplemented with successful systemic treatment.

tepa) directly into the pericardium, cardiac irradiation, and following this, successful systemic treatment with both chemotherapy and hormones. Nitrogen mustard is likely the most widely employed locally administered drug in malignant pericardial effusion and may be particularly applicable in patients with underlying lung cancer or lymphoma. Both the sclerosing and antitumor effects of nitrogen mustard can be beneficial mechanisms of action. The severity and often acute clinical picture of significant pericardial effusion or cardiac tamponade have made controlled trials of treatment essentially impossible (18). At Baylor College of Medicine to date there have been some 60 patients with a premortem diagnosis of malignant pericardial effusion or tamponade treated with local chemotherapy, radiation therapy, and pericardiocentesis. Survival times are superior in persons who receive aggressive local therapy without the need for pericardial window procedures. Such patients are often critically compromised by advanced disease and tolerate thoracic surgery poorly.

Adequate criteria of control of malignant pericardial effusion have not yet been outlined. This further complicates the assessment of treatment and response. Adequate primary control of pericardial effusion may be assumed if recurrent fluid accumulation does not necessitate pericardiocentesis or other local control maneuvers within one month of initial therapy. If future adequate descriptions of survival in appropriately staged individual tumor types can be made, the whole problem of definition of response to treatment would be simplified. At present such crucial information is not available.

Cardiac lesions as a feature of carcinoid tumors occur most frequently in the right side of the heart in patients with extensive hepatic metastases (30). Findings of pulmonary stenosis or tricuspid insufficiency are seen most often, but lesions of the mitral valve, superior vena cava, inferior vena cava, systemic veins, and coronary sinus have also been described. Carcinoid heart disease is seen in approximately half of the patients with cardinoid syndrome. Flushing, chronic plethora, and telangiectasia result from kinins, catechols, or histamine released from tumor.

Although the intermittent hypertension of pheochromocytoma is well known, it should be emphasized that tumor location may result in bizarre crises. One of our patients experienced syncope secondary to severe increase of blood pressure following urination. A pheochromocytoma attached to the bladder released catecholamines each time the organ contracted, thereby causing the unusual timing of the episodes. Similar situations may be seen when position change or swallowing cause the offending amines to be discharged into the circulation. Pheochromocytomas must also be sought during evaluation of any patient with medullary carcinoma of the thyroid. Operations on these persons are dangerous when the simultaneous occurrence of the two tumors exists. Ten percent of persons with medullary thyroid cancer will harbor a pheochromocytoma.

ARTERIAL AND VENOUS PROBLEMS IN NEOPLASTIC DISEASE

The spectrum of vascular difficulties associated with neoplasms is quite wide, although individual patient problems may be relatively as frequent. Minna et al. (31) have observed coagulation and thrombotic syndromes in 1–4% of patients with lung cancer. These include disseminated intravascular coagulation, marantic endocarditis, and migratory thrombophlebitis (see Chapter 9).

VENOUS SYNDROMES

Venous obstructive syndromes are not unusual, and in superior vena cava obstruction almost all patients have malignancies. Seventy-five percent of these patients have carcinoma of the lung and 15% will have lymphoma as underlying causes. Goiter, superior vena caval thrombosis, and mediastinal fibrosis are the nonmalignant causes of the syndrome most frequently considered in differential diagnosis (32,33).

Inferior vena caval obstruction is a frequent consequence of invasion from a hypernephroma from the renal vein. Such thromboses may extend into the right atrium and obstruct blood flow to the right ventricle. Other intra-abdominal tumors from a variety of sites may compress the large vein causing peripheral edema and venous collateralization but no ascites.

Hepatic vein thrombosis can cause rapidly increasing size of the liver and spleen, accompanied by ascites. Death occurs within one to seven weeks from liver failure. Hypernephroma and hepatoma are the most usual causative tumors.

Portal hypertension usually results from extensive metastatic liver involvement. The natural course of disease here is considerably longer than the more acute evolution of hepatic vein occlusion. Mesenteric or splenic vein thromboses are rare complications of intra-abdominal tumors. When they are seen, pathogenesis is from compression and/or local extension of regional disease.

Rarely, other obstructive problems arise. One of our patients with an advanced osteogenic sarcoma experienced positional syncope and was found to have a large tumor thrombus extending from the superior vena cava into the right atrium. Ball valve action of the tumor thrombus transiently obstructed flow from the right atrium to the right ventricle and resulted in findings similar to that of atrial myxoma.

MARANTIC ENDOCARDITIS

Marantic endocarditis continues to be an enigma in terms of pathogenesis, diagnosis, and treatment (34–39). The diagnosis is made at the bedside most frequently in patients with advanced disease when scattered neurologic deficits occur abruptly. Embolic signs may be seen in the spleen and extremities or when hematuria is found. Cardiac signs, including murmur, may be lacking. Electrocardiography, echocardiography, and cardiac catheterization often fail to demonstrate the small endocardial plaques. Anticoagulant therapy is disappointing, and, at present, no adequate treatment is available. Autopsy findings are often dramatic. Our most recent patient had carcinoma of the lung with extensive thromboemboli in all coronary arteries as well as multiple thromboemboli in many smaller arteries of the brain. Rosen and Armstrong's group (34) of 75 patients included 14 patients with suspected cardiovascular accident and 5 thought to have myocardial infarction as causes of death. Myocardial infarction as a consequence of nonbacterial thrombotic endocarditis is found at autopsy with greater frequency than clinical detection during life. Compression of coronary arteries or ostia of these vessels can also cause cardiac ischemia (35–38).

ARTERIAL SYNDROMES

Rarely, peripheral arterial ischemia is seen in the hands, a most unusual anatomic site because of its extensive collateral circulation. Cryoglobulins, most often associated with lymphoma or multiple myeloma, can cause gangrenous digital changes (Chapter 10). Occasionally, allergic angiitis can cause digital ischemia and chronic Raynaud's phenomena as a consequence of chemotherapy (40). This has been described as a result of treatment with mithramycin. Granulomatous arteries associated with Hodgkin's disease can cause local central nervous system ischemia responsive to steroid treatment. Ecthyma gangrenosa (Fig. 1-9) is seen in patients with gram-negative septicemia and is most often caused by septic emboli of *Pseudomonas* or other necrotizing gram-negative organisms. Needle aspiration of the necrotic, black embolic cutaneous bullous lesions yields the responsible bacteria. The usual underlying neoplasms are leukemia or lymphomas. If these lesions are identified, antibiotic therapy can be initiated while cultural results are awaited.

Arterial tumor emboli may rarely be seen as metastases within atheromatous plaques. One such patient in our hospital had surgery for severe aortic atherosclerosis, and a microscopic tumor within atheromatous plaque was seen on frozen section. A thorough intraoperative search of the abdomen failed to disclose the source of the tumor embolus. The postoperative examinations did not identify the primary. The patient died two years later with widespread metas-

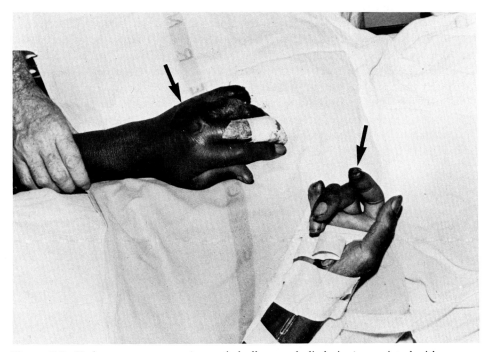

Figure 1-9. Ecthyma gangrenosa (necrotic bullous embolic lesion) associated with pseudomonas septicemia (upper arrow). Concomitant cryoglobulinemia causing gangrene (lower arrow) in a patient with lymphocytic lymphoma.

tases. The tissue of origin of the poorly differentiated carcinoma could not be discerned.

OTHER VASCULAR SYNDROMES

Venous tumor emboli can also cause lethal outcome when larger lesions lodge in the pulmonary arteries as a consequence of rapidly proliferating malignancy. Choriocarcinoma is the most likely underlying tumor in this unusual situation (Chapter 2).

Mucus secreting carcinomas of the pancreas, ovary, colon, and breast or carcinoma of the lung have long been known to cause simple pulmonary emboli (41). A procoagulant has been sought but never identified.

Arteriovenous communication is manifested in many tumors and may be used in diagnosis when arteriography is employed, particularly in the study of lesions of the kidney, liver, or brain. Virtually any anatomic site of malignancy may show neovascularization phenomena, including the "tumor blush" seen when dye is injected into the arteries supplying the affected area.

If arteriovenous communication is extensive, bruits can be heard over lesions, and if shunting within the tumor reaches enormous proportions, high-output cardiac failure may follow. Hypernephroma, both primary and metastatic, is by far the most frequent neoplasm at fault. A patient we observed had a metastatic sternal lesion associated with a loud bruit. High-output failure responded only to radiation therapy control of the metastatic lesion. When the tumor recurred locally several weeks following radiotherapy, the bruit reappeared and ensuing recurrent cardiac failure led to death. Biopsy procedures of vascular neoplasms may be quite hazardous and should be undertaken with appropriate caution.

Hyperviscosity syndrome as a complication of myeloma can cause hypertension through increased cardiac work, and peripheral vascular "sludging" of blood leads to "box-car" abnormalities seen in retinal veins. In this syndrome, the cardiovascular consequences are due to large quantities of abnormal globulins accumulating in the circulation, and they can be relieved promptly by plasmaphoresis (42).

REFERENCES

1. Thurber DL, Edwards JE, Achor WP: Secondary malignant tumors of the pericardium. *Circulation* 26:228, 1962.
2. DeLoach JF, Haynes JW: Secondary tumors of the heart and pericardium. *Arch Intern Med* 91:224, 1953.
3. Goldman BS, Pearson FG: Malignant pericardial effusion. *Can J Surg* 8:157, 1965.
4. Young JM, Goldman IR: Tumor metastases to the heart. *Circulation* 9:220, 1954.
5. Hanfling SM: Metastatic cancer to the heart. *Circulation* 22:474, 1960.
6. Javier BV, Yount WS, Crosby DT, et al: Cardiac metastasis in lymphoma and leukemia. *Dis Chest* 52:481, 1957.
7. Shelburne SA, Aronson HS: Tumors of the heart. *Ann Intern Med* 14:728, 1940.
8. Strauss BL, Matthews MJ, Cohen MH, et al: Cardiac metastases in lung cancer. *Chest* 71:607, 1977.

9. Quraishi MA, Costanzi JJ, Hokanson J: Natural history of lung cancer with pericardial metastases. *Cancer* 51:740, 1983.

10. Lewis TN, Kligerman MM: Pericardial and myocardial involvement by lymphomas and leukemia. *Cancer* 25:1103, 1970.

11. Smith FE: Malignant melanoma. *Cancer Chemother* 2:257, 1981.

12. Cardozo PL: A critical analysis of 3000 cytologic examinations of pleural, ascitic and pericardial fluid. *Acta Cytol* 10:455, 1966.

13. Lokich JJ: The management of malignant pericardial effusion. *JAMA* 224:1401, 1973.

14. Mitchell-Heggs P: Intra-thoracic lymphoma associated with atrial arrhythmias and A-V conduction defects. *Br J Dis Chest* 72:71, 1978.

15. Gupte S: Acute leukemia with complete heart block. *Am J Dis Child* 131:926, 1977.

16. Wanless IR: Mesothelioma of the AV node with long standing complete heart block. *Am J Clin Pathol* 63:377, 1975.

17. Terry LN, Kligerman MM: Pericardial and myocardial involvement by lymphomas and leukemias. *Cancer* 25:1002, 1970.

18. Smith FE, Lane M, Hudgins PT: Conservative management of malignant pericardial effusion. *Cancer* 33:47, 1974.

19. Feigenbaum H, Weldhausen JA, Hyde LP: Ultrasound diagnosis of pricardial effusion. *JAMA* 191:711, 1965.

20. Goldschlager AW, Freeman LM, Davis PJ: Pericardial effusions and echocardiography: False results with ultrasound reflection method. *NY State J Med* 67:1854, 1967.

21. Casarella WJ, Schneider BO: Pitfalls in the ultrasonic diagnosis of pericardial effusion. *Am J Roentgenol, Radiat Therapy and Nucl Med* 10:760, 1972.

22. Ratshin RA, Smith MK, Hood, WP: Possible false-positive diagnosis of pericardial effusion by echocardiography in the presence of large left atrium. *Chest* 65:112, 1974.

23. D'Cruz I, Prabhu R, Cohen HC, et al: Potential pitfalls in quanification of pericardial effusions by echocardiography. *Br Heart J* 39:529, 1977.

24. Charkes ND, Sklaroff DM: Radioisotopic photoscanning as a diagnostic aid in cardiovascular disease. *JAMA* 186:920, 1963.

25. Biran S, Hochman A, Levig IS, et al: Clinical diagnosis of secondary tumors of the heart and pericardium. *Dis Chest* 55:202, 1969.

26. Wood EH: New vistas for the study of structural and functional dynamics of the heart, lungs and circulation by non-invasive numerical tomographic vivisection. *Circulation* 56:506, 1977.

27. Lipton MJ, Brundage BH, Doherty PW, et al: Contrast medium-enhanced computed tomography for evaluating ischemic heart disease. *Cardiovasc Med* 4:1219, 1979.

28. Tomada H, Hoshiai IM, Furuya H, et al: Evaluation of cardiac diseases with computed tomography. *Jpn Heart J* 51:149, 1980.

29. Isner JM, Carter BL, Bankoff MS, et al: Computed tomography in the diagnosis of pericardial heart disease. *Ann Intern Med* 97:473, 1982.

30. Smith FE, Lane M: Carcinoid tumor and carcinoid syndrome, in Conn HF, Conn RB (eds): *Current Diagnosis.* Philadelphia, Saunders, 1980, p 783

31. Minna JD, Higgins, GA, Glatstein EJ: Principals and practice of oncology, in DeVita VT, Hellman S, Rosenberg SA (eds), *Cancer*, Philadelphia, Lippincott, 1982, p 414.

32. Schechter MM: The superior vena cava syndrome. *Am J Med Sci* 227:46, 1954.

33. Lokich JJ, Goodman RL: Superior vena cava syndrome. *JAMA* 231:58, 1975.

34. Rosen P, Armstrong D: Bacterial thrombotic endocarditis in patients with malignant neoplastic diseases. *Am J Med* 54:23, 1973.

35. Fayemi AO, Deppsich LM: Coronary embolism in myocardial infarction associated with nonbacterial thrombotic endocarditis. *Am J Clin Pathol* 69:393, 1977.

36. Rohner RF, Prior JT, Sipple JH: Mucinous malignancies, venous thromboses and terminal endocarditis with emboli: A syndrome. *Cancer* 19:1805, 1966.

37. Bryan CS: Non-bacterial thrombotic endocarditis with malignant tumors. *Am J Med* 46:787, 1969.

38. Ray-Chaudhuri M: Non-bacterial thrombotic endocarditis in association with mucous secreting adenocarcinomas. *Br J Dis Chest* 65:98, 1971.

39. Hoffer WD: Hypercoagulability in verrucous endocarditis associated with adenocarcinoma of the lung. *Ann Thoracic Surg* 6:181, 1968.

40. Margileth DA, Smith FE, Lane M: Arterial occlusion associated with mithramycin therapy. *Cancer* 31:708, 1973.

41. Trousseau A: Phlegmasia Alba Dolens. Clinique medicale de l'Hotel-Dieu de Paris. London: *The New Sydenham Society* 3:94, 1865.

42. Russell JA, Toy JL, Powles RL: Plasma exchange in malignant paraproteinemias. *Exp Hematol* 5:105, 1977.

2
The Pulmonary System and Malignant Disease

Garrett Rushing Lynch

The respiratory tract is a frequent site to manifest the complications of cancer and its therapy for two reasons. First, carcinoma of the lung is the second most frequent cause of cancer, skin excluded, in this country. Second, due to its rich vascular and lymphatic supply, the respiratory system is a common site of cancer metastases.

The respiratory manifestations of cancer are often detected by chest roentgenography obtained during the evaluation of cough, dyspnea, fever, and chest pain, or during routine screening and evaluation procedures. The approach to the pulmonary complications of cancer in this chapter will, therefore, be based on their roentgenographic manifestations.

THE SOLITARY PULMONARY NODULE

The solitary pulmonary nodule is a major diagnostic problem in medicine; in all cases, the diagnosis of cancer must be excluded. The solitary pulmonary nodule is often an incidental finding on a chest x-ray obtained at the time of a routine physical examination or patient follow-up. The patient may have a variety of complaints, including cough, hemoptysis, pain, wheezing, or systemic symptoms such as malaise, fever, or weight loss. On the other hand, the patient is often asymptomatic.

The physical examination may give a clue to the nature of the lesion. Cachexia, clubbing of the fingers, supraclavicular adenopathy, or hepatomegaly may suggest malignancy; these findings, however, may be present with infections or other nonmalignant diseases. The presence of telangectasia of the skin and mucous membranes may suggest an arteriovenous malformation. Examination of the lungs may reveal a localized wheeze or rhonchus; a rub may be audible if the lesion abuts the pleura. On the contrary, the chest examination may be entirely normal. A careful breast examination in women patients, head and neck evaluation in smokers, and rectal examination in all patients is also in order.

The chest x-ray film may give clues to the cause of the lesion, but it is seldom diagnostic. A lesion with ill defined margins and eccentric calcification is often, but not always, malignant. The converse does not hold true; perfectly circum-scribed lesions are not necessarily benign. A solitary nodule associated with bone destruction may imply malignancy, as may an elevated hemidiaphragm or ate-lectasis. Mediastinal or hilar enlargement may suggest lymph node involvement.

The differential diagnosis of a solitary pulmonary nodule includes primary and metastatic carcinoma, hamratoma, benign teratoma, arteriovenous malfor-mation, collagen-vascular disease, including rheumatoid nodules, Wegener's granulomatosis, or an infectious process. Infections that can occur in this manner include tuberculosis, histoplasmosis, coccidiomycosis, aspergillosis, and other fungal infections (1,2).

Evaluation of a solitary lesion should include a review of previous x-ray films; if these reveal that the lesion has been present and stable in size over a period of 18 months, it is likely benign. Otherwise, if the lesion has increased in size or no old films are available, a tissue diagnosis should be obtained. Since less than 2% of solitary nodules are malignant in patients younger than age 30, many investigators recommend watchful waiting in this group, while applying vigorous work-up in older patients (2). If telangiectasias of the skin and mucous mem-branes are noted, it is imperative to obtain a pulmonary arteriogram, thus avoid-ing a dangerous biopsy procedure in patients with arteriovenous malformations.

There are several ways to obtain a tissue diagnosis. Three sputum samples for cytologic analysis should be obtained; lesions communicating with the bronchus may have a positive cytology. If the nodule is peripheral and greater than 2 cm, a fluoroscopic or CT-directed needle biopsy may provide a cytologic diagnosis (3). Bronchoscopy with brushings, biopsy, and postbronchoscopy sputum sam-ples may yield the diagnosis in more centrally located lesions (4). Adequate cytologic evaluation may provide a diagnosis of malignancy in 90–95% of cases and the specific cell type in 70% of cases. If needle biopsy and bronchoscopy fail to yield the diagnosis, thoracotomy is in order. In patients with pure solitary nodules with or without radiographic mediastinal enlargement, mediastinoscopy is indicated. If mediastinoscopy is unrevealing, careful inspection of the me-diastinum at the time of thoracotomy, with biopsies of enlarged or abnormal appearing lymph nodes, is necessary.

In patients without a past history of cancer, 90–95% of malignant solitary nodules are primary lung tumors. In patients with a history of cancer in another anatomic area, it is important not to assume that the lesion is due to metastatic disease. In some series up to 50% of solitary pulmonary nodules in patients with a history of cancer are primary lung tumors and not metastases from the pre-viously diagnosed malignancy (5).

If a metastatic solitary nodule is documented by needle aspiration or bron-choscopic biopsy, consideration of surgical resection of the lesion is in order. A series from Memorial Sloan–Kettering Cancer Center concluded that surgical therapy of metastatic pulmonary nodules is justifiable if the primary site is controlled or controllable, no metastatic extrapulmonary sites are demonstrable, a long interval from the diagnosis of the primary and the diagnosis of the metastases is present, there is good surgical risk, and no effective therapy is available by nonsurgical means (6). The preferred surgical treatment is wedge resection (7). A median five-year survival of 21% was obtained in 188 cases in the Memorial series. The highest five-year survival was noted in head and neck cancer (43%) (6).

MULTIPLE PULMONARY NODULES

A common radiographic pattern of tumors metastatic to the lung is that of multiple pulmonary nodules. Tumor emboli 8–12 u in diameter are easily entrapped in the pulmonary capillaries; they may then grow into nodular form. Tumor emboli can be entrapped in the pulmonary lymphatics as well. Tumors frequently metastasizing to the lung in this manner include head and neck cancer (both squamous cell and adenoid cystic varieties); carcinoma of the thyroid, breast, testes, bladder, colon, liver, and lung; melanoma; and osteogenic and soft tissue sarcomas (Figs. 2-1 and 2-2). This pattern, however, has been described with all tumors, including lymphomas. Occasionally, this is the manner of presentation of a primary lung tumor, particularly alveolar cell carcinoma.

Multiple pulmonary nodules are often bilateral and of varying size and shape. Nonmalignant conditions should be considered in the differential diagnosis,

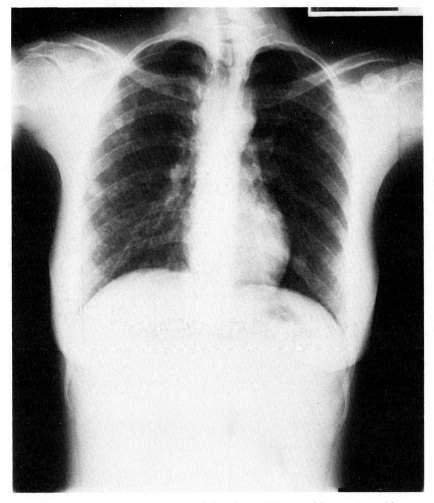

Figure 2-1. Multiple pulmonary nodules in a 21-year-old woman with gestational choriocarcinoma.

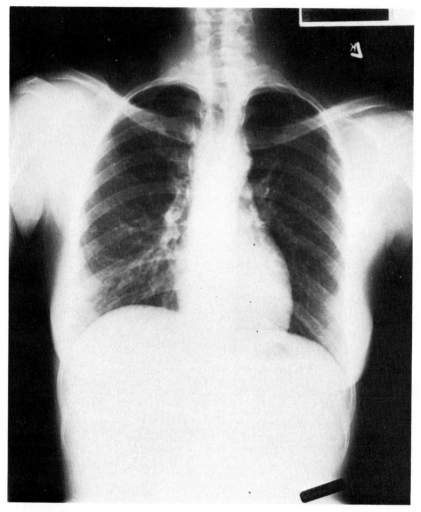

Figure 2-2. Resolution of the pulmonary nodules with methotrexate, actinomycin D, and chlorambucil chemotherapy.

including multiple pulmonary emboli, collagen-vascular disease, and infections, especially of the fungal variety. Infections and multiple pulmonary emboli often produce lesions with indistinct margins, while lesions secondary to metastatic malignancy tend to be well-defined.

Although pulmonary metastases represent disseminated disease, in some cases their presence does not portend a poor prognosis. In thyroid and adenoid cystic carcinoma, the lesions may have a very slow growth rate; 20-year survival with metastatic pulmonary lesions in these entities has been frequently reported (8). In patients with testicular carcinoma, the persistence of pulmonary nodules after chemotherapy does not necessarily imply persistent metastatic disease and a poor prognosis; such nodules are not infrequently converted into benign teratomas after chemotherapy (9,10). Such persistent nodules should be considered for wedge resection.

Patients with osteogenic sarcoma often have small pulmonary nodules not visible on plain radiograph. These patients should undergo whole lung tomography or CT scanning before commencing primary or adjuvant chemotherapy (11). Pulmonary metastases from osteogenic sarcoma are occasionally subpleural and may present as a spontaneous pneumothorax.

In a patient with a history of cancer and accessible metastatic sites elsewhere, such as skin, subcutaneous tissue, and lymph nodes, histologic diagnosis of these sites may be all that is necessary to document disseminated disease. If there is no other evidence of metastatic disease, an attempt at histologic documentation of the pulmonary nodular lesions is in order. Such documentation may be obtained by sputum cytology, bronchoscopy, and thin-needle percutaneous aspiration. Although only 5% of sputum specimens for cytologic analysis are positive with metastatic lesions, if they are positive, this may be very helpful. Tumors with a propensity for endobronchial metastases have the highest yield for a positive sputum cytology; these include breast carcinoma, hypernephroma, lymphoma, melanoma, and cervical carcinoma.

Wedge resection may be indicated in patients with a small number of lesions, a long disease-free interval, and no superior therapy otherwise available. A 15% five-year survival was noted with wedge resection of multiple pulmonary metastases (12).

The presence of multiple pulmonary lesions usually indicates the need for systemic therapy. Hormonal therapy or chemotherapy may produce excellent responses; complete responses of over 20 years duration have been reported with oophorectomy for breast cancer (13). Radioactive iodine may be indicated in selected thyroid cancers that take up the radionuclide. In patients with very slow growing tumors, such as adenoid cystic carcinoma, observation alone may be in order.

PLEURAL EFFUSIONS

Pleural effusions are a common complication of malignancy and are not infrequently the presenting manifestation. Effusions may be secondary to a primary pleural tumor (mesothelioma), metastatic disease, or a benign process. Although pleural effusions may be a manifestation of almost any neoplasm, they are more commonly associated with certain malignancies, including lung, breast, and ovarian carcinoma.

The pathophysiology of malignant effusions is varied (14). One mechanism involves direct implantation of the pleura by tumor and the associated inflammation, which results in increased capillary permeability. Other causes include obstruction of the lung or pleural lymphatics by tumor, resulting in impaired resorption of fluid and protein and obstruction of pulmonary veins by tumor, with subsequent elevation of the capillary hydrostatic pressure and reduction in the gradient between the parietal and visceral pleura. The superior vena caval syndrome and pericardial effusions may cause pleural effusions by the latter mechanism. A pleural effusion is, in fact, the most common radiographic manifestation of a pericardial effusion. Central impairment of lymphatic flow due to thoracic duct or mediastinal involvement by tumor may produce a pure chylous effusion.

Pleural effusions may have an asymptomatic presentation. Patients commonly have progressive dyspnea. Chest pain, chiefly pleuritic in nature, is often a major complaint. Cough and fever are also frequently associated symptoms.

Radiographic manifestations of pleural effusions range from fluid in a major or minor fissure, an appearance of an elevated hemidiaphragm or blunted costophrenic angle, to obliteration of an entire hemithorax. A concomitant pleural or lung mass may be present. Enlarged hilar and mediastinal lymph nodes may suggest lymphatic obstruction as the cause.

A pleural effusion in a cancer patient is not always malignant. Cardiac, hepatic, and renal disease, as well as infectious processes, must be ruled out. Especially important is eliminating the possibility of an effusion on a tuberculous basis.

All new pleural effusions in patients with cancer should be evaluated with thoracentesis and analysis of the fluid. The following studies should be obtained: glucose, protein, and LDH determinations; bacterial, fungal, and acid-fast stains and cultures; and cytologic analysis. Pleural fluid cytology may be positive if the effusion is due to direct implantation of tumor; the cytology is often negative in effusions due to other mechanisms. The yield of cytologic analysis varies with the type of tumor (15). Cytology is positive in 85% of effusions in breast cancer. In lung cancer, one-third of patients will have no tumor cells in the fluid; in these cases, a reactive inflammatory pattern is present. Effusions secondary to ovarian cancer may be positive in 90–95% of cases. If the first cytologic analysis is negative for malignancy, a second thoracentesis and cytologic analysis increases the yield of positive fluid by only 4%. If the diagnosis of malignancy is questionable, a pleural biopsy is in order rather than multiple repeat thoracenteses and cytologic determinations of the pleural fluid (16).

Hypoglycemia may be present in effusions due to infection and malignancy. The total protein is usually elevated in malignant effusions, even if direct implantation of tumor cells is not present. LDH values in neoplastic effusions are usually elevated and are higher than the corresponding serum levels.

There are several therapeutic options in managing neoplastic pleural effusions. Treatment should be directed at the underlying disease. Thus hormonal therapy or chemotherapy may completely control the pleural effusions associated with breast cancer, while chemotherapy may erradicate effusions associated with ovarian cancer, oat cell carcinoma, lymphomas, and other tumors. Occasionally, radiation of enlarged hilar and mediastinal lymph nodes in patients with lymphoma or lung cancer may alleviate such effusions, which are secondary to central lymphatic obstruction.

More often than not, effusions are symptomatic and need relief before hormonal therapy or chemotherapy have a chance to control the effusion. Thoracentesis may yield a diagnosis as well as provide immediate symptomatic relief. However, 80–90% of effusions treated with thoracentesis alone recur within an average of four to seven days (17). Instillation of a sclerosing agent is not as effective following simple thoracentesis as following tube thoracostomy; the failure of simple thoracentesis is probably related to poor opposition of the pleural surfaces.

Once a malignant effusion has been diagnosed, tube thoracostomy may be in order. Tube thoracostomy alone may control 50–65% of malignant effusions (18).

A number of sclerosing agents have been used to treat malignant effusions; these include nitrogen mustard, tetracycline, quinacrine hydrochloride, bleomycin, and thiotepa. The mechanism of action of the sclerosing agents is their vesicant and mesothelial destructive effects rather than any specific antitumor activity. Most of these agents have been reported to have a 40–75% response rate. Tetracycline has been shown to have the highest response rate, being in the range of 70–80% (19,20). All of the sclerosing agents can cause fever and pleuritic chest pain; in addition, the chemotherapuetic agents can be absorbed systemically with resulting myelosuppression. Although tetracycline causes the greatest degree of pleuritic chest pain, it is probably the drug of choice because of its high response rate, ease of administration, lack of systemic toxicity, and cost effectiveness. It is important to completely drain the pleural space before and after instillation of the sclerosing agent in order to maximize opposition and subsequent fibrosis of the pleural surfaces.

Occasionally, decortication may be indicated in patients with a reasonable life expectancy whose effusions have not been controlled by other means. In a Memorial Sloan-Kettering series of 106 patients treated with pleurectomy, none of the effusions recurred; the median survival of patients was 16 months (21).

MEDIASTINAL AND HILAR ENLARGEMENT

Mediastinal and/or hilar adenopathy is a common abnormality in patients with cancer. Enlargement of the area may represent benign disease, a primary mediastinal tumor, or cancer metastatic to the mediastinal lymph nodes. Mediastinal and hilar enlargement may be the only radiographic abnormality, or, more commonly, it may be associated with solitary or multiple lung masses, a pleural effusion, or interstitial and alveolar infiltrates.

Patients with a mediastinal or hilar mass may be totally asymptomatic. They may, however, have cough, chest pain, and shortness of breath, or systemic symptoms such as fever, night sweats, or weight loss. Right hilar masses may cause superior vena caval obstruction; patients with this entity may experience headache, confusion, dyspnea, and swelling of the face and upper extremities. Dysphagia may occur if there is esophageal compression. Likewise, tracheal compression may produce cough and stridor. Arrythmias and signs of cardiac tamponade may occur secondary to direct extention of the tumor to the pericardium. Other complications of mediastinal masses include pleural effusions due to retrograde flow from blocked lymphatics, hoarseness secondary to recurrent laryngeal nerve involvement, and hiccups secondary to phrenic nerve involvement.

The differential diagnosis of benign mediastinal and hilar enlargement includes sarcoidosis, tuberculosis, syphilis, Wegener's granulomatosis, histoplasmosis, and occasionally other infections. Other entities to consider are aneurysms of the thoracic aorta and bronchogenic and pericardial cysts.

It is best to consider primary mediastinal and hilar neoplasms in terms of which tumors cause enlargement of a given area (22). Lesions that may cause enlargement of the anterior mediastinum include a substernal thyroid gland, benign and malignant teratomas and other germ cell tumors, and thymomas. The mediastinum is second to the testes as the leading site of germ cell tumors; mediastinal germ cell tumors should be treated aggressively with a regimen similar to that used for testicular tumors of similar histology (23,24). Posterior mediastinal tumors are most often neurogenic tumors arising in the intercostal or sympathetic nerves. These can be benign or malignant, such as malignant schwannoma, pheochromocytoma, and ganglioneuroblastoma (25).

The most common neoplasms arising in the middle mediastinum are lymphomas. Two lymphomas typically occur in this manner. One, lymphoblastic lymphoma, is a T-cell neoplasm, occurring most commonly in adolescent males (26). The disease is typically associated with mediastinal masses and has a propensity for bone marrow and central nervous system involvement. This lymphoma has a very aggressive natural history and should be treated with chemotherapeutic regimens used to treat acute lymphocytic leukemia. The other lymphoma is Hodgkin's disease, especially the nodular sclerosis variety; a mediastinal mass is a very common feature of Hodgkin's disease in young women (27). Mediastinal Hodgkin's disease is often associated with subclinical disease involving the pulmonary parenchyma (28). It is important to evaluate the pulmonary parenchyma in patients with mediastinal masses and Hodgkin's disease with lung tomography or CT of the mediastinum before beginning treatment or local failure at the margin of the radiation therapy port will ensue. Patients with large mediastinal masses should receive radiation therapy before laparotomy, as the risk of intubation and anesthesia is great in these patients (29). When large hilar masses are to be irradiated, the incidence of radiation pneumonitis is high. This has been minimized with the shrinking fields technique, in which after 1,500 rads of radiation are given, a rest period is allowed for the masses to shrink; subsequently, radiation therapy is given to the smaller tumor volume. Despite advances in therapy, Hodgkin's disease often relapses at sites of bulk disease, such as the mediastinum (30).

Primary carcinomas of the trachea, main stem bronchus, or esophagus may appear as mediastinal enlargement, usually with early symptoms of stridor or dysphagia.

The most common cause of mediastinal enlargement in patients with tumors is metastases of the tumor to the mediastinal lymph nodes. Although lung cancer is the most common malignancy to metastasize to mediastinal and hilar lymph nodes, virtually all tumors may do so. This is especially common with breast cancer, seminomas, lymphomas, and esophageal and gastric carcinomas. Of the various pathologic types of lung cancer, oat cell carcinoma uniformly involves these nodes (Figs. 2-3 and 2-4). Squamous cell carcinomas and adenocarcinomas of central and midlung fields also involve these lymph nodes (31). With the exception of ipsilateral hilar lymph node involvement, mediastinal or hilar metastases signify nonresectability. Occasional cures have been noted, however, when microscopic mediastinal metastases have been resected.

Evaluation of patients with a mediastinal mass should include a history and physical examination, routine blood count and chemistries, and a thorough evaluation of the remainder of the chest x-ray film for clues to the cause of the

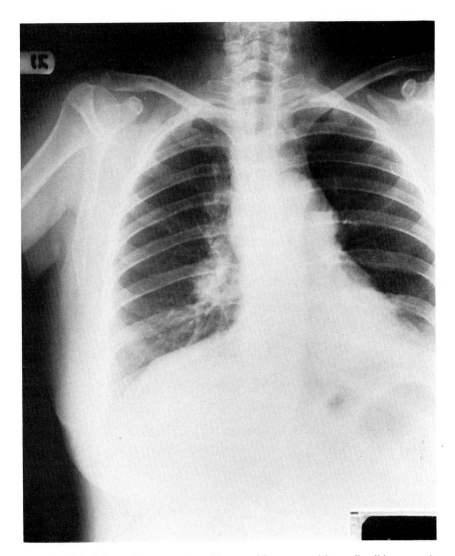

Figure 2-3. Right hilar enlargement in a 62-year-old woman with small cell lung carcinoma.

mediastinal process. Sputum should be obtained for cytologic analysis and tuberculous smears and cultures. Consideration should be given to biopsy of abnormal lymph nodes, especially in the supraclavicular area; if the x-ray film reveals a pulmonary mass, biopsy via bronchoscopy or fine-needle aspiration is indicated. If the chest x-ray pattern suggests sarcoidosis, a transbronchial biopsy may yield the diagnosis in up to 92% of cases. Other diagnostic studies may be in order. A barium swallow may define the relationship of the mass to the esophagus. A CT scan of the chest may delineate the exact location of the mass and its density and contiguity with other structures. A tissue diagnosis, however, will ultimately be necessary. For lesions of the upper or right mediastinum, mediastinoscopy may be considered. If there is any suspicion of a vascular lesion or if the lesion is in the left mediastinum, a median sternotomy will be necessary

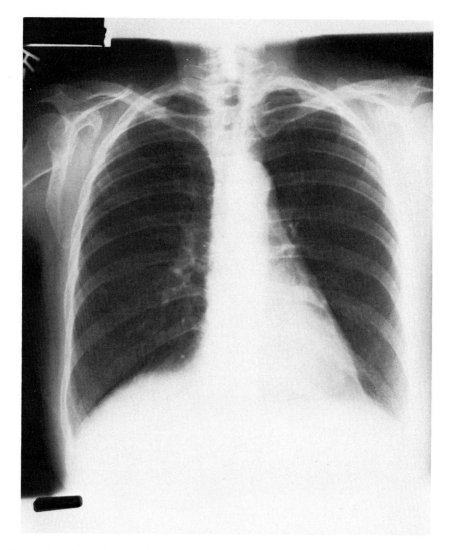

Figure 2-4. Complete resolution of hilar enlargement after two cycles of chemotherapy with Cytoxan, Oncovin, and Adriamycin.

to obtain the diagnosis. In addition, touch preparations for lymph node histology and tissue for T- and B-cell markers and electron microscopic evaluation may be helpful in some cases.

Occasionally, a pathology report may merely reveal a poorly differientiated tumor. In such cases, it is important to exclude the diagnosis of small cell carcinoma, lymphoblastic lymphoma, and mediastinal germ cell tumors, as these are highly treatable entities in which very specific therapies are available.

INTERSTITIAL INFILTRATES

Another common roentgenographic pattern in patients with cancer is that of a diffuse interstitial infiltrate. This infiltrate may occur without other radiographic abnormalities or may occur in association with a lung mass, mediastinal widening, an effusion, or an alveolar infiltrate. The differential diagnosis of this process includes both benign and malignant lesions, including idiopathic pulmonary fibrosis, collagen vascular disease, the pneumoconioses, sarcoidosis, radiation pneumonitis, drug-induced pulmonary disease, lymphangitic spread of tumor, pulmonary hemorrhage, leukoagglutinin reactions, and infectious processes such as bacterial, viral, parasitic, fungal, and tuberculous processes (32). It is important to make a concerted effort to establish a diagnosis in patients with a diffuse interstitial process, as a number of them, especially infections, are treatable, and successful management may alter the prognosis.

Several interstitial processes in the cancer patient deserve further discussion. Most of this section will be devoted to actual complications of cancer rather than to its treatment. The first of these is lymphangitic carcinomatosis. Although discussions of lymphangitic spread of cancer were originally weighted to cases of gastric cancer, this entity has been described with virtually every neoplasm (33). In all series, however, breast, lung, pancreatic, gastric, and colonic lesions predominate. In a series of 23 cases of lymphangitic spread of cancer from the Massachusettes General Hospital, one-half were secondary to breast cancer (34).

Originally, lymphangitic spread of cancer was felt to be due to retrograde spread from the hilar lymph nodes involved with tumor. Although this pattern has been seen with breast cancer and lymphoma, it is rare; in the Massachusettes General Hospital series, only 1 out of 23 patients had hilar lymph node involvement and thus lymphangitic spread on this basis. It is now felt that the cause of lymphangitic spread is tumor entrapment in pulmonary capillaries; the tumor emboli then invade pericapillary lymphatics and spread along these channels to invade the perivascular and peribronchial lymphatics (34). This form of spread produces an "interstitial fibrotic" pattern. Occasionally, the tumor emboli grow in a nodular fashion, producing a reticulonodular pattern on chest x-ray films.

The most common clinical presentation of lymphangitic spread is progressive dyspnea (35). Cough is present in up to 60% of patients. Other symptoms include chest pain, fever, weakness, and weight loss; occasionally, the patient may be asymptomatic. The physical examination may vary from a negative physical examination to a cyanotic patient who is in a coma secondary to hypoxia. The most common physical finding is moderately coarse, bibasilar rales. Wheezing may be present. Late in the course, signs of right heart failure may be present.

Radiographically, lymphangitic carcinomatosis appears as increased interstitial markings, often radiating to the hilum; the interstitial markings may vary in length and thickness (36,37). Kerley A and B lines may be present, as well as a reticulonodular pattern. Much of the radiographic picture is related to interstitial edema and inflammatory reactions around tumor-stuffed lymphatics. On occasion, the chest x-ray examination results have been negative in cases in which lymphangitic spread has been documented pathologically.

The exact diagnosis of lymphangitic spread of cancer requires histologic proof. Bronchoscopy with transbronchial biopsy is the easiest diagnostic approach; biopsy may reveal tumor-filled lymphatics. Occasionally, open lung biopsy will be needed to make the diagnosis.

Treatment of lymphangitic spread of tumor is directed at palliation of acute symptomatology and control of the specific disease entity. By controlling associated edema and inflammatory reactions, steroids may provide early relief of symptoms and may be lifesaving. Hormone therapy and/or chemotherapy may produce remissions in patients with breast cancer (Figs. 2-5 and 2-6). In patients who relapse after therapy or who do not respond to therapy, supportive care with oxygen, pain medications, antitussives, and steroids are in order. The response of the lung to lymphangitic spread of tumor is a fibrotic reaction; thus in spite of a pathologically documented antitumor response, symptoms and radiographs may not necessarily improve.

Overall, the prognosis of patients with lymphangitic spread of tumor is poor. Of 62 patients in one series, 50% were dead in 3 months, and only 8 of 62 patients survived 6 months. Of the 8 patients surviving longer than 6 months, 7 lived 6 to 20 months, and one lived 72 months (36). Although the overall survival rate is poor, occasional patients survive for a long period of time after aggressive treatment with hormonal or chemotherapy (38,39).

Another entity in the differential diagnosis of increased interstitial markings on chest x-ray film is radiation pneumonitis. Of the interstitial pneumonitides,

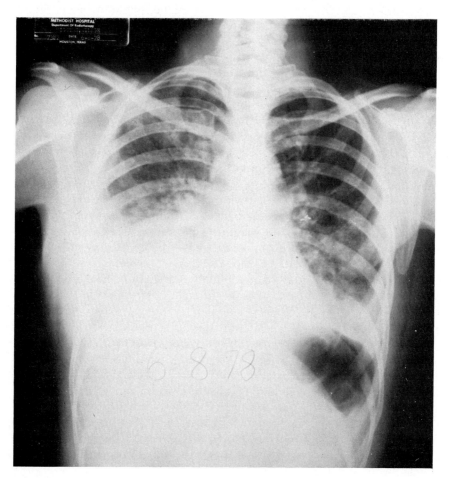

Figure 2-5. A woman with breast cancer with dyspnea and a PO$_2$ of 40. Lymphangitic carcinomatosis was documented on transbronchial lung biopsy.

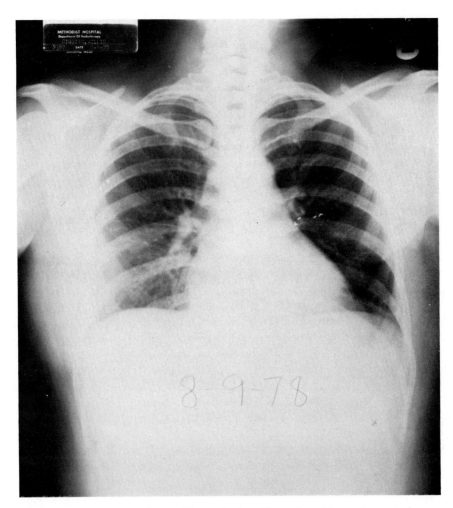

Figure 2-6. Clinical and radiographic resolution of lymphangitic carcinomatosis occurred after two months of Adriamycin chemotherapy.

this is one of the easiest to diagnose, as its location corresponds to that of previous radiation therapy treatment ports. There are two varieties of radiation pneumonitis: acute and late.

The acute form of radiation pneumonitis occurs within one to six months of receiving radiation therapy. Patients may have fever, a nonproductive cough, and dyspnea. Physical findings may include an elevated temperature and coarse rales; radiation skin changes over the area of pneumonitis may be present. A leukocytosis may be present. The chest x-ray film may show acute infiltrates and increased interstitial markings. Pathologically, the lesion consists of interstitial and capillary edema, as well as ballooning of the alveolar lining cells.

Acute radiation pneumonitis may resolve spontaneously or may proceed to chronic radiation fibrosis. Patients with chronic radiation penumonitis may, however, not have a history of an antecedent acute illness. These patients may present with progressive fatigue and dyspnea. The chest x-ray film may reveal diminishing lung volumes in addition to increased interstitial markings.

Radiation pneumonitis is most often seen in patients irradiated for breast and lung cancer; in most series, the incidence of pneumonitis approaches 5% of patients with these two entities who are irradiated (40). Patients treated to large lung volumes have a higher incidence of radiation pneumonitis; likewise, patients whose radiation dose exceeds 2000 rad in two to three weeks are at increased risk (41). Concomitant chemotherapy with drugs toxic to the lung, especially bleomycin, may increase a given patient's risk.

The best treatment of radiation pneumonitis is prevention. Careful patient selection and limitation of dose and volume of treatment are necessary (42). For individual cases, supportive care with supplemental oxygen and antibiotics for superimposed infection are in order. Steroids may be acutely beneficial and occasionally lifesaving in severe cases. A flare in symptomatology notoriously occurs when steroids are abruptly tapered; patients with radiation pneumonitis should be withdrawn from steroids very slowly (43). Flares in previously unsuspected pneumonitis have occurred with MOPP chemotherapy for Hodgkin's disease after cycles of therapy containing prednisone.

A number of cancer chemotherapeutic agents have been implicated in drug-induced lung disease associated with increased interstitial markings and fibrosis. The clinical course of lung disease related to the chemotherapeutic agents ranges from acute, self-limited interstitial pneumonitis to a progressive and occasionally fatal interstitial fibrosis. The agents most commonly associated with a pulmonary interstitial reaction include bleomycin, busulfan, BCNU (carmustine), and methotrexate. Other agents that have occasionally been reported to cause interstitial lung disease include mercaptopurine, procarbazine, melphalan, leukeran, mitomycin C, and cytoxan (44).

Pulmonary hemorrhage may produce acute interstitial infiltrates. Thrombocytopenia due to the underlying disease or its therapy and disseminated intravascular coagulation may be the cause of bleeding. The clinical course may vary from self-limited pneumonitis to a pattern of a "white-lung," respiratory failure, and subsequent death. Survivors may have residual fibrosis in the area of hemorrhage.

Diffuse interstitial infiltrates associated with a clinical picture of acute dyspnea, hemoptysis, and severe hypoxemia have complicated the use of granulocyte transfusions; this reaction is fatal in a significant proportion of patients. Pathologically, diffuse intra-alveolar hemorrhage has been observed in these patients. A recent study has shown that the incidence of this pulmonary reaction is higher when amphotericin B is given with or shortly after the granulocyte transfusion; the combined use of amphotericin B and granulocytes was associated with a 64% incidence of interstitial pulmonary reactions, while granulocyte transfusions alone were associated with a 6% incidence of the pulmonary reactions (45). The cause of this reaction is unknown. It has been postulated that amphotericin B may cause lysis of granulocytes that were trapped in small pulmonary vessels; neutrophil proteases are subsequently released, causing the pulmonary damage.

Infectious processes are a frequent cause of interstitial infiltrates in patients with neoplastic disorders. Although patients may be febrile and may manifest physical findings suggestive of an infectious pulmonary process, these patients may be immunosuppressed and may not manifest a febrile response. The course and pattern of the infection may be very atypical. There is often a lag between the physical findings and chest x-ray results; this is especially true in the case of viral and *Pneumocystis carinii* pneumonias. Infections may produce a variety of radiographic patterns, including lobar consolidation, segmental or diffuse interstitial infiltrates, or alveolar infiltrates. Patients with a low granulocyte count may be unable to develop a radiographic picture of lobar consolidation (46).

A wide variety of infections may produce a pattern of diffuse interstitial infiltrates. Bacterial infections, including pneumococcal, streptococcal, pseudomonas, and *Klebsiella* pneumonias may occur in this manner; Gram's stain and cultures of sputum and bronchoscopic specimens may reveal the diagnosis in these cases. A bacterium that may also produce pulmonary infection in the compromised host is *Nocardia asteroides;* nearly 50% of patients with *Nocardia* infections are being treated with steroids or are immunocompromised on the basis of their underlying disease (47). The clinical pattern may range from no symptoms to fever, cough, malaise, and pleuritic chest pain. The radiographic picture may include segmental or lobar infiltrates, necrotizing pneumonia, pulmonary nodules, lung abscesses, or empyema. It is often difficult to grow *Nocardia* from routine sputum cultures; more invasive procedures, such as transbronchial or open lung biopsy, may be necessary to make the diagnosis. Due to its propensity to involve the central nervous system and skin, as well as the lung, a search for *Nocardia* infection is indicated in the patient with infection involving these sites.

Tuberculosis must also be considered in the differential diagnosis of interstitial infiltrates in patients with neoplastic disease. The incidence of both *Mycobacterium tuberculosis* infections and infections with atypical mycobacteria is increased in the compromised host. A series from Memorial Sloan-Kettering Cancer Center demonstrated that prevalence rates were highest in patients with Hodgkin's disease, non-Hodgkin's lymphoma, and cancer of the lung (48). In this series, patients whose active tuberculosis developed after treatment for the underlying neoplasm more often had diffuse infiltrates or disseminated disease; untreated patients with cancer developed classic upper lobe infiltrates and cavities. The overall mortality rate from tuberculosis was 17% in the Memorial series; in the subgroup with lymphoma, it was 48%.

Fungal infections may also cause pulmonary infection in patients with malignancy; among the fungi causing such infection are cryptococcus, aspergillus, phycomycetes, *Candida,* histoplasmosis, coccidioidomycoses, and *Torulopsis glabrata* (Fig. 2-7). Cryptococcal infection is seen in association with Hodgkin's disease; it may also complicate steroid therapy (49). Symptoms may include cough, chest pain, fever, and hemoptysis; in one series 32% of patients were asymptomatic. The radiographic pattern may include single or multiple mass lesions, lobar consolidation, hilar adenopathy, or diffuse interstitial infiltrates that are indistinguishable from a variety of other pulmonary infections (50). Diagnosis requires demonstrating the organism in lung tissue. It is important to aggressively diagnose and treat pulmonary cryptococcosis, as early amphotericin therapy may prevent central nervous system dissemination.

Aspergillus species, especially *Aspergillus fumigatus,* have a propensity to involve the lung. *Aspergillus* infection is characterized by vascular invasion, with necro-

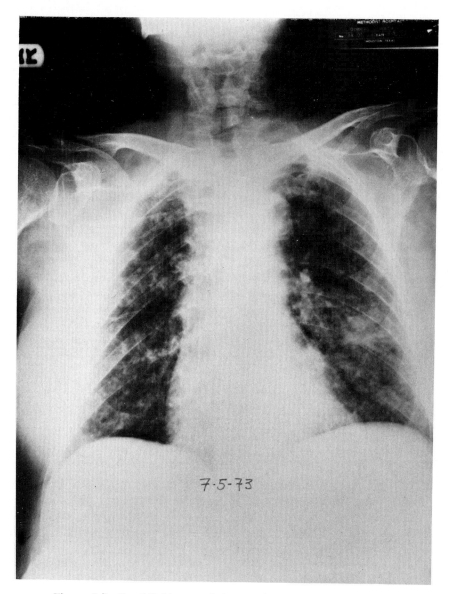

Figure 2-7. Coccidioidomycosis in a patient with lymphoma.

tizing pneumonia and pulmonary infarction being common clinical patterns. Thus, pleuritic pain, cough, and fever are frequent symptoms. Radiographically, nodular lesions, cavities, wedge-shaped densities abutting the pleura, and diffuse infiltrates may be present (51). Diagnosis requires both cultural growth and demonstration of tissue invasion.

Infection with phycomycetes is also characterized by blood vessel invasion with subsequent infarction. Pulmonary rather than nasal involvement is more common in patients with malignancy. Symptoms are often those of pulmonary infarction, as seen with aspergillosis. The radiographic pattern includes infiltrates, nodular densities, and lobar consolidation (52). Sputum cultures are usually negative; the demonstration of the organism in tissue is needed to establish the diagnosis.

Candida infections, especially with *Candida albicans*, are not infrequent pulmonary infections in the compromised host. Predisposing features include treatment with steroids and immunosuppressive chemotherapeutic agents, indwelling catheters, and prolonged use of antibiotics (46). The chest x-ray pattern includes extensive bronchopneumonia, abscess formation, and diffuse infiltration; an M. D. Anderson Hospital and Tumor Institute series, however, demonstrated no evidence of radiographic manifestations in 46% of patients at the onset of *Candida* infection involving the lungs (53). Diagnosis of *Candida* infection based on sputum culture is unreliable due to the high incidence of contamination; demonstration of the organism in lung tissue is needed to establish the diagnosis.

Viruses are often a cause of diffuse interstitial infiltrates in the immunocompromised patient; cytomegalovirus, herpes simplex, and herpes zoster are frequent offenders (Fig. 2-8). Acute and convalescent sera for viral titers may be beneficial in the diagnosis of these disorders, as may viral cultures. The diagnosis is most quickly established by demonstration of the pathognomonic intranuclear inclusions in the infected cells.

Pulmonary infection with herpes simplex virus may range from tracheobronchitis to pneumonia. Herpetic ulcerations of the mouth and upper respiratory or gastrointestinal tract may point to the diagnosis. The chest x-ray pattern may range from lobar bronchopneumonia to diffuse interstitial pneumonia.

Cytomegalovirus pulmonary disease often presents with fever, nonproductive cough, and progressive dyspnea leading to respiratory failure. The physical examination may reveal tachypnea, coarse rales and rhonchi, and later cyanosis and hypoxemic coma. As in other viral pneumonias, there may be a lag between the physical examination and radiographic manifestations, which may range from an apparently normal chest x-ray pattern to alveolar and interstitial infiltrates; multiple pulmonary nodules may also be seen (54).

Varicella zoster pulmonary infection is an often fatal pulmonary disease in patients with malignancy. This infection most commonly complicates Hodgkin's disease, recent irradiation, and recent treatment for leukemia (55). Physical findings involving the lung are often minimal and are discordant with the severe radiographic pattern; however, the characteristic vesicular rash usually precedes pulmonary involvement and points to the diagnosis (56). The radiographic pattern is one of a peribronchiolar, nodular infiltrate with a predilection for the lower lung fields. Prevention of this infection is very important; isolation of patients with malignancy from those with chicken pox and herpes zoster is mandatory.

Pneumocystis carinii is a protozoan causing diffuse interstitial lung disease in the compromised host; it typically occurs in patients who have recently been tapered off corticosteroids (Fig. 2-9). Symptoms may include fever, cough, hemoptysis, and progressive dyspnea. The physical examination may reveal bronchial breath sounds and diffuse rales, or it may be entirely normal. Likewise, the radiographic pattern may range from an occasionally negative chest x-ray film to a more typical pattern of diffuse interstitial infiltrates radiating from the hilum (57). The diagnosis may occasionally be established by demonstrating the

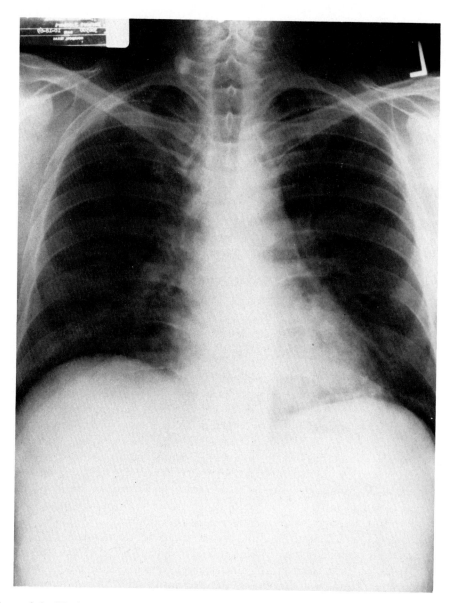

Figure 2-8. Viral pneumonitis proven by percutaneous lung biopsy. PO_2 was 45 mm Hg at the time of the chest x-ray.

offending organism on Gram' and Wiegert's stain or methenamine silver stain of the sputum or bronchial brushings. More frequently, stains obtained from an open lung biopsy specimen are needed to make a diagnosis.

Other organisms that may cause pulmonary disease in the compromised host include the protozoan *Toxoplasma gondii* and *Strongyloides stercoralis*, a nematode. Both may produce a pattern ranging from pulmonary consolidation to diffuse interstitial infiltrates.

In all cases in which infection is the suspected cause of pulmonary disease in patients with malignancy, the specific etiology must be aggressively pursued so that appropriate therapy may be given when available. Demonstration of the offending organism should not stop short of open lung biopsy when indicated. When bacterial pathogens are established as the cause of infection, the appropriate antimicrobial is given. If pulmonary tissue invasion by fungi is demonstrated, amphotericin B is the drug of choice. Therapy for viral infections consists of supportive care at this time; interferon and antiviral agents are being studied at some centers. Trimethoprim-sulfamethoxazole is thought to be as effective as pentamidine in the treatment of *Pneumocystis carinii* infections (58). Ease of

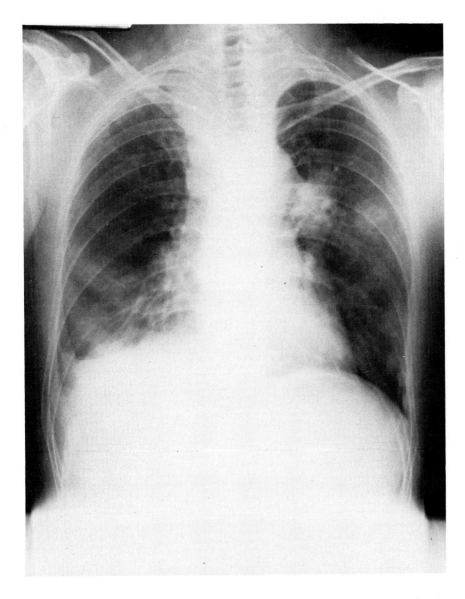

Figure 2-9. Pneumocystis carinii pneumonia. Diagnosis was made by transbronchial biopsy.

administration has led to trials of the prophylactic use of trimethoprim-sulfa-methoxazole in patients being tapered off steroids; early reports indicate a reduction in the number of cases of *Pneumocystis* infection in patients so treated (59).

PNEUMOTHORAX

Spontaneous pneumothorax has been noted to complicate subpleural metastases. It is a notable complication of adjuvant chemotherapy for osteogenic sarcoma. During treatment, spontaneous pneumothorax may occur as a result of tumor lysis of a previous subclinical pulmonary metastases. Small (<15%) pneumothoracies in this setting are treated by observation; larger or symptomatic ones are best treated with tube thoracostomy.

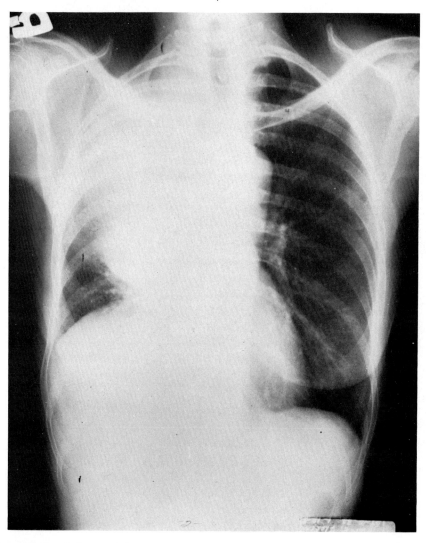

Figure 2-10. Collapse of the right upper and middle lobes in a 55-year-old woman with small cell carcinoma.

ATELECTASIS

Collapse of a lobe or segment of the lung suggests bronchial obstruction (Figs. 2-10 and 2-11). Symptoms include fever, cough, and occasionally, chest pain and purulent sputum production. Radiographically, the lesion may present with obscuration of the diaphragm or heart border; an air bronchogram may be present. The mediastinum may be shifted to the affected side.

The differential diagnosis includes a mucus plug, foreign body obstruction, bronchogenic carcinoma, and endobronchial metastases from other tumors. Tumors with a propensity for endobronchial metastases include breast cancer, hypernephroma, melanoma, lymphoma, and metastases from lung cancer. Endobronchial metastases have been described, however, with virtually all tumors, including carcinoma of the uterine cervix. Sputum cytology may be positive for

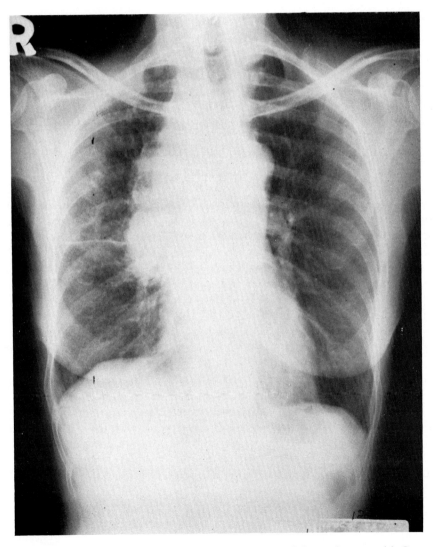

Figure 2-11. Resolution of lobar collapse after one cycle of chemotherapy with Cytoxan, Adriamycin, and Oncovin.

the metastatic tumor; this is especially true in the case of endobronchial metastases from malignant melanoma.

When patients suffer collapse of a lung segment, a diagnosis of cancer must be vigorously excluded. Bronchoscopy may be both diagnostic and curative in cases of foreign objects and mucus plugs. In other cases, bronchoscopic brushings and cytologic analyses should be obtained. In patients with primary lung tumors who have no nodal or distant metastases, resection may be in order. In patients with metastatic bronchogenic carcinoma and patients with endobronchial metastases from other tumors, radiation therapy may relieve the obstruction.

MISCELLANEOUS PULMONARY COMPLICATIONS OF CANCER

There are several other pulmonary complications of cancer that defy strict categorization in terms of their radiographic presentation.

PULMONARY EMBOLISM

Pulmonary embolism is a common occurrence in malignancy; its cause in cancer patients is multifactorial. Immobilization from debilitating illness, pathologic fractures, and surgery predispose the patient to deep vein thrombosis and pulmonary embolism. Likewise, cancer patients may be predisposed to pulmonary emboli on a mechanical basis. Pelvic and intra-abdominal tumors may cause vena cava compression and compression of vascular structures; such compression may cause thrombosis and subsequent emboli. Occasionally, renal tumors may invade the renal vein and extend into the vena cava. Pulmonary embolus of actual tumor or secondary vascular clot may occur. This has also been seen with choriocarcinoma and hepatoma. Renal vein and subsequent inferior vena cava thrombosis may complicate the nephrotic syndrome associated with malignancy.

A third and very important mechanism of pulmonary emboli involves venous thrombosis secondary to hypercoagulable states associated with cancer. Trousseau described the syndrome of migratory thrombophlebitis in association with pancreatic cancer. This syndrome has been described with a wide variety of neoplasms but most frequently with mucin-producing adenocarcinomas such as pancreatic, gastric, and ovarian cancer (60). It is presumed that mucin and other thrombogenic materials in the tumor cells activate factor X, with subsequent initiation of the clotting cascade. In acute promyelocytic leukemia, clotting may be initiated by release of thromboplastin from promyelocytic granules (61).

Pulmonary embolus presents as it does in patients without malignancy; tachypnea, tachycardia, cough, hemoptysis, and low-grade fever are frequent manifestations. In cancer patients, primary neoplasia involving the lung, superimposed infection, and pulmonary complications of chemotherapy and radiotherapy may be present and may mask the symptoms of pulmonary embolus; a high suspicion for this diagnosis is, therefore, very important.

Radiographically, pulmonary embolus may appear as a wedge-shaped density, a pleural effusion, or fleeting infiltrates; likewise, the chest x-ray pattern may be normal.

Once the diagnosis of pulmonary embolism is suspected, it must be confirmed. Although a ventilation-perfusion lung scan showing mismatching of ventilation and perfusion makes the diagnosis of pulmonary embolism highly likely, the ultimate diagnostic test is a pulmonary arteriogram.

Once the diagnosis is made, anticoagulation with heparin is in order. Anticoagulation in cancer patients may be quite hazardous due to altered mucosal barriers and tumors that are susceptible to bleeding; thrombocytopenia secondary to the neoplasm or its therapy, or occasional primary fibrinolytic states such as those occurring in prostate carcinoma, may increase the bleeding tendency. If the risk of bleeding is great, umbrella placement or inferior vena cava ligation may be in order.

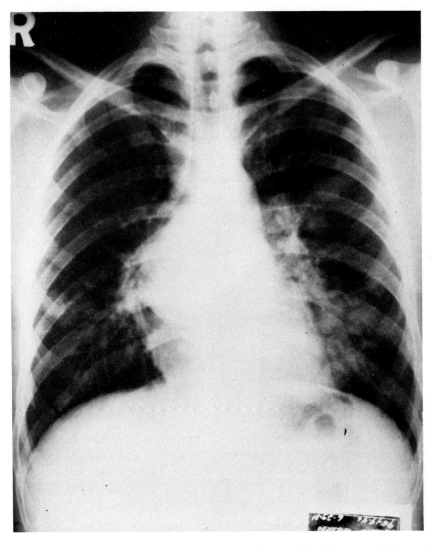

Figure 2-12. Multiple pulmonary nodules and an enlarged right hilum in a 27-year-old with testicular carcinoma.

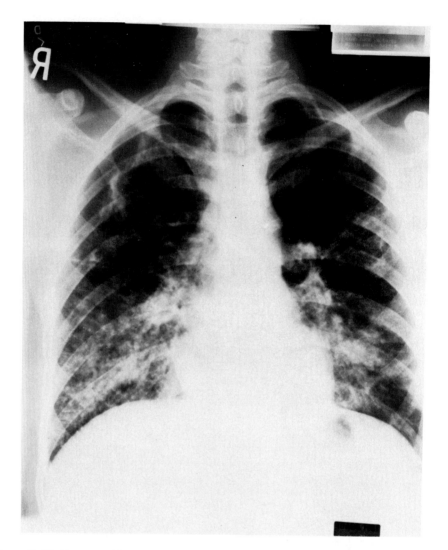

Figure 2-13. Pneumonitis secondary to rupture of a bronchus after two cycles of chemotherapy with *cis*-platinum, vinblastine, and bleomycin. Rapid tumor lysis caused rupture of the right bronchus.

BRONCHIAL RUPTURE

Treatment of metastatic testicular cancer with aggressive chemotherapy has produced bronchial rupture in a patient secondary to lysis of a central bronchial tumor (62) (Figs. 2-12 and 2-13). The patient subsequently suffered a severe pulmonary infection; upon recovery, the patient underwent subsequent courses of chemotherapy without difficulty.

FISTULA FORMATION

Bronchopleural and tracheoesophageal fistulas may complicate neoplastic diseases and their treatment. Tracheoesophageal fistulas may complicate lung carcinoma, esophageal carcinoma, lymphomas, and metastases to the mediastinum. They are most commonly due to direct tumor extension; however, tumor lysis from radiation therapy and chemotherapy may produce tracheoesophageal fistulas (63). Tracheoesophageal fistulas often appear with cough after eating or drinking and as aspiration; they can be diagnosed by use of barium swallow, demonstrating a communication between the trachea and esophagus. Bronchopleural fistulas often have recurrent pleural effusions and occasional empyemas; these fistulas most often complicate surgery and radiation for carcinoma of the lung.

REFERENCES

1. Higgins G, Shields T, Keehn R: The solitary pulmonary nodule. *Arch Surg* 110:570, 1975.

2. Ray R, Lawton B, Magnin G, et al: The coin lesion story: Update 1976. *Chest* 70:332, 1976.

3. Lolli A, McCormack L, Zelch M, et al: Aspiration biopsies of chest lesions. *Radiology* 127:35, 1978.

4. Wilson J, Eskridge M, Scott E: Transbronchial biopsy of benign and peripheral lung lesions. *Radiology* 100:541, 1971.

5. Reynolds R, Pajak T, Greenberg B, et al: Lung cancer as a second primary. *Cancer* 42:2887, 1978.

6. McCormack P, Bains M, Beattie E, Martini N: Pulmonary resection in metastatic carcinoma. *Chest* 73:163, 1973.

7. Dongen J, von Slooten E: The surgical treatment of pulmonary metastases. *Cancer Treat Rev* 5:29, 1978.

8. Conley J, Dingman D: Adenoid cystic carcinoma of the head and neck (cylindroma). *Arch Otolaryngol* 100:81, 1974.

9. Hong W, Wittes R, Hajdu S, et al: The evolution of mature teratoma from malignant testicular tumors. *Cancer* 40:2987, 1977.

10. Donahue J, Einhorn L, Perez J: Improved management of non-seminomatous testicular cancer. *Cancer* 42:2903, 1978.

11. Jeffree G, Price C, Sissons H: The metastatic pattern of osteosarcoma. *Brit J Cancer* 32:87, 1975.

12. Vincent R, Choksi L, Takita H, et al: Surgical resection of the solitary pulmonary metastases, in Weiss L, Gilbert H (eds): *Pulmonary Metastases*. Boston, GK Hall and Co, 1978.

13. Legha S, Davis H, Nuggia F: Hormonal therapy of breast cancer: New approaches and concepts. *Ann Intern Med* 88:69, 1978.

14. Leff A, Hopewell P, Costello J: Pleural effusion from malignancy. *Ann Intern Med* 88:532, 1978.

15. Cardozo P: A critical evaluation of 3,000 cytologic analyses of pleural fluid, ascitic fluid, and pericardial fluid. *Acta Cytol* 10:455, 1966.

16. Von Hoff D, Li Valsi V: Diagnostic reliability of needle biopsy of the parietal pleura. A review of 272 biopsies. *Ann J Clin Pathol* 64:200, 1975.

17. Lambert C, Shah H, Urshel H, Paulson D: The treatment of malignant pleural effusions by closed trocar drainage. *Ann Thorac Surg* 3:1, 1967.

18. Leininger B, Barker W, Lanston H: A simplified method for management of malignant pleural effusions. *J Thorac Cardiovasc Surg* 58:758, 1969.

19. Wallach H: Intrapleural tetracycline for malignant pleural effusion. *Chest* 68:510, 1975.

20. Robinson R, Balooki H: Intrapleural tetracycline for control of malignant pleural effusions. *South Med J* 65:847, 1972.

21. Jensik R, Cagle J, Milloy F, et al: Pleurectomy in the treatment of pleural effusion due to metastatic malignancy. *J Thorac Cardiovasc Surg* 46:322, 1963.

22. Silverman N, Sabistan D: Primary tumors and cysts of the mediastinum. *Curr Probl Cancer* 2:1, 1977.

23. Martini N, Golbey R, Hajdu S, et al: Primary mediastinal germ cell tumors. *Cancer* 33:763, 1974.

24. Reynolds T, Yagoda A, Vugrin D, et al: Chemotherapy of mediastinal germ cell tumors. *Semin Oncol* 6:113, 1979.

25. Gale A, Lelihovsky T, Grant F, et al: Neurogenic tumors of the mediastinum. *Ann Thorac Surg* 17:434, 1974.

26. Simone J, Verzosa M, Rudy J: Initial features and prognosis in 363 children with acute lymphoblastic leukemia. *Cancer* 36:2099, 1975.

27. Kaplan H: *Hodgkin's Disease*, ed 2. Cambridge, Harvard University Press, 1980.

28. March P, Goodman R, Hellman S: The significance of mediastinal involvement in early stage Hodgkin's disease. *Cancer* 42:1039, 1978.

29. Piro A, Weiss D, Hellman S: Mediastinal Hodgkin's disease: A possible danger for intubation anesthesia. *Int J Radiol Oncol Biol Phys* 1:415, 1976.

30. Young R, Cannellos G, Chabner B, et al: Patterns of relapse in advanced Hodgkin's disease treated with combination chemotherapy. *Cancer* 42:1001, 1978.

31. Goldberg E, Shapiro C, Glickman A: Mediastinoscopy for assessing mediastinal spread in clinical staging of lung carcinoma. *Semin Oncol* 1:205, 1974.

32. Faire A, Greenberg S, O'Neal R, et al: Diffuse interstitial fibrosis of the lung. *Am J Clin Pathol* 59:636, 1973.

33. Hauser T, Stern A: Lymphangitic carcinomatosis of the lung: Six case reports and a review of the literature. *Ann Intern Med* 34:881, 1951.

34. Janower M, Blennerhasselt J: Lymphangitic spread of metastatic cancer to the lung: A radiologic-pathologic classification. *Radiology* 101:267, 1971.

35. Harold J: Lymphangitis carcinomatosa of the lungs. *Q J Med* 21:353, 1952.

36. Yang S, Lin C: Lymphangitic carcinomatosis of the lungs: The clinical significance of its roentgenologic classification. *Chest* 62:179, 1972.

37. Trapnell D: Radiological appearance of lymphangitis carcinomatosa of the lung. *Thorax* 19:251, 1954.

38. Schimmel D, Julien P, Gamsu G: Resolution of pulmonary lymphangitic carcinoma of the breast. *Chest* 69:106, 1976.

39. Schwartz M, Waddell L, Dombeck D, et al: Prolonged survival in lymphangitic carcinomatosis. *Ann Intern Med* 71:779, 1969.

40. Levene H, Harris J, Hellman S: Treatment of carcinoma of the breast by radiation therapy. *Cancer* 39:2840, 1975.

41. Wara W, Phillips T, Margolis L, Smith V: Radiation pneumonitis: A new approach to the derivation of time-dose factors. *Cancer* 32:547, 1973.

42. Gross N: Pulmonary effects of radiation therapy. *Ann Intern Med* 86:81, 1977.

43. Castellino R, Glastein E, Turbow M, et al: Latent radiation injury of lungs or heart activated by steroid withdrawal. *Ann Intern Med* 80:593, 1974.

44. Wilson J: Pulmonary toxicity of antineoplastic drugs. *Cancer Treat Rep* 62:2003, 1978.

45. Wright D, Robichaud K, Pizzo P, et al: Lethal pulmonary reactions associated with the combined use of amphotericin B and leukocyte transfusions. *New Engl J Med* 304:1185, 1981.

46. Williams D, Krick J, Remington J: Pulmonary infection in the compromised host. *Ann Rev Resp Dis* 114:359, 595, 1976.

47. Young L, Armstrong D, Blevins A, et al: *Nocardia asteroides* infection complicating neoplastic disease. *Am J Med* 50:356, 1971.

48. Kaplan M, Armstrong D, Rosen P: Tuberculosis complicating neoplastic disease. *Cancer* 33:850, 1974.

49. Goldstein E, Rambo O: Cryptococcal infection following steroid therapy. *Ann Intern Med* 56:114, 1962.

50. Warr W, Bates J, Stone A: The spectrum of pulmonary cryptococcosis. *Ann Intern Med* 69:1109, 1968.

51. Meyer R, Young L, Armstrong D, et al: Aspergillosis complicating neoplastic disease. *Ann J Med* 54:6, 1973.

52. Meyer R, Rosen P, Armstrong D: Phycomycosis complicating leukemia and lymphoma. *Ann Intern Med* 77:871, 1972.

53. Bodey G: Fungal infection complicating acute leukemia. *J Chronic Dis* 19:667, 1966.

54. Ho M: Cytomegalovirus infections and diseases. *Disease-a-Month* 24:1, 1978.

55. DoRin R, Reichman R, Mazur M, et al: Herpes zoster-varicella injection in immunosuppressed patients. *Ann Intern Med* 89:375, 1978.

56. Triebwasser J, Harris R, Bryant R, et al: Varicella pneumonia in adults. *Medicine* 46:409, 1967.

57. Hughes W: *Pneumocystis carinii* pneumonia. *New Engl J Med* 297:1381, 1977.

58. Winston D, Law W, Gale R, et al: Trimethoprimsulfamethoxazole for the treatment of *Pneumocystis carinii* pneumonia. *Ann Intern Med* 92:762, 1980.

59. Hughes W, Kuhn S, Chaudhory S, et al: Succesful chemoprophylaxsis for *Pneumocystis carinii* pneumonitis. *New Engl J Med* 297:1419, 1977.

60. Sack G, Levin J, Bell W: Trousseau's syndrome and other manifestations of chronic disseminated coagulopathy in patients with neoplasms: Clinical, pathophysiologic, and therapeutic features. *Medicine* 56:1, 1977.

61. Gralnick H, Tan H: Acute promyelocytic leukemia: A model for understanding the role of malignant cells in hemostatis. *Hum Pathol* 5:661, 1974.

62. Doty J, Lynch G, Smith F, et al: Bronchial rupture complicating chemotherapy for testicular cancer. Submitted for publication.

63. Wara W, Mauch P, Thomas A, et al: Palliation for carcinoma of the esophagus. *Radiology* 121:717, 1976.

3

Genitourinary Complications of Cancer

Mary Anne Zubler

There are numerous direct and indirect gynecologic and urinary tract manifestations of cancer. The natural course and disease processes of patients with primary renal, ureteral, bladder, cervical, ovarian, and uterine cancer have been discussed elegantly in other texts and will not be reiterated here (1–4). However, the secondary effects of any type of cancer on the structure or function of these organs will be examined. Neoplastic disease affects the genitourinary (GU) system in several ways, including direct involvement by the primary or metastatic process and functional impairment due to local or remote tumor processes. The clinical features, the diagnosis and differential diagnosis, and general approaches to the treatment of complications of cancer in this system will be examined.

METASTASES TO THE KIDNEY

Klinger reviewed the subject of tumor metastases to the genitourinary system in 142 patients selected from an autopsy series of 5,000 (5). In this survey, the most common tumors to metastasize to the GU tract were the lymphoma-leukemia group. The second most common were primaries in the respiratory tract, followed by stomach, breast, pancreas, ovary, esophagus, and the biliary system (Figs. 3-1 to 3-3). He excluded those cancers that are well known to spread to the GU system by contiguity, such as those of the lower large bowel and the female generative tract. This group exerts its effects by compression and direct spread.

In more than one-half of the cases, there were multiple sites of metastases. The solid tumors tended to be seen as nodular deposits, while the lymphomas and leukemias tended to infiltrate the organs. Bilateral renal involvement was the most common pattern seen, but unilateral renal metastases and bladder metastases were also common. Rarely, there was vas deferens and urethral involvement and penile involvement (which presented as priapism).

Urinary abnormalities were found in 86 of 142 patients. Forty-eight had no

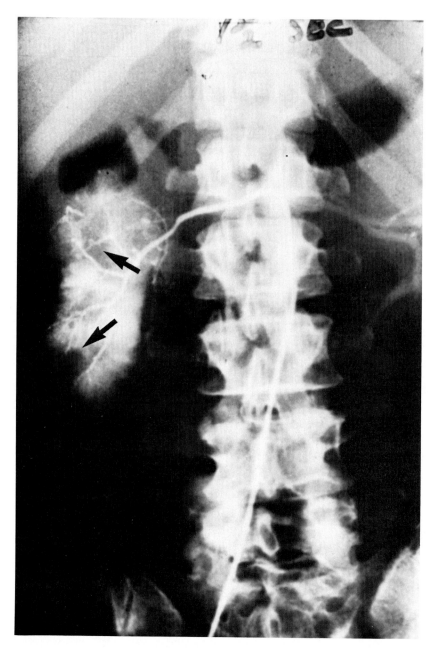

Figure 3-1. Angiographic demonstration of metastatic lung cancer involving most of the upper pole (arrow), part of the midportion, and lower pole (arrow). Massive hematuria and secondary ureteral colic responded well to focal radiation.

urinary abnormalities, and, of these, three had extensive infiltration of the kidneys by leukemia. Twenty-eight patients, about 20%, had hematuria, usually microscopic. In this series, renal insufficiency was not an important feature unless the renal destruction was extreme, combined with ureteral obstruction, or there was a superimposed disorder. It was most commonly seen in the lymphoma-

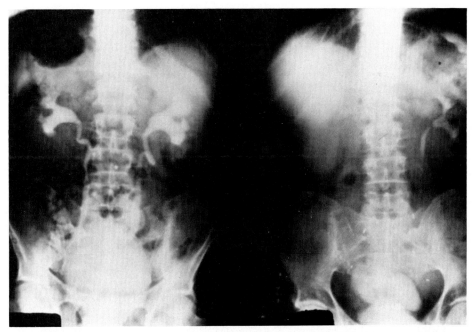

Figure 3-2. *Left:* Bilateral, nodular renal lymphocytic lymphoma, retroperitoneal adenopathy, and obstructive uropathy on IVP. *Right:* Improvement in left kidney findings after radiation and combination chemotherapy. Radiation treatment to the right kidney was not given simultaneously, resulting in local disease progression and nonfunction.

leukemia group, where there was direct renal destruction. On the other hand, in lymphomas and leukemias there were also found patients with heavy and widespread infiltration of the kidneys without any evidence of renal failure.

Conn et al. described hypertension resulting from a primary renal tumor that produced renin (6). Hypertension secondary to tumor may also be seen in renal cell cancer and Wilms' tumors (7,8). Tumor metastases causing hypertension are rare, but they have been reported.

METASTATIC DISEASE
OF GYNECOLOGIC ORGANS

Although Krukenberg's tumor is the best known of metastatic deposits in gynecologic organs, other tumors also invade these organs. In 357 cases of metastatic disease of the ovary, gastrointestinal tract primaries account for three-fourths according to one study done in 1975 (9). There is also a high incidence of metastatic disease from breast primaries, but these statistics may be due to the previous practice of oophorectomy at the time of mastectomy (10). Most of these metastases were asymptomatic and were not visible grossly (11). On the other hand, metastases from colon carcinoma tend to be large, cystic, and hemorrhagic (12). In those patients who have primary surgery for intestinal carcinoma, about 20% are found to have involvement at the time of surgery or

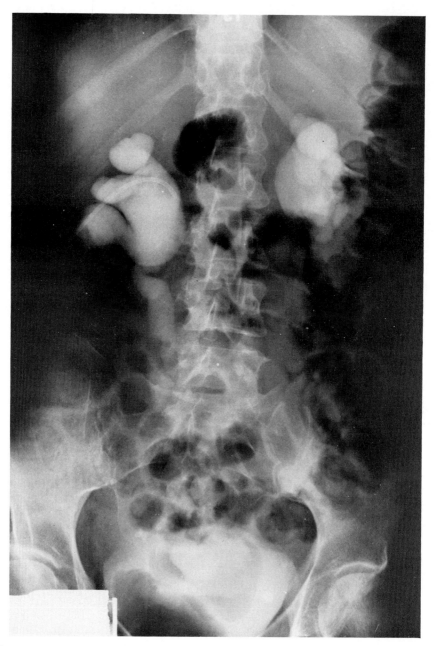

Figure 3-3. Bilateral obstructive uropathy and metastatic renal tumor from primary carcinoma of the breast proven at laparotomy. The patient survived four years as a consequence of nephrostomy, radiation therapy, hormonal therapy, and combination drug treatment.

metastases to the ovary within five to six years (13,14). Most ovarian metastases develop in postmenopausal women, with the exception of breast cancer, where almost 90% occur in premenopausal women (9). Only about 20% of patients with ovarian metastases will have vaginal bleeding; a few will have ascites or pleural effusion, but the majority are not symptomatic (15).

Cervical metastases from both breast cancer and stomach cancer have been reported (16). These usually manifest themselves as vaginal bleeding, but are occasionally discovered as an exphytic growth on the cervix (17).

Uterine metastases are most commonly from a primary melanoma, but others, such as pancreatic metastasis, have been reported (17–18). Again, the symptoms are most often vaginal bleeding, with uterine enlargement (19).

Vaginal metastases are uncommon but have been reported from primaries in the colon, cecum, pancreas, and kidney (20–22). These metastases may be asymptomatic, can be the only site of metastasis, and are often compatible with a long survival (20,21). In contrast metastases to the vulva, which have been seen in cervical, endometrial, vaginal, urethral, ovarian, renal, and breast cancer, are usually an ominous symptom of terminal disease, and death occurs within one year in most cases (23).

RADIATION

Radiation effects on the kidneys have been well characterized, and the limits of radiation in fields involving the kidneys are well known. Luxton and Kunkler classified the effects of radiation on the kidney into five categories: (1) acute radiation nephritis; (2) chronic radiation nephritis; (3) asymptomatic proteinuria; (4) essential hypertension; and (5) late developing malignant hypertension (24). The effects of radiation depend on the type of radiation, the dose, fractionation, and the prior function of the kidney. Gup et al. and Avioli et al. showed no changes in dogs and in humans, respectively, in common renal function tests when giving up to 2400 rads total dose in fractions of 100 to 1000 rads (25,26). However, a decrease in renal plasma flow was found with as little as 400 rads, and continued to accrue with each successive dose. Glomerular function showed a transient increase, probably a result of transient hyperemia, followed by a rapid decrease to below normal and subsequent gradual but incomplete improvement. Generally, doses higher than 2300 rads both experimentally and clinically produce damage to both tubules and glomeruli.

Since Assher and Anson's studies on accelerated atherosclerotic changes that occur in irradiated blood vessels, the pathophysiology of the damage is fairly well understood (27). After a single dose of irradiation, hypergranulation of the juxtaglomerular cell can be seen in about 90 days. In approximately five months in rats, hypertension is present and necrosis of the "sensitized" arteries develops. Light microscopy in chronic radiation nephritis shows marked tubular destruction with interstitial fibrosis and glomerular hyalinization and subendothelial fibrous connective tissue proliferation in the medium and smaller arteries.

The clinical picture of acute radiation nephritis consists of proteinuria, hematuria, acute hypertension, anemia, and cardiomegaly. Although recovery may occur, the usual course is one of permanent damage to the kidneys. Treatment consists of supportive measures: antihypotensive drugs, careful fluid and dietary management, rest, and transfusion as needed.

Chronic radiation nephritis may develop from months to years after treatment and usually occurs over a period of time. It may develop in the absence of an acute episode of radiation nephritis. In the study by Kunkler et al., 40% of patients who received 2500 to 3250 rads in three to six weeks developed renal damage and seven died secondary to this damage (28). Twenty-four patients developed chronic radiation nephritis from months to years later, although nine remained normotensive for eight years. Usually, however, the picture of chronic glomerulonephritis with hypertension, telescopic urine sediment, and abnormal renal function tests develops, with the progression to small fibrotic kidneys. An important point is made in the article by Crummy et al. on renal radiation damage in a patient with unilateral dysfunction causing hypertension cured by nephrectomy (29). If the damage is known to be unilateral, nephrectomy should be considered.

The hemolytic-uremic syndrome, with its characteristic blood picture of hemolytic anemia, red cell fragmentation, thrombocytopenia, and increased fibrin split products, as well as hypertension and renal failure, has also been described, mainly in children, as a sequela to radiation, with or without chemotherapy (30). Some feel that chemotherapy may increase the susceptibility of the kidney to radiation.

The description by Keane et al. of the electron microscopic changes in acute radiation nephritis with splitting of the glomerular basement membrane and subendothelial dense deposits is similar to those found in cases of the hemolytic-uremic syndrome, thrombocytopenic purpura, and renal allograft rejection (31). They theorized that endothelial cell damage following irradiation and the subsequent death of these cells within a number of months resulted in a platelet–basement membrane interaction and subsequent local activation of the coagulation system.

Several courses have been suggested to avoid renal damage: (1) limitation of doses to no more than 2000 rads in two weeks, or its biological equivalent; (2) redefining fields after the initial shrinkage to exclude the kidneys where possible; (3) selective infusion of the renal artery with vasoconstrictors during treatment; or (4) surgical repositioning of the kidney to a site not in the radiation fields. At present, it is still experimental to consider the use of anticoagulants or antiplatelet drugs in the management of the microangiopathy associated with radiation nephritis.

RADIOTHERAPY-RELATED COMPLICATIONS IN GYNECOLOGIC CANCER

While radiotherapy is a very effective tool in the management of gynecologic cancers, it has disadvantages and complications. Acute effects occur when the radiotherapy, acting on local tissues that are normal as well as the tumor tissues, causes necrosis or inflammation of these normal structures. Some anatomic factors predispose patients to such injuries. For example, a narrow vagina causes an increase in the normal dose administered for treatment of cervical cancer and leads to necrosis of vaginal walls and resulting fistulas (32).

Bulky disease of the cervix or endometrium with tumor extending over a wide area requires high doses for effective treatment, and normal tissue tolerances may be exceeded.

Secondary inflammatory responses to the radiation may cause inflammation in the fallopian tubes and later development of adhesions to adjacent structures. This is a particular problem when normally mobile bowel becomes fixed to a spot near the radiation source. Fistulous leak into the peritoneum with secondary peritonitis will occur regularly.

In patients with either acute or chronic pelvic infection, the radiation effect of decreasing host resistance makes such sites a ready culture. The vasculitis that occurs with radiotherapy and the destruction of local blood supply makes these types of infections difficult to treat, since the drugs do not easily reach the source of sepsis. Radiation therapy must be discontinued while infection is treated and should include drainage, if possible. Unfortunately the time–dose relationships that are interrupted may make the radiotherapy treatment less effective.

Chronic effects of radiation are due to fibrosis and late tissue necrosis. Post-irradiation ureteral stricture due to fibrosis is reported in less than 1% of all patients treated with radiation for carcinoma of the cervix. However, radiation may cause obstruction through other means, such as tubo-ovarian abscess and lymphocyst. The most common cause of ureteral obstruction after therapy is failure of therapy to control the disease, and subsequent recurrence.

Radiation ureteritis has been studied pathologically and found to fall into three separate stages. There is a reversible acute stage seen about three weeks after the completion of therapy. This is the cause of the transient hydronephrosis seen in about 50–60% of patients. On histologic examination, there is hyperemia and edema of the ureter, with epithelial degeneration, necrosis, and proliferation. This stage can progress to a subacute and then to a chronic stage, which occurs from six months to ten years after radiotherapy. The subacute stage shows continued epithelial degeneration, subendothelial fibrosis, medial vascular fibrosis, and inflammatory infiltration. The chronic stage is characterized by deterioration of fine vasculature, endothelial obliteration, epithelial and muscular atrophy, connective tissue proliferation, and contracture of fibrous tissue.

The most common point of obstruction is where the ureter passes through the broad ligament, 3–6 cm from the UV junction. However, Skarloff et al. report two distinct types of structure: a localized form in the distal ureter, and a long threadlike proximal form due to the pelvic connective tissue fibrosis, which can occur from 13 months to 11 years following surgery (33). Patients with ureteral obstruction may have complaints of a dull constant ache in the lower lumbar region or groin, occasionally referred to the lower abdomen, thigh, or leg. A number of patients will have symptoms of obstruction and secondary uremia. The evaluation of ureteral obstruction should include an intravenous pyelogram (IVP), barium enema, cystoscopy, cystometrogram, proctosigmoid-oscopy, and pelvic venogram or angiogram if necessary. A computed tomographic scan of the abdomen may be helpful in determining recurrence but does not usually determine the cause, only the presence of obstruction. It has been said that surgical trauma will activate radiation ureteritis.

Surgical exploration is sometimes necessary for documentation of radiation fibrosis, at which time the necessary procedures can be used to allow free flow or urine. It is important to maintain a high index of suspicion of this entity in order to save those few patients who suffer this problem, since it is treatable in a patient otherwise free of cancer.

Nevertheless, in the study by Dean and Lytton, only 2.5% out of 203 urologic problems (cystitis, hematuria, fistula, obstruction) in 964 gynecologic cancer patients were secondary to radiation therapy (34). Most of the symptoms occurred within 30 months of treatment, but there was a wide range of time. Cystitis secondary to radiation occurred in about 1% of the patients, hematuria was noted in less than 1%, and obstruction due to radiation was found in only one patient out of 964. In the majority of patients who were found to have symptoms due to radiation, a relationship to dose could be constructed. It appeared that a dose of 6000 or 6500 rad predisposed the patient to radiation changes.

ENTERITIS

Radiation enteritis occurs in many patients receiving radiotherapy for gynecologic tumors. The strip irradiation technique for cancer of the ovary, as well as external beam therapy for cancer of the uterus and intracavitary therapy for cervical cancer, can all affect the bowel. The small bowel is more subject to this complication, being more sensitive to radiotherapy than the large bowel. The small bowel also tends to develop adhesions to the pelvic floor, which has been denuded of peritoneum intraoperatively. Thus this normally mobile organ is subject to higher doses of radiation in one spot. Most patients will have symptoms of malabsorption such as diarrhea, but they can also have delayed transit time, increased intestinal secretions, and symptoms suggesting partial small bowel obstruction, such as intermittent nausea and vomiting. Late radiotherapy effects include ulceration and fibrosis as well as adhesions. Both the large and small bowels not uncommonly develop ulcerations and perforations because of the high dose of combined external and intracavitary radiation used in the treatment of cervical cancer.

GLOMERULOPATHIES

The association of apparently immune-related glomerular disease and neoplasms in many patients has intrigued both the oncologist and the nephrologist for many years. Eagen and Lewis classify the immunopathologic features of the glomerular lesions associated with carcinoma as (1) tumor-associated antigens; (2) reexpressed fetal antigens; (3) viral antigens; and (4) autologous nontumor antigens and their respective antibodies (35). Their review summarizes the work in antigen–antibody systems described in tumor-related immune complex glomerulopathy. They found that membranous glomerulonephritis was the most common lesion in association with many carcinomas: lung, colon, stomach, gall bladder, adrenal, head and neck, skin, breast, testicular, and renal. In Hodgkin's disease, multiple myeloma, melanoma, and benign solid tumors, lipoid nephrosis and minimal changes disease have been reported to be more common. Such terms as lobular glomerulonephritis and minimal focal glomerulonephritis have also been used in the description of renal findings in association with cancer. A decrease in the size of the tumor load has been directly related to a decrease in the functional injury to the kidney in many cases. Although most of the researchers interested in this problem have eluted an antibody or found an antigen, no single study has identified both antigen and antibody. In the studies of Lee et al. and Row et al. 11% of adult patients with a glomerulopathy subsequently develop a malignancy (36,37). The activity of the renal lesion not infrequently waxes and wanes with the activity of the tumor. A decrease in proteinuria may occur even with radiation to a nonrenal primary, and relapse may be heralded by worsening renal function.

The overall significance of this immune-related disease has not been established. It appears that the prognosis is worse in those patients with carcinoma who developed a glomerulopathy, while this is not true in those with Hodgkin's disease. It is theorized that the glomerular lesion may be the host's response to the tumor antigen, and there is evidence to support the theory that the glomerular deposits are tumor-associated antigen–antibody complexes (38–42).

With the knowledge of host–tumor interactions in mind, researchers have made several attempts at modulation of the host immune system through administration of both specific and nonspecific immune stimulation in order to encourage host rejection of the tumor. A comprehensive review of these complex relationships has been done by Klein and Klein (43). In clinical practice, however, these theories have not been useful, and this avenue of treatment not successful. In some cases it has created problems of its own. Nephrotoxicity from cancer immunotherapy has been described following intravenous immunotherapy with *Corynebacterium parvum* in three patients whose renal biopsies showed a proliferative glomerulonephritis with subendothelial basement membrane deposits (44). Renal failure resolved in these patients spontaneously after the cessation of *Corynebacterium parvum* immunotherapy.

HYPERURICEMIA

Hyperuricemia has been described as an acute and chronic cause of renal failure in patients being treated for malignancies especially of the lymphoproliferative type (45,46). It is a complication well known to those who regularly treat patients with large amounts of tumor that are very sensitive to treatment. The rapid increase in uric acid production following cytolytic therapy may cause urate crystal deposition within the renal tubules or uric acid stone formation within the renal pelvis or ureter. Pathologic examination of the kidneys at this time will show hyperemia, edema, and tubular damage. Renal function tests usually show a transient decrease in tubular function, and the return to normal is usually rapid without any sequelae, although fatal acute renal failure has occurred. The prophylactic use of allopurinol has relieved some of these problems. Liberal fluid administration with alkalinization of the urine is a useful, although temporary, maneuver. Careful selection of patients is advised when using allopurinol due to the toxicity in the form of toxic epidermal necrolysis. Chronic hyperuricemia can also contribute to renal failure by the development of interstitial fibrosis, lymphocytic infiltration, and nephrosclerosis; but this is a rare problem in patients with most malignancies, since the purine content of the diet is usually so low.

NEPHROTIC SYNDROME

The nephrotic syndrome has been associated with neoplasia since 1922, when Galloway first noted it in a patient with Hodgkin's disease. It is well known as an accompanying syndrome for Hodgkin's disease, signifying activity of the disease and/or recurrence in those who develop it, first described by Cornig in 1939 (47). As previously mentioned, it has been associated with many different neoplastic diseases.

It has been postulated that the etiology of the antigen–antibody complexes is an oncogenic virus, and indeed evidence exists in animal models to support this. Immune complex depositions in the glomeruli have been found after infection with oncogenic viruses (48). Circulating viral antibodies, as well as immune complexes in the kidneys, have been noted by Hirsch, in BALB/C mice infected with Maloney leukemia virus (49). Clinical support for these postulates comes from Sutherland and Mardney, who discovered a mammalian oncornavirus-related antigen in the kidney in two patients with acute myeloblastic leukemia and immune complex disease (50). A viral cause has long been suspected in lymphomas and leukemias as well as in sarcomas and carcinomas of the cervix, nasopharynx, breast, and liver (51–57).

Shalhoub has proposed a theory suggesting a disorder of T-cell function. Lipoid nephrosis in patients with malignancies may be related to the known dysfunctions of T cells in neoplastic states, particularly in lymphomas and leukemias (58).

The treatment of this disorder before the malignancy is identified is similar to other etiologic types of nephrosis. It is important to realize, however, that some investigators believe this may be a prodrome, and, particularly in older patients presenting for the first time with immune complex nephritis or lipoid nephrosis, one must be conscious of the possible development of malignancy (59). Those whose syndromes appear concomitantly with, or following, discovery of the tumor may be most efficiently treated by definitive therapy of the tumor. The general treatment of both may be in many cases the same, utilizing steroid therapy and alkylating agents. Relapse of tumor is generally associated with the recurrence of the renal disease, but it is not known if the presence of renal disease in association with the tumor leads to a better or worse overall prognosis.

Further support for the concept of immune complex injury to the kidney is seen in the example of the immune response of the host to components of the tumor or its catabolic products. This gives rise to what appears to be a collagen vascular disorder, such as dermatomyositis, or rheumatoid arthritis. This concept was proposed in order to explain the otherwise unusual association of these syndromes with the development of neoplasms.

LYMPHORETICULAR DISORDERS

Two disease entities deserve special mention due to their well-known and frequent association with renal complications: multiple myeloma and lymphoma.

Several reports have covered the topic of multiple myeloma thoroughly. Martinez-Maldonado et al. studied 47 patients with multiple myeloma and found 15 renal abnormalities associated with this disease (60). They found that abnormal urine sediments occurred in about 30% of these patients. Most of these were pyuria related to infection; hematuria was rare. Hyperviscosity syndrome in this disease causing renal failure is uncommon but a well-known and treatable complication. The increase in viscosity is related to both the amount and type of abnormal protein present in the plasma. The treatment for immediate relief of symptoms is plasmapheresis, although long-term relief must depend on the control of the disease. Hypercalcemia, often seen in myeloma, can also cause, or contribute to, renal failure. Hypercalcemia occurs in 30–60% of patients with multiple myeloma at some time during their course, and the duration and level of calcium influences the degree of renal impairment. It is, however, a reversible cause of renal insufficiency if treated adequately. Uric acid production as a result of excessive cell turnover may result in tubular precipitation of uric acid leading to obstruction and renal failure. The critical level for renal damage is thought to be about 20 mg%, although some degree of renal impairment may occur at much lower levels. The use of hydration, alkalinization of the urine, and allopurinol have much decreased the renal toxicity from this cause and should be begun before starting treatment for myeloma. Renal compromise following intravenous pyelograms have in the past been attributed to a reaction between abnormal globulins and the contrast media; but this was never actually able to be shown, and it is now felt that this phenomenon is related to the dehydrating preparation procedures for an IVP. Although the occurrence is unusual, it is recommended that patients suspected of having renal failure secondary to myeloma be well hydrated before the procedure. Proteinuria was a common finding, present in the urine of 60–90% of the patients, and was related to the type of chains being produced. D-myeloma patients had proteinuria 90% of the time, while it was found in only 20% of the A-myeloma patients. "Myeloma kidney," a specific pathologic appearance, has been variously reported to occur in 35–70% of patients with D-myeloma and thus thought to be related to the degree of proteinuria. The tubular casts in this entity are of interest to pathologists because of their singular appearance. They are glassy, eosinophilic, sometimes lamellar casts associated with varying degrees of giant cell reaction, tubular dilation, atrophy, and interstitial fibrosis. These casts may extend the entire length of the nephron and may block or directly injure the renal tubules and ultimately lead to renal insufficiency. Border has described four cases of patients with the acute onset of renal failure, and renal biopsy showed typical myeloma kidney. None of these patients had physical or historical evidence of myeloma nor did they have serum protein gammopathy or bone lesions at the time of diagnosis, although they did have bone marrow evidence confirmatory of multiple myeloma.

Amyloid disease has an increased association with multiple myeloma and may lead to hypertension in patients with this disease. Deposits of amyloid are found in about 10% of autopsied cases. Nephrotic syndrome in the presence of multiple myeloma is not common but has been reported; the relationship is not clear. As with other instances of nephrotic syndrome in the presence of a neoplastic disease, it has been theorized that the proteinuria is related to immune complex deposits in the glomeruli. Plasma cell invasion of the kidney has been described in autopsy specimens, but is of no clinical importance. Plasma cells have been identified in the urinary sediment of patients with myeloma, and the urine should be examined for these cells in all patients with unexplained renal failure.

Pyelonephritis is a significant complication and may be secondary to other processes involving the kidney, such as protein casts, nephrocalcinosis, renal stones, or neurogenic bladder. The incidence in myeloma patients may be higher due to their increased susceptibility to infection.

The Fanconi syndrome, or proximal tubular dysfunction, has been reported in association with rod-shaped crystal deposits in plasma cells and proximal tubular cells (61). It has been suggested that these are precipitates of Bence Jones proteins. Other investigators believe that the abnormality is the result of absorption of abnormal L-chains.

Distal renal tubular acidosis has been reported but poorly documented in multiple myeloma patients. The Fanconi syndrome has also been reported in solid tumors (62).

The hyperviscosity syndrome as a cause for renal failure is an uncommon but well-known and treatable complication. The increase in viscosity is related to both the amount and type of abnormal protein present in the plasma, and the treatment of choice for immediate relief is plasmapheresis.

Since lymphoma so frequently involves the kidney, some of its special features will be mentioned here. In a sense, the renal complications of lymphoma may serve as a model for the renal complications of malignancies, for they are quite characteristic, although relatively more frequently, in lymphomas than in other cancers.

RENAL COMPLICATIONS OF LYMPHOMA

Anatomic
    Primary renal lymphoma
    Metastatic invasion of parenchyma
    Hydronephrosis from retroperitoneal adenopathy
    Compression of the renal pedicle
Electrolyte abnormalities
    Hypercalcemic nephropathy
    Uric acid nephropathy
Immunologic abnormalities
    Nephrotic syndrome
    Amyloidosis
    Retroperitoneal fibrosis

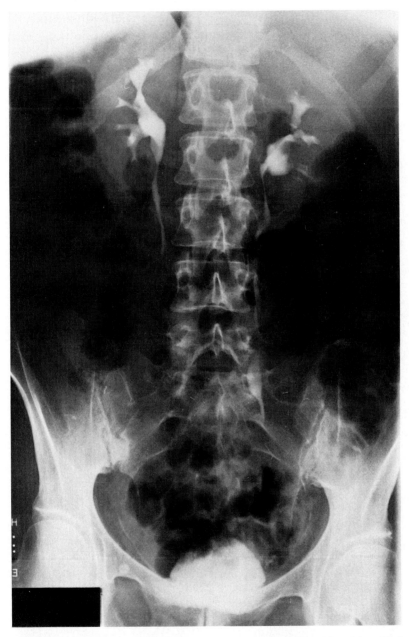

Figure 3-4. Bilateral renal lymphocytic lymphoma causing functional insufficiency at initial examination. Percutaneous kidney biopsy showed diffuse involvement. All other clinical staging tests for lymphoma were negative.

Primary renal lymphoma is extremely rare. One case with unilateral involvement has been reported that did well after treatment with nephrectomy (63). Bilateral involvement was seen in one of our own patients with no other involvement by physical or laboratory examination (Fig. 3-4). Treatment with radiation therapy was given but death resulted from renal failure, with no clinical evidence of other disease. Many authors are skeptical that primary renal involvement occurs. Metastatic disease, however, is quite common. Single or multiple cortical lesions are seen most often, but a diffuse or circumscribed invasion may be seen. The cortical lesions will be seen on IVP as multiple bulges, while the diffuse picture

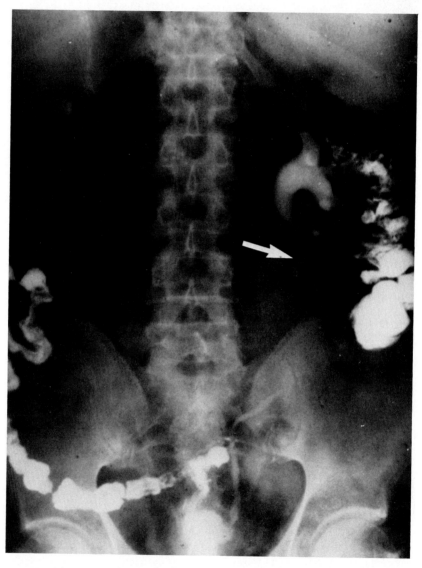

Figure 3-5. Nonfunctional right kidney and partially obstructed left ureter due to ret-roperitoneal adenopathy in a patient with lymphocytic lymphoma. The arrow points toward the "step ladder" left ureter.

may show only enlargement with hydronephrosis. With extensive retroperitoneal disease the kidneys may become encased and the tumor may spread into the cortex (Fig. 3-5). Both situations may be palliated by radiation therapy to the kidneys and, therefore, recognition is important. Compression of the renal pedicle or ureter from retroperitoneal adenopathy may lead to hypertension or hydronephrosis, respectively. These complications may likewise be treated successfully with focal radiation. Return of renal function to normal may occur with treatment even if the obstruction has been present for weeks.

Hypercalcemia in conjunction with lymphoma may be a result of the synthesis of a parathyroid hormonelike substance by the tumor, but more often is a result of bone destruction; thus treatment must be aimed at identification and treatment of the involved bones, in addition to the usual measures for control of hypercalcemia. Hypercalcemic nephropathy and uric acid renal damage occurs in lymphoma as it does in myeloma. In addition, fever associated with lymphoma and the vomiting associated with treatment may further increase the precipitation of uric acid in the renal tubules by contributing to a metabolic acidosis and may also impair the excretion of calcium. Hydration, alkalinization of the urine, and pretreatment with allopurinol may alleviate or avoid the development of these problems.

The nephrotic syndrome in conjunction with lymphomas is probably more common than has been appreciated and often requires no treatment other than the treatment of lymphoma itself. It has been theorized that the well-known immunologic abnormalities in lymphomas are also the cause or at least contribute to the development of this syndrome.

Amyloidosis in association with lymphoma has been recognized for over a century. It is suggested that renal insufficiency with proteinuria in the presence of renal enlargement is a clue to diagnosis. Renal amyloidosis has a poor prognosis, and it is important to differentiate the nephrotic syndrome secondary to an idiopathic cause from that secondary to amyloidosis, as the prognosis in the two conditions is vastly different.

Occasional lymphomas may be accompanied by a marked firbrotic reaction, and rare lymphomas have appeared as idiopathic retroperitoneal fibrosis without peripheral lymphadenopathy. It is important to establish the cause in such cases, since at the present time most lymphomas are highly treatable.

HEMORRHAGE

Sudden massive vaginal bleeding in patients with cancer is a life-threatening event requiring prompt diagnosis and treatment. It is most common in patients with cancer of the cervix, but it also occurs in endometrial and ovarian cancer and choriocarcinoma. Twenty-five percent of patients with choriocarcinoma will have some acute complication requiring surgical intervention even though the primary treatment is chemotherapy (Figs. 3–6 and 3–7). Bleeding may occur spontaneously or as a sudden breakdown of tumor during response. It can also occur as a result of operative injuries in highly friable tumor beds or may be an effect of radiation, infection, or recurrent tumor. Perivascular infection in pelvic

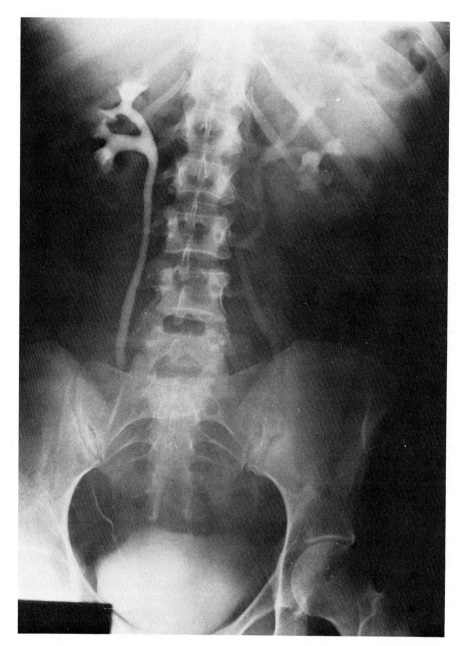

Figure 3-6. Gestational choriocarcinoma causing pelvic mass and bilateral ureteral and calyceal dilatation. Pulmonary metastases were present.

or femoral vessels postoperatively may result in thrombosis of the vasa vasorum and avascular necrosis of the vessel walls. Recurrent tumor through major vessels.

Sudden intracranial bleeds have been associated with metastatic deposits of choriocarcinoma in the brain, which, when treated with radiation and surgery, give patients a fair chance of survival. Bleeding into the peritoneum from metastatic deposits in the liver has also been reported.

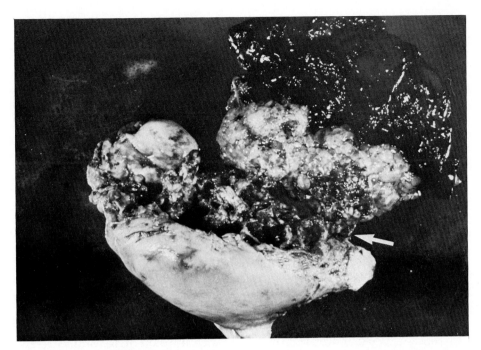

Figure 3-7. Operative specimen of spontaneously ruptured uterus in the patient shown in Figure 3-6 10 days after IVP. The arrow points toward the perforation area. Gonadotropin titers and pulmonary metastases responded to combination chemotherapy postoperatively. The patient was disease free four years later.

Rapid dissolution of tumor as a result of successful treatment of cervical cancer with bleomycin infusion has been described at Memorial Hospital, and is a potential problem with any successful therapy in a highly vascular tumor. This complication also contributes to the appearance of fistulas and cavitation in this area. Plastic surgical procedures in attempts to close fistulas have been the subject of small numbers of experimental studies, but are no longer generally attempted due to poor results. It is important to determine if the fistula is a result of tumor dissolution or tumor recurrence before decisions are made as to the justification of further therapy.

Flap necrosis after radical vulvectomy has been associated with massive bleeding from the femoral vessels. Transposition of the sartorius muscle across the femoral triangle at the time of initial surgery is a useful technique to avoid this problem.

The biological effect of chemotherapy causing thrombocytopenia is a common cause of bleeding in patients on chemotherapy. The platelet count must be determined in all patients who come in for evaluation of bleeding. Necrotic tumors will bleed from friable tissue when platelets are low or poorly functioning as a result of treatment, but usually respond well to matched platelet transfusions. Progestins may be used where there is a question of dysfunctional uterine bleeding, for example, in estrogen therapy for treatment of breast cancer. In patients with ovarian cancer a hypercoagulable state has been described, which is associated with thrombosis-disseminated intravascular coagulation. This can also occur with other gynecologic cancers. An activated factor X has been described in a patient with bleeding who had on ovarian cancer (64). Disseminated intravascular coagulation is always a threat in the presence of gram-negative sepsis, to which postoperative patients and patients with advanced disease are subject. It is in fact the most common cause of bleeding and should be considered before other more rare problems are investigated.

Bleeding can also occur secondary to metastatic cancer to the uterus and vagina. Breast cancer is one of the more common cancers seen with metastases to these sites, and, in the presence of bleeding in a patient with a known history of breast cancer, differentiation between a metastatic and primary lesion can often only be made by biopsy.

THROMBOSIS

There are several known cases of thrombotic events in gynecologic cancers. Radiotherapy has been said to be related to accelerated atherogenesis, thus leading to an increased rate of vascular occlusion or narrowing in an irradiated field. Thus one may see pelvic or femoral vascular occlusion in these patients, which may occur as pelvic pain or leg pain, which is sometimes ascribed to recurrence of pelvic tumor with pressure or an invasion of sacral nerves. Dye studies of the involved vessels or CT scans of the area give much information regarding the cause. The previously mentioned hypercoagulable state noted with gynecologic cancers predispose these patients to pulmonary emboli and is always a source of concern in those patients with acute shortness of breath, chest pain, or other suggestive diagnosis. The awareness of this problem, especially in patients who are immobilized postoperatively, has led to the finding that perioperative and postoperative low-dose heparin is an effective preventive.

INTESTINAL OBSTRUCTION

A common complication in the course of patients with gynecologic cancer, especially ovarian cancer, is that of obstruction of the intestines. Although the patient may first appear with obstruction, it is most commonly seen in patients who have been already heavily pretreated with surgery, radiotherapy, and chemotherapy. It thus becomes a therapeutic dilemma usually only resolved by a surgical operation. Complications of surgery or radiotherapy, such as fibrosis or adhesion, may be adequately handled with decompressive surgery in patients with extensive intra-abdominal disease causing obstruction or perforation. There may be benefit to gain from chemotherapy, since there are effective first-line as well as second-line drugs available. Palliative relief can be obtained by decompressive suction. In a review by Brown et al. the 30-day mortality of patients with advanced ovarian cancer after palliative surgery was 32% and the median survival was 3.2 months with a range of 1 to 12 months (65). However, since new drugs are showing promise, it may be that these figures are somewhat pessimistic for today's multimodality therapies.

INFERIOR VENA CAVA OBSTRUCTION

Inferior vena cava obstruction in its middle third as a result of tumor can appear as hematuria, albuminuria, or the nephrotic syndrome, simulating primary renal disease. Of all middle third inferior vena cava obstructions, 16% are due to invasion by tumor. The most common tumor to cause this is renal cancer, comprising about 10% of the nephrectomy specimens. Involvement of the inferior vena cava by other tumors is usually associated with retroperitoneal metastases. Those that have been reported include cervix, uterus, fallopian tube, prostate, testicle bladder, colon, lymphoma, adrenal, and pancreas.

Once suspected on the basis of other clinical information, such as lower extremity or scrotal edema or symptoms of retroperitoneal disease, the diagnosis is easily made with an inferior venacavogram. A competent radiologist should perform this procedure, as the vena cava, with its large diameter and slow blood flow rate, low pressure, and multiple venous tributaries, may give rise to such problems as diversion of the contrast material into the paracaval venous system, streaming of nonopaque blood venous tributaries into the vena cava, and lavering of contrast material in slow moving blood. A CT scan of the abdomen may give more information about the primary tumor or may be used in patients who cannot have venacavograms.

Radiotherapy is useful in a few selected cases, but for the most part treatment should be directed at the primary tumor. In many cases, especially genitourinary cancers, this event occurs in the very late stage of disease and therapy must best be supportive.

HYPERTENSION

Tumor metastases causing hypertension are rare, but have been reported. External compression of the renal artery causing a Goldblatt effect has been reported with several local tumors, such as pheochromocytoma and ganglioneuroma, but metastasis from a carcinoma of the lung was first reported in 1964 by Jenning et al. (66). In this patient, labile hypertension was the symptom, and it responded to nephrectomy. Although the pathologic diagnosis was made at the time of nephrectomy, no clinical or radiologic evidence of bronchogenic carcinoma was ever present. In most instances of hypertension associated with urinary tract metastases, the renal failure preceding the hypertension is the result of metastases. Other causes of hypertension are hypercalcemia, pheochromocytoma, and Cushing's syndrome, all of which may be seen in this group of patients.

Diagnosis and treatment of this disorder is no different than the general approach to hypertension unless specific causes are determined. Long-term control is dependent on the prognosis of the underlying disease.

HYPERCALCEMIA IN GYNECOLOGIC CANCERS

An increase in serum calcium is seen in both urologic and gynecologic cancers, most commonly in cervical and renal cancer. There are several mechanisms.

Skeletal metastasis due to invasion of the bone by tumor is probably the most common cause, and thus should be suspected when the patient develops bony metastases. This in itself is unusual in this group of patients since these tumors tend to be local invasions. Squamous cell cancers of any origin, including the cervix, and adenocarcinoma of the kidney have been associated with a parathyroid hormone or parathyroid hormonelike factor that causes increased levels of serum calcium with its attendent symptoms. This is described at length in another chapter.

CORD COMPRESSION AND MENINGEAL CARCINOMATOSIS IN GYNECOLOGIC CANCERS

Spinal cord compression secondary to gynecologic tumors is an unusual complication, occurring in about 2.5% of patients. In renal cancer this problem is more frequent, with an incidence of about 6%. A discussion of this problem will be found in Chapter 6. A rarer problem is meningeal spread of cancer, seen very uncommonly in gynecologic tumors and uncommonly in urinary tract cancers, most often in hypernephromas. Further discussion of this topic will also be found in Chapter 6.

MENINGEAL CARCINOMATOSIS

Spread of cancer to meninges has been reported with many types of cancer, most commonly breast and lung cancers, but only very rarely with gynecologic cancers. The presentation of this complication is that of central nervous system (CNS) dysfunction, with change in personality, headaches, confusion, nausea, seizures, cranial nerve dysfunction, or asymteric polyneuropathies. Weed and Creasman reported meningeal carcinomatosis from advanced squamous cell cancer of the cervix (67). Their patient developed her symptoms three years after the diagnosis of the primary was made and died two weeks after the diagnosis of CNS disease was made, as a result of therapy.

PAIN

Pelvic and lower extremity pain in patients with genitourinary cancer remains a significant and prevalent problem. Since these cancers tend to be locally invasive, there are several ways in which they can produce pain. The most common of these is the pain related to invasion or compression of nerves in the pelvis or nerve roots supplying the lower extremities. This is often seen with cervical cancer, but also with uterine, bladder, and renal cancer, uncommonly with ovarian. The cancer in this case tends to spread down the pelvic sidewalls and encompasses the nerves in the pelvis as it advances. Patients may complain of some nonspecific intra-abdominal discomfort, or the pain may be sharp and unrelenting with characteristics that suggest nerve involvement, such as a burning or tingling quality. It is usually poorly relieved by the usual analgesics. Another type of pain is caused by distended viscera, such as seen in bowel obstruction that occurs with ovarian cancer. In both postoperative and radiotherapy patients infection is an ever present threat and causes pain secondary to abscess formation and peritonitis. The pain caused by the growth of the tumor itself is usually insidious in onset, at first a discomfort much like that noticed at the beginning of the disease. It is usually progressive, and its cause is easily diagnosed by patient history and physical and, occasionally, abdominal and pelvic CT scans. Pain due to the collection of ascites is usually not severe when first noted, but the gross distention with tense ascites seen in late stages of ovarian cancer can be very uncomfortable and occasionally painful.

URETERAL OBSTRUCTION

The most common cause of death in patients with gynecologic tumors is renal failure due to ureteral obstruction. The natural history of these diseases is local growth. It is common to allow this complication to proceed to its natural end, since this is usually a terminal event, occurring in patients who are debilitated and have undergone most forms of effective surgery and radiotherapy. However, some authors have advocated the use of nephrostomy, ureterostomy urinary diversion, urinary conduit diversion, or ureteral stents in delaying the onset of renal failure. These measures are effective and warranted in those patients in whom salvage measures are available to control the primary problem (i.e., the growth of the cancer). In a study by Delgado and Smith, urinary conduit diversion was used successfully in 15 patients with advanced gynecologic malignancies with improvement of their renal status before therapy for the primary tumor (68). In the group in which there was little or no response to the therapy for the cancer, survival was not affected by the diversionary procedure. In those who responded to therapy, the quality of life was improved, and time was gained in order to administer the treatment. In Chua's study of 12 patients who underwent nephrostomies or ureterostomies for advanced cervical cancer and ureteral obstruction, there was no difference in the survival of the two groups. Ureteral stents are preferred by some urologists, since it is a simple procedure. It can be placed cystoscopically and it requires no incision or external appliance. In the group of 15 patients studied by Pellman et al., 11 stents in 10 patients were passed through this method (69). The stents remained in place from four to 14 months, but required replacement in several patients because they were expulsed and expelled. Although the stents did not prolong survival, they did prolong comfortable life and in several instances procured enough time to begin the patient on an effective course of therapy.

FISTULAS

Fistulous tracts continue to be a significant problem in patients with gynecologic cancer. Although a small number of them are secondary to radiation, the development of fistulas usually indicates recurrent disease.

Some, however, such as enteroperineal fistulae, usually are seen following radiotherapy, due to the adherence of heavily irradiated intestine to the denuded pelvic floor. The small bowel fistula is particularly serious, with operative mortality rates of about 50% and nonoperative management resulting in a mortality of close to 100%. Berman et al. reported a ten-point program of management of patients with such fistulas with good results in four patients (70). This program included preoperative diagnostic x-rays, small bowel drainage, hyperalimentation, and antibiotics; operative procedures to isolate the damaged segment, create a mucocutaneous fistula, and the preparation of an enterocolostomy and an ileostomy; and finally continuation with postoperative hyperalimentation and drainage, allowing the damaged areas to heal.

Vaginal fistulas are a more common problem and are seen most frequently in patients with carcinoma of the cervix. They are rarely due to radiotherapy and then may be suspected by calculation of the doses in various areas of the vagina. Patients with narrow vaginas will sometimes receive higher than normal doses due to the overlap of radiation fields. The anterior surface is most subject to this problem, and thus vesicovaginal fistulas are a recurrent and difficult problem. This complication is not handled successfully by anything less than urinary diversion procedures, which the patient may be in too poor a condition to tolerate. Rectovaginal fistulas also occur, although with less frequency. These may also be handled by diversionary procedures. Surgical repair of the vagina itself has been singularly unsuccessful due to the poor tissue that remains in the vaginal wall after radiotherapy and the usual presence of tumor in this area.

Arterioenteric fistulas have been reported as a course for rectal bleeding in patients with previous radiation for gynecologic cancer; the first symptoms are those of rectal bleeding. For the most part, however, patients with fistulas do not have rectal bleeding as a symptom of a fistula. Rather, as one would expect, the symptoms are urine or feces per vagina, or, in the case of enteric fistulas, an acute chronic abdomen.

NONBACTERIAL THROMBOTIC ENDOCARDITIS

Marantic endocarditis is occasionally seen in patients with gynecologic tumors (68). As with other types of tumors, it is usually a postmortem diagnosis and is usually associated with a mucin-producing cancer. However, squamous cell cancer of the cervix has been reported in association with marantic endocarditis in one case. Its premortem presentation is similar to that in other types of cancer; patients have evidence of embolic phenomena and a heart murmur. In the setting of widespread disease, these symptoms should strongly suggest this diagnosis. Some authors have noted in addition the association of an intravascular coagulopathy with this entity. Treatment at this time, however, is still unknown, and most patients die of the disease. Some workers have used heparin with short-term effects.

UREMIA

Insufficient renal function or frank renal failure complicates the course of disease in many patients with pelvic cancer at some time during their diagnosis or treatment. There are several causes for this, the most common being the tumor itself impinging the path of the ureters and causing obstruction and subsequent renal failure. Usually this is seen with recurrent tumor, although it may appear in far advanced cervical cancer. Radiotherapy may initiate renal obstruction by edema or fibrosis of the ureters. This is usually a late complication, although it has been seen early as three months. Occasionally this complication may occur as late as five years after initial diagnosis. Some currently used chemotherapy drugs, such as *cis*-platinum, are renal toxic and, when used in the face of previously inadequate renal function, can be associated with fatal renal toxicity. Retrograde catheters can be used for temporary relief of ureteral obstruction but have a high association with infection. If laparotomy is not planned for delineation of the source of the obstruction, then permanent nephrostomies, ureterostomies, or conduit diversion may be considered to stabilize renal function. Nevertheless, if the source of the obstruction is a recurrent tumor, as may be surmised by the presence of tumor growth elsewhere, some clinicians feel that prolongation of a painful death is not warranted through the use of urinary diversion.

SECOND MALIGNANCIES

The question of the delayed toxicity of chemotherapeutic agents is one that becomes more important as patients have increasing survival from more effective therapy. There is some evidence to suggest that these patients have an inherent susceptibility to develop malignancy, which is allowed expression with increased survival. A genetic predisposition to develop cancer may predispose these patients to a second spontaneous tumor or make them more susceptible to carcinogens. Nevertheless, it is well documented that chemotherapeutic agents are in themselves mutagenic, some agents more than others.

Leukemia developing after treatment for malignancy is well documented in the literature. It has also been reported in ovarian cancer, breast cancer, Hodgkin's lymphoma, and multiple myeloma, bladder cancer, and non-Hodgkin's lymphoma (71–76). Data are sometimes conflicting. Smith and Rutledge reported in 1972 on 494 patients treated with melphalan from 1960 to 1969 and found no cases of the development of leukemia, while Reimer et al. found 13 cases of acute leukemia out of 5455 patients treated with L-PAM (77,71). Patients treated with combined therapy (radiotherapy and chemotherapy) for Hodgkin's disease and possibly for oat cell cancer of the lung appear to be at an increased risk of developing another malignancy. Radiation may also contribute to second malignancies in these patients. Scheffey stated that irradiation does not affect the development of malignant neoplasms of the uterus (78). However, Palmer and Spratt concluded that malignant tumors occurred in the pelvis after radiotherapy of cervical cancer and in women irradiated for castration, and they believed that this was related to small doses of irradiation (79). They later concluded that the sources used for the therapy of cervical cancer did not increase the risk of development of other cancers. In Cezesnin and Wronkowski's study there were 8043 patients with cervical cancer treated between 1948 and 1966 (80). Of this group 28, or 0.34%, developed another cancer in the irradiated area. The time of occurrence after radiotherapy ranged from 1.5 to 22 years, with a mean of 8.8 years. The most frequent type of second neoplasm in this study was uterine corpus, then ovarian, vulvar, and bowel cancers. The observed incidence of the second neoplasms were lower than the expected rates for those with uterine corpus cancer, ovarian cancer, and colon and rectal cancer and almost the same for those with urinary bladder cancer. The observed incidence rates were significantly higher for uterine corpus sarcoma and cancers of the skin and soft tissue in the irradiated area. Other epidemiologic studies have not confirmed these findings. Fehr and Prem found uterine cancer more likely to develop, as did Morton and Villasanta and Seydel. Schoenberg et al. found colon and rectal cancer more common in patients developing second malignancies, and Bailar and Newell et al. found urinary bladder cancer most common (81–86). The reason for such discrepancies is not clear.

INFECTION

Bacteremia with secondary sepsis is a continuing threat in patients with gynecologic cancers. Since the predominant flora in the pelvic area includes anaerobes as well as aerobes, particular care should be taken to order appropriate antibiotics in the face of suspected infection. Guidelines for prophylactic antibiotics are summarized in the review by Ledger et al. (87). Prophylactic antibiotics should be used when the operation carries a significant risk of postoperative site infection and significant bacterial contamination. The antibiotic used for prophylaxis should have laboratory evidence of effectiveness against some of the contaminating micro-organisms. Antibiotics should be present in the wound in effective concentrations at the time of the incisions, and only short-term, low toxicity antibiotics should be used. Antibiotics needed to combat resistant infections should be reserved and not used for prophylaxis. The benefits of prophylactic antibiotics must outweigh the dangers of their use.

The first time infection may be encountered is postoperatively, where necrotic tumor and poor preceding nutrition contribute to the susceptibility of the host. Thereafter, radiotherapy may incite previously quiescent infection, such as old pelvic inflammatory disease, diverticulitis, or postoperative cellulitis. Loculated abscess formation is not an uncommon occurrence, particularly when the uterus is unable to drain, causing pyometrium. Occurrence of significant fever during radiotherapy interrupts natural barriers and should mandate discontinuing therapy and immediate evaluation for the source of the fever. After radiotherapy and surgery, intestinal, bladder, and vaginal necrosis may sometimes be seen, and may or may not be related to the presence of recurrent tumor. Biopsy specimens of the involved areas will often clarify this and is important for prognosis and decisions relating to other medical and supportive care. Hyperalimentation is sometimes used in these instances with success, to rest the bowel while healing occurs, but is in itself a potential source of sepsis.

REFERENCES

1. De Vita V Jr, et al (eds): *Cancer: Principles and Practice of Oncology.* Philadelphia, Lippincott, 1982, pp 732, 823.

2. Holland JF, Frei E (eds): *Cancer*. Philadelphia, Lea & Febiger, 1982, pp 1880, 1957.

3. Rutledge F, Borrow RC, Wharton JT (eds): *Gynecologic Oncology*. John Wiley & Sons, 1976, pp 3, 97, 159, 213, 259.

4. Rieselbach RE, Garnick MB (eds): *Cancer and the Kidney*. Philadelphia, Lea & Febiger, 1982, p 707.

5. Klinger ME: Secondary tumors of the genitourinary tract. *J Urol* 65:144, 1951.

6. Conn JW, Cohen EL, Lucas CP, et al: Primary reninism: Hypertension, hyperreninemia, and secondary aldosteronism due to renin-producing juxtaglomerular cell tumors. *Arch Intern Med* 130:682, 1972.

7. Hollifield JW, Page DL, Smith C, et al: Renin-secreting clear cell carcinoma of the kidney. *Arch Intern Med* 135:859, 1975.

8. Ganguly A, Bribble J, Tune B, et al: Renin-secreting Wilms' tumor with severe hypertension. *Ann Intern Med* 79:835, 1973.

9. Webb MJ, Decker DG, Mussey E: Cancer metastatic to the ovary: Factors influencing survival. *Obstet Gynecol* 45:391, 1975.

10. Gastleman B, Kibbee BV: Case presentation, Mass. Gen. Hosp. #46501. *New Engl J Med* 263:1251, 1960.

11. Marone C, Beretta-Piccoli C, Wiedman P: Acute hypercalcemic hypertension in man: Role of hemodynamics, catecholamines and renin. *Kidney Int* 20:92, 1980.

12. Luxton RW, Kunkler PB: Radiation nephritis. *Acta Radiol (Ther)* 2:169, 1964.

13. Gup AK, Schelegel JV, Caldwell T, et al: Effect of irradiation on renal function. *J Urol* 97:36, 1967.

14. Scully RE, McNeely BU: Case presentation, Mass. Gen. Hosp. *New Engl J Med* 292:521, 1975.

15. Castleman B, McNeeley, BU: Case presentation, Mass. Gen. Hosp. *New Engl J Med* 276:519, 1967.

16. Esposito JM, Zarou DM, Zarou CS: Extragenital adenocarcinoma metastatic to the cervix uteri. *Am J Obstet Gynecol* 92:792, 1965.

17. Daw E: Extragenital adenocarcinoma metastatic to the cervix uteri. *Am J Obstet Gynecol* 114:1104, 1972.

18. Casey JH, Shapiro RF: Metastatic melanoma presenting as a primary uterine neoplasm: A case report. *Cancer* 33:729, 1974.

19. Lefkovitz L, Letsch SD, Weiss DR, et al: Metastatic melanoma presenting as abnormal uterine bleeding: A case report. *Mt Sinai Med J* 43:180, 1976.

20. Raider L: Remote vaginal metastasis from carcinoma of the colon. *Am J Roentgenol* 97:944, 1966.

21. Weitzner S, Dressner SA: Vaginal metastasis from adenocarcinoma of pancreas. *Am Surg* 40:256, 1974.

22. Mulcahy J, Furlow WL: Vaginal metastasis from renal cell carcinoma: Radiographic evidence of possible route of spread. *J Urol* 104:50, 1970.

23. Dehner LP: Metastatic and secondary tumors of the vulva. *Obstet Gynecol* 42:47, 1973.

24. Luxton RW, Kunkler PB: Radiation nephritis. *Acta Radiol (Ther)* 2:169, 1964.

25. Gup AK, Schelegel JV, Caldwell T, et al: Effect of irradiation on renal function. *J Urol* 97:36, 1967.

26. Avoili LV, Lazor MZ, Cotlove E, et al: Early effects of radiation on renal functions in man. *Am J Med* 34:329, 1963.

27. Assher AW, Anson SC: Arterial hypertension and irradiation damage to the nervous system. *Lancet* 2:1343, 1962.

28. Kunkler PB, Farr RF, Luxton RW: The limit of renal tolerance to x-rays. *Br J Radiol* 25:190, 1952.

29. Crummy AB, Hellman S, Starrnel HC, et al: Renal hypertension secondary to unilateral radiation damage relieved by nephrectomy. *Radiology* 84:108, 1965.

30. Steele BT, Lirenman DS: Acute radiation nephritis and the hemolytic-uremic syndrome. *Clin Nephrol* 11:272, 1979.

31. Keane WF, Crosson JT, Staley NA, et al: Radiation induced renal disease. A clinicopathological study. *Am J Med* 60:127, 1976.

32. Kagan AR, DiSaia PJ, Wollin M: The narrow vagina, the antecedent for irradiation injury. *Gynecol Oncol* 4:291, 1976.

33. Skarloff DM, Cananeswaran P, Skarloff RB: Postirradiation ureteric stricture. *Gynecol Oncol* 6:538, 1975.

34. Dean RJ, Lytton B: Urologic complications of pelvic irradiation. *J Urol* 119:64, 1978.

35. Eagen JW, Lewis, EJ: Glomeruliopathies of neoplasia. *Kidney Int* 11:297, 1977.

36. Lee JC, Yamanchi H, Hopper J Jr: The association of cancer and the nephrotic syndrome. *Ann Intern Med* 64:41, 1966.

37. Row PG, Cameron JS, Turner DR et al: Membranous nephropathy: Long-term follow-up and association with neoplasia. *Q J Med* 44:207, 1975.

38. Gilboa N, Durante D, Guggenheim S, et al: Immune deposit nephritis and single-component cryoglobulinemia associated with chronic lymphocytic leukemia. *Nephron* 24:223, 1979.

39. Baldwin RW, Price MR: Tumor antigens and tumor-host relationships. *Ann Rev Med* 27:151, 1976.

40. Synder HW, Hardy WD, Zucherman EE, et al: Characterization of a tumor-specific antigen on the surface of feline lymphosarcoma cells. *Nature* 257:656, 1978.

41. Hellström I, Hellström KE: Cell-mediated immune reactions to tumor antigens with particular emphasis on immunity to human neoplasms. *Cancer* 34:1461, 1974.

42. Fahey JL, Brosman S, Ossorio RC, et al: Immunotherapy and human tumor immunology. *Ann Intern Med* 84:454, 1976.

43. Klein C, Klein E: Immune surveillance against virus-induced tumors and nonrejectability of spontaneous tumors: Contrasting consequences of host vs. tumor evolution. *Proc Natl Acad Sci USA* 74:2121, 1977.

44. Dosik CM, Gutterman JV, Hersh EM, et al: Nephrotoxocity from cancer immunotherapy. *Ann Intern Med* 89:41, 1978.

45. Conger JD, Falk SA: Intra-renal dynamics in the pathogenesis and prevention of acute urate nephropathy. *J Clin Invest* 59:786, 1977.

46. Reiselbach RC, Bertzel CJ, Cotlove E, et al: Uric acid excretion and renal function in acute hyperuricemia of leukemia: Pathogenesis and therapy of uric acid nephropathy. *Am J Med* 37:872, 1964.

47. Cornig HJ: Une forme nouvelle de la maladie de Hodgkin's lymphogranulomatose maligne à type de nephrose lipoidique: Thèse de Paris 1939, no. 517, cited by Tapice J, Laporte J, Ricalen S: *Syndrome nephrotique au cours de la maladie de Hodgkin*. Sternberg, Presse Med. 65 287, 1967.

48. Pascal RR, Rollwagen FM, Harding TA, et al: Glomerular immune complex deposits associated with mouse mammary tumor. *Cancer Res* 35:302, 1975.

49. Hirsch MS: Activation of C-type viruses during skin graft rejection in the mouse: Interrelationships between immune suppression and immune stimulation. *Int J Cancer* 15:493, 1975.

50. Sutherland JC, Mardney MR: Immune complex diseases in the kidneys of leukemia-lymphoma patients: The presence of an oncornavirus-related antigen. *J Natl Cancer Inst* 50:633, 1973.

51. de The G, Geser A, Day NE, et al: Epidemiological evidence for causal relationship between Epstein-Barr virus and Burkitt's lymphoma from Ugandan prospective study. *Nature* 275:756, 1978.

52. Berard CW, Gallo RC, Jaffe ES, et al: Current concepts of leukemia and lymphoma: Etiology, pathogenesis and therapy. *Ann Intern Med* 85:351, 1976.

53. Balduzzi P, Morgan HR: Mechanism of oncogenic transformation by Rous sarcoma virus. 1: Intracellular inactivation of cell transforming ability of Rous sarcoma virus by 5-bromodeoxy-uridine and light. *J Urol* 5:470, 1970.

54. Rawls WE, Tompkins WAF, Melnick JL: The association of herpes type 2 and carcinoma of the uterine cervix. *Am J Epidemiol* 89:547, 1969.

55. Ho JHC: An epidemiologic and clinical study of nasopharyngeal carcinoma. *Int J Radiol Oncol Biol Phys* 4:183, 1978.

56. Moore DH, Charney J, Kramarshy G, et al: Search for a human breast cancer virus. *Nature* 229:611, 1971.

57. Szmuness W: Hepatocellular carcinoma and the hepatitis B virus: Evidence for a causal relationship. *Prog Med Virol* 24:40, 1978.

58. Shaloub RJ: Pathogenesis of lipoid nephrosis: A disorder of T-cell function. *Lancet* 2:556, 1974.

59. Ghosh LB, Muehrehe RC: The nephrotic syndrome: A prodrome to lymphoma. *Ann Intern Med* 72:279, 1970.

60. Martinez-Maldonado M, Yium J, Suki WN: Renal complications in multiple myeloma: Pathophysiology and some aspects of clinical management. *J Chronic Dis* 24:221, 1971.

61. Engle RI, Wallis LA: Multiple myeloma and the adult Fanconi syndrome. *Am J Med* 22:5, 1957.

62. Megerson RM, Pastor BH: The Fanconi syndrome and its clinical variants. *Am J Med Sci* 228:378, 1954.

63. Knoepp LF: Lymphosarcoma of the kidney. *Surgery* 39:510, 1956.

64. Siegman-Igra Y, Flatau E, Deligdish L: Chronic diffuse intravascular coagulation in non-metastatic ovarian cancer. *Gynecol Oncol* 5:92, 1977.

65. Brown PW, Terz JJ, Lawrence J, et al: Survival after palliative surgery for advanced intraabdominal cancer. *Am J Surg* 134:575, 1977.

66. Jenning RC, Shaikh VAR, Allen WMC: Renal ischemia due to thrombosis of renal artery resulting from metastasis from primary carcinoma of the bronchus. *Br Med J* 2:1053, 1964.

67. Weed JC, Creasman WT: Meningeal carcinomatosis secondary to advanced squamous cell cancer of the cervix: A case report. *Gynecol Oncol* 3:201, 1975.

68. Delgado G, Smith JP: Gynecological malignancy associated with non-bacterial thrombotic endocarditis. *Gynecol Oncol* 3:203, 1975.

69. Pellman C, Sall S, Calanog A: The relief of ureteral obstruction by internal ureteral stent in patients with gynecological cancer. *Gynecol Oncol* 5:2, 1965.

70. Berman M, LaCasse LD, Watring WG, et al: Enteroperineal fistulae following pelvic exenteration: A 10 point program of management. *Gynecol Oncol* 4:360, 1976.

71. Reiner RR, Hoover R, Fraumeni JF Jr, et al: Acute leukemia after alkylating-agent therapy of ovarian cancer. *New Engl J Med* 297:177, 1977.

72. Lerner J: Second malignancies diagnosed in breast cancer patients while receiving adjuvant chemotherapy at the Pennsylvania Hospital *Proc AACR-ASCO* 18:340, 1977.

73. Arseneau JC, Sponzo RW, Levin DL, et al: Non-lymphomatous malignant tumors complicating Hodgkin's disease. *New Engl J Med* 287:1119, 1972.

74. Bergsagel TE, Bailey DJ, Langley CR, et al: The chemotherapy of plasma-cell myeloma and the incidence of acute leukemia. *New Engl J Med* 301:743, 1979.

75. Wall RL, Clausen KP: Carcinoma of the urinary bladder in patients receiving cyclophosphamide. *New Engl J Med* 293:271, 1975.

76. Rosner F, Grunwald HW, Zarrabi MH: Acute leukemia as a complication of cytotoxic chemotherapy. *Int J Radiol Oncol Biol Phys* 5:1705, 1979.

77. Rutledge FN, Burns BC: Pelvic exenteration. *Am J Obstet Gynecol* 91:692, 1965.

78. Scheffey LC. Malignancy subsequent to irradiation of the uterus for benign conditions. *Am J Obstet Gynecol* 44:925, 1942.

79. Palmer JP, Spratt DW: Pelvic carcinoma following irradiation for benign gynecological diseases. *Am J Obstet Gynecol* 72:497, 1956.

80. Cezesnin K, Wronkowski Z: Second malignancies of the irradiated area in patients treated for uterine cervix cancer. *Gynecol Oncol* 6:309, 1978.

81. Fehr PE, Prem KA: Post-irradiation sarcoma of the pelvic girdle following therapy for squamous cell carcinoma of the cervix. *Am J Obstet Gynecol* 116:192, 1973.

82. Villasanta V: Complications of radiotherapy for carcinoma of the uterine cervix. *Am J Obstet Gynecol* 114:717, 1972.

83. Seydel HG: The risk of tumor induction in man following medical irradiation for malignant neoplasms. *Cancer* 35:1641, 1975.

84. Schoenberg BS, Greenberg RA, Eisenberg H: Occurrence of certain multiple primary cancers in females. *J Natl Can Inst* 43:15, 1969.

85. Bailar JC: The incidence of independent tumors among uterine cancer patients. *Cancer* 16:842, 1963.

86. Newell GR, Krementz KT, Roberts JD: Excess occurrences of cancer of the oral cavity, lung and bladder following cancer of the cervix. *Cancer* 36:2155, 1975.

87. Ledger WJ, Gee C, Lewis WP: Guidelines for antibiotic prophylaxis in gynecology. *Am J Obstet Gynecol* 121:1038, 1975.

4
Selected Gastrointestinal Difficulties in Neoplastic Disease

Frank E. Smith

Primary gastrointestinal neoplasms are common and are discussed extensively in many writings (1). Repeated discussions of primary tumors in this system is unnecessary, but selected consequences of malignancy in enteric sites direct attention to less frequently described problems requiring the physician's attention. When extensive disease or an acute medical situation initially suggests a difficult outlook, the attending physician may take a negatively biased view of events. Despite the poor outcome of many advanced neoplasms within the abdomen, successful definitive treatment or palliation is often possible. The masquerade of malignancy may lead the physician to view a potentially treatable situation as one in which no favorable outcome is likely. The emphasis of the following discussion reiterates the simple necessity of individual patient evaluation in clinical situations that can be difficult to assess diagnostically and therapeutically. Neoplasms involving gastrointestinal organs continue to be great challenges in diagnosis and treatment.

ESOPHAGUS

Carcinosarcomas, sarcomas, and metastatic carcinomas follow primary carcinoma of the esophagus in frequency of incidence (2). These lesions are usually located submucosally and eventually cause symptoms of obstruction, bleeding, perforation, or aspiration.

Lung cancer frequently locally extends from the mediastinum and causes esophageal symptoms (3). Our most unusual example experienced perforation of the esophagus with fistulous communication to the pericardium. The more common formation of bronchoesophageal fistulas cannot be treated successfully with any currently available modality. Extrinsic esophageal compression can be treated easily with radiation therapy. If lymphoma or oat cell carcinoma is the

offending disease, combination chemotherapy and/or radiation therapy can relieve symptoms quite rapidly.

Metastatic breast carcinoma can cause dysphagia by direct infiltration or nodal
compression. The unusual capacity of breast lesions to stimulate fibrosis, either
in primary or metastatic lesions, may complicate biopsy interpretation since
individual tumor cells or small nests of cells may be quite scattered. Patients with
this disorder may erroneously receive a pathologic diagnosis of radiation fibrosis
or achalasia. Figure 4-1 shows the barium swallow in a patient with metastatic
breast cancer associated with excessive fibrous tissue deposition. When there is
involvement of the esophagus and paraesophageal structures treatment with
radiotherapy, chemotherapy, or hormonal maneuvers may improve swallowing
somewhat, but the underlying predominant histology of fibrotic reaction prevents a complete response. These patients frequently require long-term nasogastric feeding tubes or placement of an intragastric feeding device, since survival

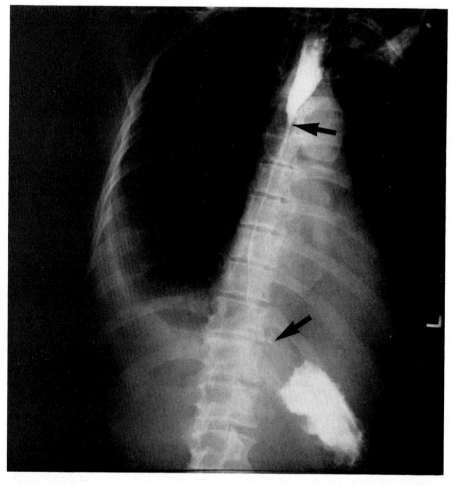

Figure 4-1. Esophageal obstruction with metastatic breast cancer. Marked fibrotic reaction was present on biopsy with scattered small nests of malignant cells.

can often be measured in years. The patient in Fig. 4-1 was successfully treated for widespread disease some five years after the discovery of esophageal involvement. Successful local treatment to the esophagus and concomitant systemic therapy resulted in a 24-pound weight gain.

Melanoma must also be considered when esophageal symptoms develop in patients with metastatic disease. Lymphomas often involve structures surrounding the esophagus, but radiation and chemotherapy is so effective that local difficulties seldom exist for any significant length of time.

Candida esophagitis can also be a major difficulty for many cancer patients (4). For those who fail treatment with oral antifungals, a short course of amphotericin B for several days may result in dramatic improvement. In these instances the very thickness of the fungus coating of the esophageal wall probably inhibits penetration of topical oral preparations.

STOMACH

Metastatic malignancy may involve the stomach in patients with carcinoma of the lung, breast carcinoma, or melanoma. Of particular interest is the capacity of breast cancer to mimic primary gastric tumor. A picture essentially identical to that of linnitus plastica or "benign" gastric ulcer can be seen (Figs. 4-2 and 4-3). Delayed patterns of recurrence are not unusual in the natural course of breast cancer; thus a pathologic diagnosis of "primary" adenocarcinoma of the stomach may be made if the pathologist is unaware of a previous mastectomy. The patients depicted in Figures 4-2 and 4-3 received a diagnosis of gastric carcinoma because the pathologist did not know of previous breast cancer in both patients. Bleeding from upper gastrointestinal breast cancer metastases is frequently massive and fatal (5).

Lymphomas may be primary or secondary gastric neoplasms (6,7). Weingrad observed 76 instances of gastric lymphoma in a total of 104 patients with primary gastrointestinal lymphomatous disease. Local resection followed by radiation treatment reduced hemorrhage and perforation from 22% to 12% when compared to treatment with radiation alone in this report on primary gastrointestinal lymphoma. The presence of tumor at resection margins did not decrease survival in this group of patients (8). It should be noted that lymphoma, leiomyoma, and leiomyosarcoma are the most numerous primary tumors of the stomach following gastric cancer (8,9,10) (Fig. 4-4).

DUODENUM AND SMALL BOWEL

Although carcinoma of the duodenum and small bowel is the most common primary malignancy of these structures, metastatic cancer is not unusual. Non-Hodgkin's lymphoma can cause longer segmental involvement of the duodenum than carcinoma examined by an upper gastrointestinal series (11). Extension of pancreatic carcinoma may widen the duodenal loop or cause the "reversed 3 sign" to form (Fig. 4-5). Duodenal extension of tumor may occur with cancer of the stomach, pancreas, kidney, or colon (12–15).

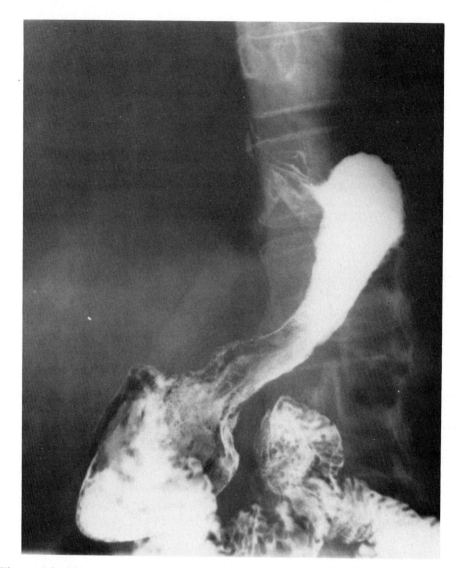

Figure 4-2. Metastatic breast cancer mimicking linnitus plastica. Biopsy was obtained endoscopically.

Small bowel metastases can be seen in patients with carcinoma of the breast, ovary, or lung as well as in malignant melanoma (Fig. 4-6). Gastrointestinal involvement in patients with melanoma is detected in 10% of the patients during life, while at autopsy examination 36% of persons suffering from melanoma demonstrate intestinal involvement (16). Intra-abdominal carcinomas of the colon, stomach, pancreas, kidney, and testicle may also result in small bowel metastases (17,18).

In Farmer and Hawk's series 14 of 87 patients with small bowel disease were considered good surgical candidates, but none had evidence of overwhelming disease elsewhere (19). Palliative local resections were possible in 11 of 14 patients

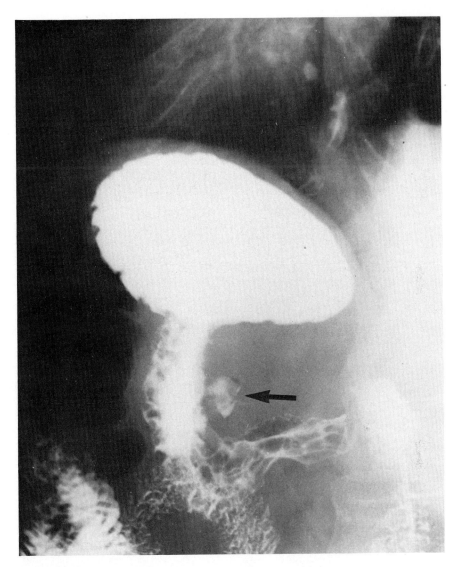

Figure 4-3. Metastatic breast cancer causing a malignant ulcer (arrow) of the lesser curvature. Biopsy was obtained endoscopically.

in this study while 3 were successfully bypassed. The average postsurgical survival was 10.2 months.

The patient whose x-ray film is shown in Figure 4-7 had metastatic breast carcinoma to the small bowel. This occurs in approximately 18% of patients dying of breast cancer (20).

Plasmacytomas have also been seen in the small bowel and stomach as unusual consequences of this disease (21).

Small bowel lymphoma may cause intussusception, obstruction, hemorrhage, or perforation (Fig. 4-8). One hundred one of 104 patients with primary gastrointestinal lymphoma described by Weingrad et al. complained of abdominal

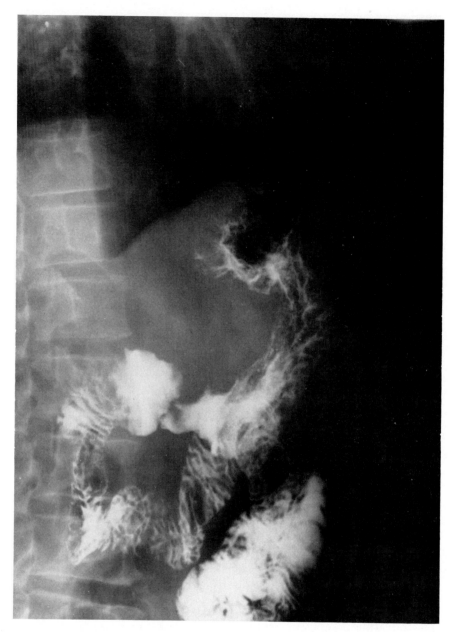

Figure 4-4. Lymphocytic lymphoma causing lower gastric, large rugal folds and an irregular, fixed antrum. Extrinsic lymphoma is compressing the second portion of the duodenum.

pain at presentation. The five-year survival for this group for all stages of lymphoma was 44% (6).

Protein losing enteropathy in malignancy may be associated with lymphomatous infiltration or chronic congestive heart failure as a result of carcinoid heart disease or constrictive disease following radiation.

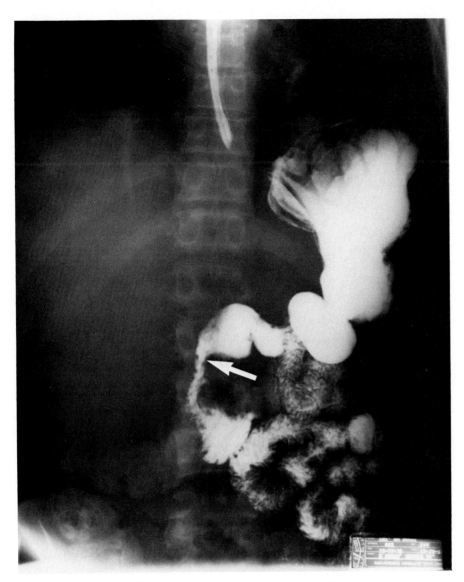

Figure 4-5. The "reversed 3 sign" of pancreatic carcinoma. The arrow points to the upper portion of the "3."

Biliary obstruction by tumors of the pancreas and biliary tree as a result of local lymphomatous disease can cause malabsorption. The malabsorption syndrome may accompany neoplasms involving the bowel (Fig. 4-9). Most cases are the result of lymphomatous infiltration, extensive bowel resection, or abdominal radiation. In patients with underlying carcinoma of the colon, lung, prostate, or pancreas, a flat mucosal pattern with simple or partial villous atrophy is seen (22,23). Rarely, widespread gastrointestinal plasma cell infiltration may cause obstruction, protein losing enteropathy, or bleeding. At times, plasma cells form multiple intestinal polyps (24).

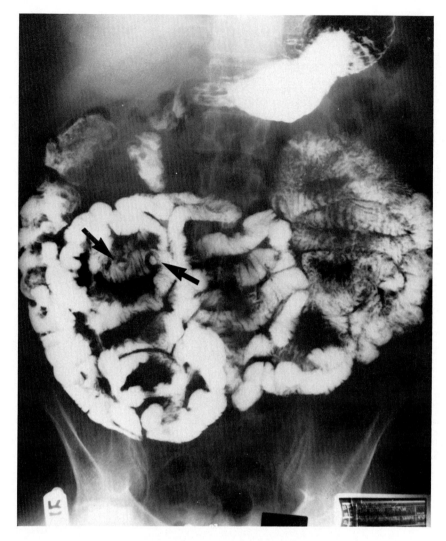

Figure 4-6. The "bull's eye" lesions of metastatic small bowel melanoma.

Intestinal pseudo-obstruction is a rare medical event associated with carcinoma of the lung. The patient of Schiffler et al. had a markedly increased gastric emptying time and a highly abnormal transit time (25). The lesion is felt to be a paraneoplastic neuropathy and is characterized histologically by degeneration of the myenteric plexus. Examination of the dorsal root ganglia shows similar changes.

COLON

Local extension from lesions of the ovary, uterus, bladder, or prostate frequently involve the colon. Large bowel metastases are much less common but may occur

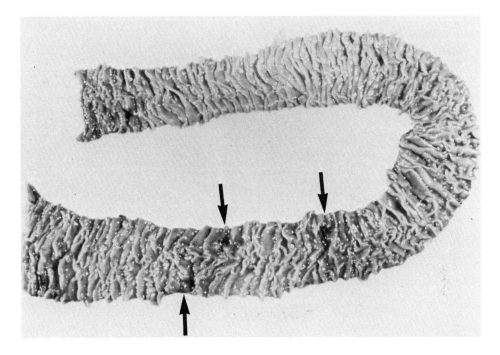

Figure 4-7. Metastatic carcinoma of the breast in small bowel. Surgical resection was done because of massive bleeding from the small lesions (arrows).

in patients with carcinoma of the lung or breast, melanoma, or lymphoma (26). Occasionally, primary lymphoma of the colon may mimic colon carcinoma. Radiographically, tumor masses, ulcers, or polyps may be seen. About 10% of primary gastrointestinal lymphoma appear as lesions of the colon. Primary lymphoma of the colon is the least frequent site of origin of all intestinal lymphomas (Fig. 4-10). Patients with disseminated lymphoma examined at autopsy show some site of enteric involvement in over half the cases (7). Plasmacytomas are a rare cause of obstruction of the colon (27).

LIVER

Liver metastases are extremely common in many patients with cancer and may cause substantial difficulty in diagnosis and assessment of response to treatment. For example, under 25% liver replacement by tumor correlates poorly when preoperative scanning is compared to laparotomy findings (28). Hepatic angiography may be helpful diagnostically or therapeutically, but many metastatic tumors are hypovascular or avascular. These include melanoma, carcinomas of the lung, breast, and endometrium, and many gastrointestinal tumors that spread to the liver. Conversely, hypernephroma, carcinoid, islet cell carcinoma, and leiomyosarcomas are often quite vascular and may be easily demonstrated by angiography.

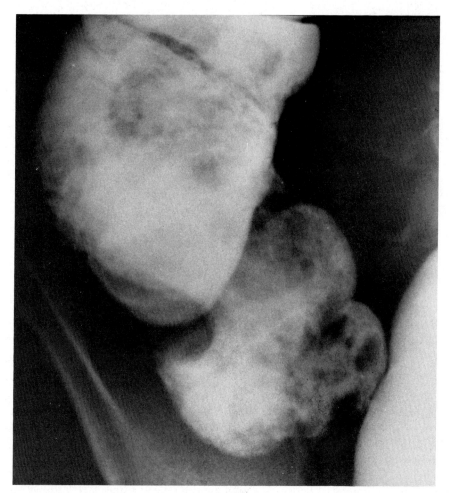

Figure 4-8. Intussusception of the cecum with primary histiocytic lymphoma of the right ovary. The lesion was reduced easily with the barium enema.

Definition of hepatic metastases can be crucial during clinical staging procedures and in judging response to treatment. The frequency of hepatic metastases in many diseases is quite high; thus staging and treatment can be altered significantly if lesions are found. For example, 15% of patients dying from breast cancer do so as a result of hepatic insufficiency (29). Approximately one-half of women dying from metastatic breast cancer have liver involvement at postmortem. Twenty-four percent of patients with melanoma develop hepatic metastases clinically, while at autopsy examination this figure increases to 77%. Small cell carcinoma of the lung with liver involvement is associated with hepatic dysfunction in 50–66% of patients (30). In most instances, abnormalities of liver function tests are quite mild. Biopsy at initial staging discloses tumor in 28% of subjects (31). The high incidence of metastases to the liver in small cell lung cancer is higher than that of any other form of carcinoma of the lung and reflects early hematogenous dissemination.

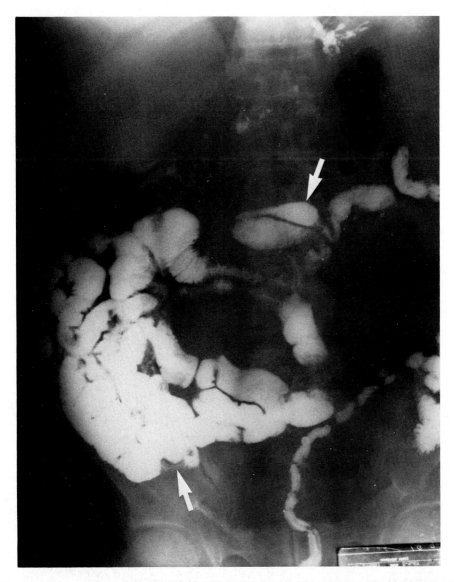

Figure 4-9. Lymphocytic lymphoma of the small bowel showing loss of intestinal folds, as well as flocculation and clumping of barium (arrows). Malabsorption syndrome and protein-losing enteropathy were present.

Several items of interest emerge in the evaluation of potential liver involvement in Hodgkin's disease:

1. Liver involvement is almost never seen in the absence of splenic disease (32). In the presence of a normal size spleen, Hodgkin's disease of the liver occurs in under 1% of all cases.
2. Hodgkin's disease within the liver is an uncommon laparotomy finding, occurring in only three of 100 patients evaluated at Stanford (33).

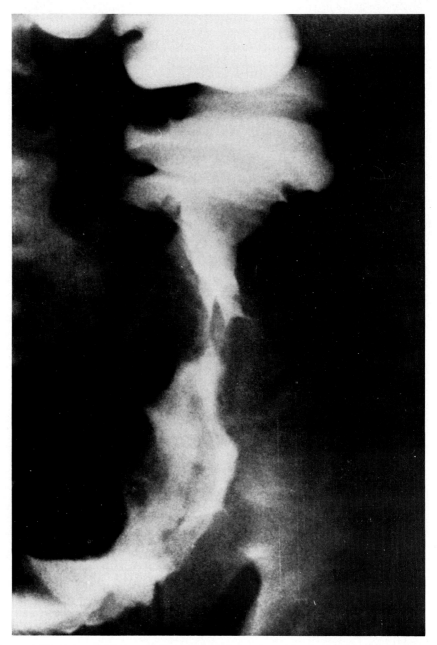

Figure 4-10. Primary histiocytic lymphoma of the sigmoid colon. The admitting clinical diagnosis, before biopsy, was "possible colon carcinoma."

3. Increasing use of peritoneoscopy successfully detects Hodgkin's disease in the liver almost as accurately as laparotomy. Only two of 110 patients were shown to have Hodgkin's disease in the liver at laparotomy after a negative preoperative peritoneoscopy (34–35).

4. Noncaseating granulomas of liver may accompany Hodgkin's disease but do not represent lymphomatous organ involvement. Similar granulomas occur in the spleen, lymph nodes, or bone marrow in 9–19% of patients with Hodgkin's disease. Reed-Sternberg cells are never seen and in actuality these granulomas may be associated with improved survival in all stages of disease (36).

In other malignancy states liver dysfunction may be present in the absence of metastatic disease. The hepatopathy associated with hypernephroma causes hepatomegaly, hypoalbuminemia, increased alkaline phosphatase, increased globulin, increased cholesterol, and increased prothrombin time, all of which may improve with removal of the renal primary. Nonspecific focal periportal inflammation is seen histologically. Liver scans fail to demonstrate space occupying lesions, and an erroneous initial clinical impression of hepatic metastases can be avoided (37,38).

Multiple myeloma infrequently causes plasma cell infiltration of portal areas resulting in perisinusoidal portal hypertension and potential esophageal variceal bleeding (39). In terminal disease 70% of patients demonstrate plasma cell hepatic infiltration. Jaundice at the time of diagnosis of myeloma occurs rarely and reflects a grim prognosis. Most patients die within three weeks. Plasma cells may also be seen in ascitic fluid, apparently the result of liver pathology (40).

Hepatic vein thrombosis in malignant disease leads to death in days to several months when hepatoma, hypernephroma, leiomyosarcoma, or adrenal carcinoma are the underlying causes. Differential diagnosis includes idiopathic fibrous obliteration of the hepatic vein, myeloproliferative disorders, paroxsymal nocturnal hemoglobinuria, pregnancy, and oral contraceptives. The poor prognosis of Budd-Chiari syndrome associated with malignancy reflects ineffective current treatment in the presence of advanced disease (41).

ASCITES

Retroperitoneal lymphoma and carcinomas of the ovary, endometrium, colon, stomach, and pancreas are responsible for approximately 80% of malignant ascites (42–45). Rarely, myeloma and melanoma cause intra-abdominal fluid accumulation (46–48). If the fluid is cytologically negative, peritoneal biopsy may be necessary for diagnosis, particularly when lymphomas are suspected. Most cases of ascites occurring in nonmalignant disease states do not increase the levels of carcinoembryonic antigen in aspirated fluid. Fifty percent of patients with malignant ascites have carcinoembryonic antigen in excess of 12 ng/ml (49). Careful evaluation of the pathogenesis of ascites in each patient is essential inasmuch as treatment and prognosis is extremely variable depending on the presence of single or multiple causes. The clinical determination of existing peritoneal implants, hepatic insufficiency, portal hypertension, retroperitoneal tumor, cardiac or renal dysfunction, or other intra-abdominal vascular compromise dictates treatment and outlook.

JAUNDICE

Jaundice in cancer patients is most frequently caused by extensive liver metastases from pancreatic, gastric, colon, lung, breast, renal, and biliary tract primaries. Malignant melanoma and advanced non-Hodgkin's lymphomas also cause jaundice. The clinical outlook may be limited unless systemic chemotherapy or hepatic artery perfusional approaches to treatment result in successful palliation. Focal

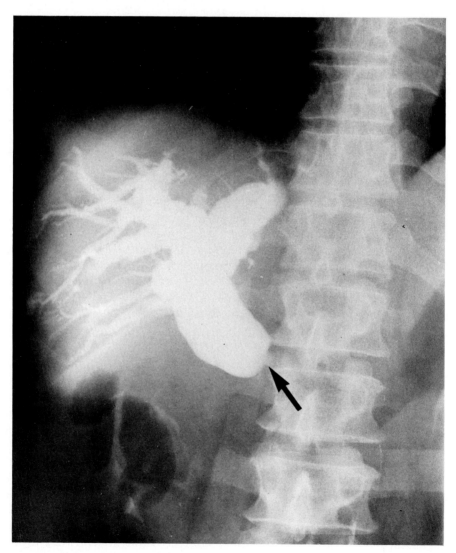

Figure 4-11. Biliary tract obstruction from lymphocytic lymphoma shown by transhepatic cholangiogram (same patient as in Fig. 4-4).

radiotherapy may relieve the pain of tumor-related capsular distention. Obstructive jaundice may be a feature of local metastases from cancer of the pancreas or stomach. By-pass operations followed by radiation therapy may be possible in selected patients.

Biliary obstruction is an unusual cause of jaundice in Hodgkin's disease but can respond well to local radiation and/or combination chemotherapy. Non-Hodgkin's lymphoma is a more frequent cause of extrahepatic obstruction and may improve with radiation therapy or chemotherapy (Fig. 4-11). Metastatic carcinoma of the breast and lung and melanoma are other tumors capable of causing biliary tract compression.

Intrahepatic obstruction may be approached by transhepatic cholangiography, making external or internal drainage of bile possible.

REFERENCES

1. Moertel CG: Alimentary tract cancer, in Holland JF, Frei E (eds): *Cancer of Medicine*, Philadelphia, Lea & Febiger, 1973, p 1519.

2. Green AE, Brogdon BG, Crowe NE, et al: Leiomyoma of the esophagus. *Am J Roentgenol* 82:1058, 1959.

3. Matthews MJ: Problems in morphology and behavior of bronchopulmonary malignant disease, in Israel L, Chaharnian P (eds): *Lung Cancer: Natural History, Prognosis and Therapy*. New York, Academic Press, 1976, p 223.

4. Levine AS, Schimpff SC, Graw RG, et al: Hematologic malignancies and other marrow failure states: Progress in the management of complicated infections. *Sem Hematol* 11:141, 1974.

5. Choi SH, Sheehan FR, Pickren JW: Gastrointestinal bleeding with metastatic breast cancer. *Cancer* 17:791, 1964.

6. Weingrad DN, Decosse JJ, Sherlock P, et al: Primary gastrointestinal lymphoma: A thirty year review. *Cancer* 49:1258, 1982.

7. Rosenberg SA, Diamond HD, Jaslowitz B, et al: Lymphosarcoma: A review of 1269 cases. *Medicine* 40:31, 1961.

8. Davis JG, Adams DD: Roentgen findings in gastric leiomyomas and leiomyosarcomas. *Radiology* 67:67, 1956.

9. Phillips GA, Linsay GA, Candall GA: Gastric leiomyosarcomas: Roentgenologic and clinical findings. *Am J Dig Dis* 15:239, 1970.

10. Sherrick DW, Hodgson JR, Dockerty MD: A roentgenologic diagnosis of primary gastric lymphoma. *Radiology* 84:921, 1965.

11. Marshak RH, Wolf BF: The roentgen findings in lymphosarcoma of the small intestine. *Am J Roentgenol* 86:682, 1961.

12. Grinell RS: Lymphatic metastases of carcinoma of the colon and rectum. *Ann Surg* 131:494, 1950.

13. Lawson LJ, Holt LP, Rooke HW: Recurrent duodenal hemorrhage from renal carcinoma. *Br J Urol* 38:133, 1966.

14. Treitel H, Meyers MA, Maza V: Changes in the duodenal loop secondary to carcinoma of the hepatic flexure of the colon. *Br J Radiol* 43:209, 1970.

15. Ngan H: Involvement of the duodenum by metastases from tumors of the genital tract. *Br J Radiol* 43:701, 1970.

16. Nathanson L: Biologic aspects of human malignant melanoma. *Cancer* 20:650, 1967.

17. Van Prohaska J, Govostis MC, Wasick M: Multiple organ resection for advanced carcinoma of the colon and rectum. *Surg Gynecol Obstet* 97:177, 1953.

18. Herbsman H, Wetstein I, Rosen Y, et al: Tumors of the small intestine. *Curr Probl Surg* 17:121, 1980.

19. Farmer RG, Hawk WA: Metastatic tumors of the small bowel. *Gastroenterology* 47:496, 1964.

20. Warren S, Witman EM: Studies on tumor metastases: The distribution of metastases in cancer of the breast. *Surg Gynecol Obstet* 57:81, 1937.

21. Godard J, Fox J, Levinson M: Primary gastric plasmacytoma. *Am J Dig Dis* 18:508, 1973.

22. Klipstein FA, Smorth G: Intestinal structure and function in neoplastic disease. *Am J Dig Dis* 14:887, 1969.

23. Troncale FJ: Distant manifestations of colonic carcinoma. *Ann NY Acad Sci* 230:332, 1974.

24. Goeggel-Lamping C, Kahn SB: Gastrointestinal polyposis in multiple myeloma. *JAMA* 239:1786, 1978.

25. Schiffler MD, Baird HW, Fleming CR, et al: Intestinal pseuo-obstruction as the presenting manifestation of small cell carcinoma of the lung. *Ann Intern Med* 98:129, 1983.

26. Wigh R, du V Tatley N: Metastatic lesions to the large intestine. *Radiology* 70:222, 1958.

27. Wing EJ, Perchick J, Hubbard J: Solitary obstructing plasmacytoma of the colon. *JAMA* 233:1298, 1975.

28. Cedermark BJ: Value of liver scan in the followup study of patients with adenocarcinoma of the colon and rectum. *Surg Gynecol Obstet* 144:745, 1977.

29. Meissner WA, Warren S: Sites of metastases at autopsy, in Anderson WAD (ed): *Pathology*. St Louis, CV Mosby, 1971, p 1538.

30. Minna JD, Higgins GA, Glatstein EJ: Principals and practice of oncology, in DeVita VT, Hellman S, Rosenberg SA (eds): *Cancer*. Philadelphia, Lippincott, 1982, p 427.

31. Hansen HH, Dombernowsky P, Hirsch FR: Staging procedures and prognostic features in small cell anaplastic bronchogenic carcinoma. *Semin Oncol* 5:280, 1978.

32. Glatstein E, Guernsey JM, Rosenberg SA, et al: Value of laparotomy and splenectomy in the staging of Hodgkin's disease. *Cancer* 24:709, 1969.

33. Kaplan HS, Dorfman RF, Nelson TS, et al: Staging laparotomy and splenectomy in Hodgkin's disease: Causes of indications and patterns of involvement in 285 consecutive unselected patients. *NCI Monograph* 36:291, 1973.

34. DeVita VT, Bagley CM, Goodell B, et al: Peritoneoscopy in the staging of Hodgkin's disease. *Cancer Res* 31:1746, 1971.

35. Bagley CM, Roth JA, Thomas LB, et al: Liver biopsy in Hodgkin's disease: Clinical pathologic correlations in 127 patients. *Ann Intern Med* 76:219, 1972.

36. Sacks EL, Donaldson SS, Gordon J, et al: Epitheloid granulomas associated with Hodgkin's disease. *Cancer* 41:562, 1978.

37. Utz DC, Warren MM, Gregg JA, et al: Reversible hepatic dysfunction associated with hypernephroma. *Mayo Clin Proc* 45:161, 1970.

38. Cronin RE, Kaehny WD, Miller PD, et al: Renal cell carcinoma: Unusual systemic manifestations. *Medicine* 55:291, 1976.

39. Brooks AP: Portal hypertension in Waldenström's macroglobulinemia. *Br J Med* 1:689, 1976.

40. Thomas FB, Clausen KP, Greenberger NJ: Liver disease in multiple myeloma. *Arch Intern Med* 132:195, 1973.

41. McMahon HE, Ball HG: Leiomyosarcoma of the hepatic and Budd-Chiari syndrome. *Gastroenterology* 61:239, 1971.

42. Osborne MP, Copeland BE: Intracavitary administration of radioactive colloidal gold (Au[198]) for the treatment of malignant effusions. *N Engl J Med* 255:1122, 1956.

43. Straus AK, Roseman DL, Shapiro TM: Peritoneal venous shunting in the management of malignant ascites. *Arch Surg* 114:489, 1977.

44. Wilbanks JD, Straus AK, Roseman DL, et al: Peritoenovenous shunting in the management of refractory ascites from a gynecological malignancy. *Proc Am Assoc Cancer Res* 20:364, 1979.

45. Wolff JP, Vignier M, Goldfarb E, et al: Ascites in cancer of the ovary. *Gynecologie* 28:517, 1977.

46. Koeffler HP, Cline MJ: Multiple myeloma presenting as ascites. *West J Med* 127:248, 1977.

47. Nutting NG, McPherson TA: Ascites in malignant melanoma after oral BCG immunotherapy. *New Engl J Med* 295:395, 1976.

48. Poth JL, George RP: Hemorrhagic ascites: An unusual complication of multiple myeloma. *Calif Med* 115:61, 1971.

49. Lowenstein MS, Rittgers RA, Feinerman AE, et al: Carcinoembryonic antigen assay of ascites and detection of malignancy. *Ann Intern Med* 88:635, 1978.

5
The Skeletal System in Malignancy

Garrett Rushing Lynch

The skeletal system is a frequent site of cancer. It is a common site of primary and metastatic tumors, and it plays a role in the paraneoplastic syndromes associated with cancer. In addition, problems involving bone may complicate the therapy for neoplastic disease.

A number of tumors occur primarily in bone. Multiple myeloma and osteogenic sarcoma are the most common, comprising 70% of primary bone tumors. Other primary bone tumors are chondrosarcoma, fibrosarcoma, Ewing's sarcoma, malignant fibrous histiocytoma, and diffuse histiocytic lymphoma of bone. Benign bone tumors, eosinophilic granuloma, and giant cell tumors of bone may appear in a similar manner as primary malignant tumors of bone.

Several factors have been shown to increase the risk of bone tumors. Paget's disease of bone predisposes to osteogenic sarcoma. These sarcomas are multicentric; they most often complicate the polyostotic variety of Paget's disease, in which case the incidence approaches 10% (1). In the past, osteogenic sarcoma was seen in workers employed to paint radium watch dials; the ingestion of radium from licking paint brushes not infrequently led to osteogenic sarcoma of the mandible. Other risk factors for the development of primary bone tumors include benign bone tumors, chronic infections of bone, a past history of radiation therapy, and osteogenesis imperfecta (2,3).

Osteogenic sarcoma has a bimodal age distribution, with peaks in late childhood and adolescence and in the sixth decade; the second peak is small, composed almost entirely of patients with Paget's disease. Osteogenic sarcoma of adolescence occurs in the metaphyseal area of long bone growth. The most commonly involved sites are the distal femur, proximal tibula, and proximal humerus (4). In osteogenic sarcoma complicating Paget's disease, the highest incidence of involvement is in the pelvis and spine, and erythema may overlie the tumor. Patients with osteogenic sarcoma complicating Paget's disease may occasionally have high output cardiac failure due to vascular shunting; in such cases, a bruit is often present (see Chapter 1). Patients with Ewing's sarcoma may have systemic symptoms, such as fever, sweats, and weight loss (5). Occasionally, patients may have pathologic fractures. Infection, anemia, bone pain, and hypercalcemic symptoms may first bring the patient with multiple myeloma to medical attention.

Laboratory evaluation should include a complete blood count (CBC), platelet count, urinalysis, liver function tests, an alkaline phosphatase determination, and chest radiographs. In osteogenic sarcoma, whole lung tomography or a CT scan of the chest is in order to look for subclinical metastases (6). Elevation of the white blood count and lactate dehydrogenase (LDH) are commonly seen in Ewing's sarcoma. Serum and urine immunoelectrophoresis are in order in multiple myeloma. In myeloma, the alkaline phosphatase may be normal, while the acid phosphatase may be elevated.

Characteristic radiographic abnormalities are seen with several primary bone tumors. Osteogenic sarcoma is often both lytic and blastic; frequently, there is an associated periosteal reaction. If the periosteal reaction occurs in a radial pattern, a characteristic sunburst appearance may be present. The periosteum is often elevated, producing a pattern known as Codman's triangle. Ossification of overlying soft tissue may occur as well. Ewing's sarcoma is characterized by lytic lesions with associated sclerosis; a layered periosteal reaction that gives an "onion-skin" appearance may be present. Multiple myeloma is a purely lytic tumor; with treatment, however, blastic healing of the lesions may occur. Characteristic "punched-out" lesions appear on the skull x-ray film.

The exact nature of a primary bone tumor is best determined by a careful open biopsy. It is imperative that the radiographic appearance of the lesion be reviewed and correlated with the biopsy specimen at the time of pathologic review. There are four major pathologic types of osteogenic sarcoma: central, telangiectatic, paraosteal juxtacortical, and periosteal (7). Of these, paraosteal juxtacortical lesions have the best prognosis and telangiectatic lesions the worst (8). Ewing's sarcoma has a pathologic pattern of a small round cell tumor and must be distinguished from lymphoma, small cell lung carcinoma, rhabdomyosarcoma, and neuroblastoma (9). Myeloma is characterized by collections of plasma cells; occasionally, it may appear as a solitary plasmacytoma (Fig. 5-1). If an apparently solitary plasmacytoma is associated with an M-spike and the M-spike does not return to normal after therapy, it is likely that the process is more extensive. Solitary plasmacytomas have a better prognosis than multiple myeloma, with treated patients living a median of 9.5 years, as opposed to 2.5 years for treated patients with multiple myeloma (10).

The major route of spread of osteogenic sarcoma is hematogenous. The lungs are the major site of metastatic disease; the tumor may spread to other sites, such as the liver, adrenal glands, and central nervous system. Ewing's sarcoma also has a propensity for widespread disease and has a predilection for lymph node, lung, and liver metastases.

A multidisciplinary approach must be taken in the management of all primary bone tumors. The classic initial therapy of most bone tumors is amputation of the affected bone, inclusive of the proximal joint; this is the primary management of osteogenic sarcoma, chondrosarcoma, malignant fibrous histiocytoma, and primary fibrosarcoma of bone. For osteogenic sarcoma limb sparing procedures, with en bloc resection and insertion of a cadaveric graft, are replacing amputation at some centers (11). Results of this procedure appear promising, but a final verdict is not yet available. Amputation is done in Ewing's sarcoma if small bones are involved. In most cases, however, radiation therapy and chemotherapy are used in lieu of surgery.

Radiation therapy plays a major role in the primary management of Ewing's

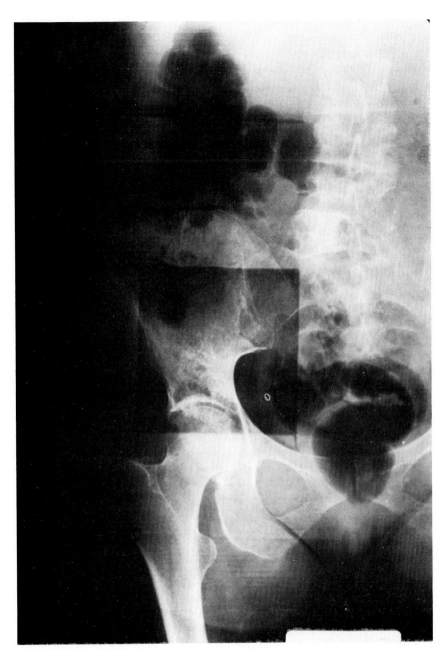

Figure 5-1. Myeloma in bone metastatic from extramedullary paratracheal plasmacytoma diagnosed two years earlier.

sarcoma, which is a very radiosensitive tumor; as stated previously, radiation in this setting is usually combined with chemotherapy (12). Radiation therapy also plays a role in the management of localized diffuse histiocytic lymphoma. In osteogenic sarcoma, chondrosarcoma, and fibrosarcoma, radiation is used to treat inoperable or unresectable tumors, as well as local recurrences.

Chemotherapy is frequently used in combination with surgery in osteogenic sarcoma. Nonrandomized trials have shown that the adjuvant use of high-dose methotrexate with citrovorum rescue, with or without Adriamycin, may increase survival in this disease to 60% at three years (13). However, a similar improvement in survival has been noted at the Mayo Clinic in patients treated with surgery alone. Some investigators feel that improvements in surgical technique may be responsible for the improved survival in the adjuvant chemotherapy series (14). A controlled, randomized trial will be needed to answer the question of the role of adjuvant chemotherapy in this disease. In Ewing's sarcoma, the addition of vincristine, Adriamycin, and Cytoxan, with or without actinomycin D, to radiation increases survival over that seen with radiation therapy alone. A study by Rosen et al. using aggressive combination chemotherapy and radiation revealed an 80% three-year disease-free survival (15). The value of chemotherapy in the adjuvant setting has not been consistently shown to prolong survival in chondrosarcoma, fibrosarcoma, and malignant fibrous histiocytoma.

For metastatic Ewing's sarcoma and osteogenic sarcoma, chemotherapy similar to that used in the adjuvant programs is used. In metastatic chondrosarcoma, malignant fibrous histiocytoma, and fibrosarcoma of bone, Adriamycin and DTIC (dacarbazine) in combination may provide palliation in the 30–40% of patients who respond to the combination (16,17). Extensive diffuse histiocytic lymphomas of bone are treated with chemotherapy regimens used for diffuse histiocytic lymphoma at other sites, such as CHOP (Cytoxan, Adriamycin, Oncovin, and prednisone), C-MOPP (Cytoxan, Oncovin, procarbazine, and prednisone), and COMLA (Cytoxan, Oncovin, methotrexate, leucovorin rescue, and cytosine arabinoside) (18).

Multiple myeloma is most often treated with Alkeran and prednisone, with up to 50% of patients obtaining an objective response. Several Southwest Oncology Group studies examined the addition of other agents to Alkeran and prednisone; the addition of vincristine increased response rates and survival. The addition of Adriamycin or procarbazine did not improve response rates or survival. Further studies by the same group failed to show an improvement in response duration or survival if maintenance therapy was given to responders after one year of induction chemotherapy (19,20). A Memorial Sloan-Kettering study using BCNU (carmustine), Alkeran, prednisone, vincristine, and Cytoxan reported a 90% objective response rate and improved survival for responders. In this study, however, historical controls were used (21).

In addition to primary bone tumors, there are two other mechanisms by which bones may be directly involved by tumor. The most common mechanism involves hematogenous spread of tumor to bone. A second less common mechanism is direct destruction of bone by adjacent tumor. Examples of this mechanism include destruction of the mandible and other cranial bones by head and neck tumors and destruction of the lumbar spine by large pelvic tumors, such as carcinoma of the uterine cervix.

Several tumors have a predilection to metastasize to bone. Solid tumors that frequently spread to bone include breast, lung, prostate, renal, and thyroid cancer (22). Other solid tumors not infrequently metastasizing to bone are melanoma and gastrointestinal cancer; of the gastrointestinal tumors, pancreatic cancer most frequently spreads to the skeletal system, while colorectal cancer does so least often. Hematologic malignancies with a propensity to metastasize to bone include Hodgkin's disease and non-Hodgkin's lymphomas, especially those of the large cell or histiocytic varieties.

Metastases to bone may be lytic, blastic, osteosclerotic, or mixed. Although certain tumors have a predilection to form one type of lesion, it is not uncommon for patients to have mixed blastic and lytic lesions. Lytic lesions are a manifestation of bone destruction, while blastic lesions result from new bone formation. Breast cancer tends to produce lytic lesions; however, up to 10% of patients may have blastic metastases (Figs. 5-2 and 5-3). The skeletal lesions of multiple myeloma are with rare exception purely lytic. Non-oat cell lung cancer also has a tendency to produce lytic lesions, as does renal and thyroid cancer. The most common tumor producing blastic metastases is prostate cancer (Fig. 5-4). How-

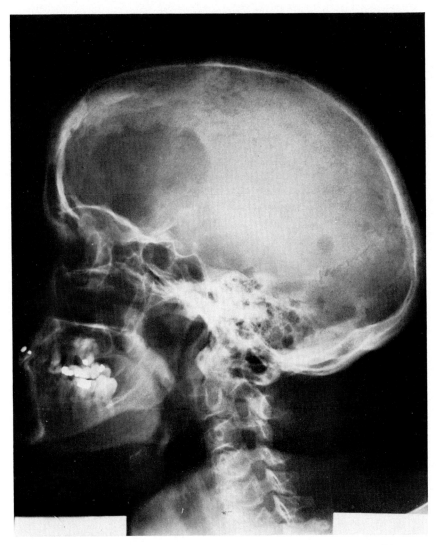

Figure 5-2. A large lytic defect in the frontal bone in a 65-year-old woman with metastatic breast carcinoma presenting with frontal headache.

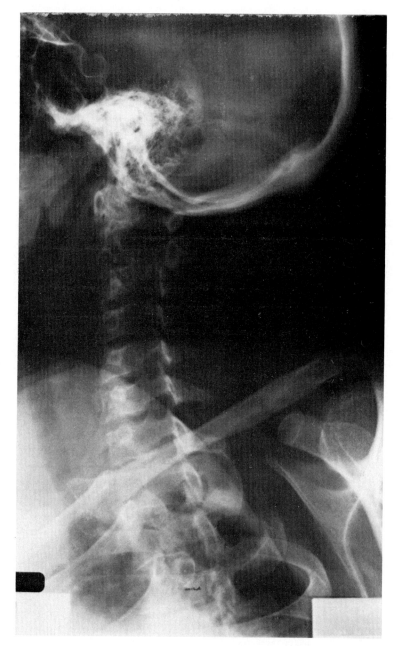

Figure 5-3. A 62-year-old woman noted instability when she moved her head. Lytic destruction of the C-2 vertebrae from metastatic breast carcinoma is shown.

ever, approximately 5% of patients with prostate cancer have purely lytic metastases. Other tumors frequently producing blastic metastases include oat cell lung carcinoma, Hodgkin's disease, non-Hodgkin's lymphoma, and carcinoid tumors. Hodgkin's disease involving bone frequently produces a blastic lesion; the term "ivory vertebrae" describes the vertebral lesion of Hodgkin's disease

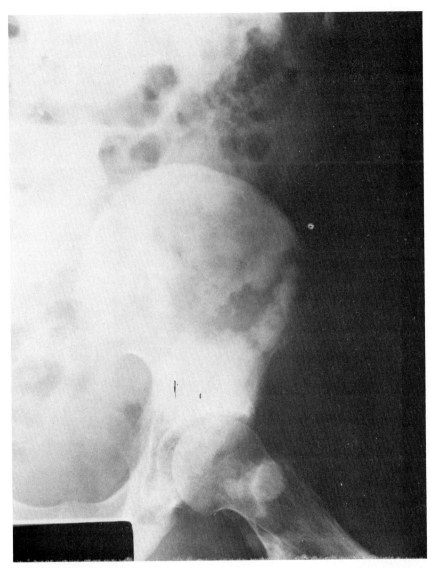

Figure 5-4. Classic osteoblastic bone lesions in a 55-year-old man with metastatic prostate carcinoma. Several lytic lesions are noted in the femur.

(23) (Fig. 5-5). Carcinoid tumors should be considered in any young patient with blastic bone lesions, as this tumor has a very high predilection for blastic metastases. Note that lesions responding to radiotherapy, chemotherapy, or hormonal therapy usually heal in a blastic fashion; thus formerly lytic lesions may become blastic with successful therapy.

Some bone metastases may be extremely vascular; this is especially true of renal and thyroid cancer. These metastases may be pulsatile, with heat and erythema of the overlying skin. It is important to keep in mind the vascularity of these tumors if operative repair is contemplated; such surgery may be associated with significant blood loss (24).

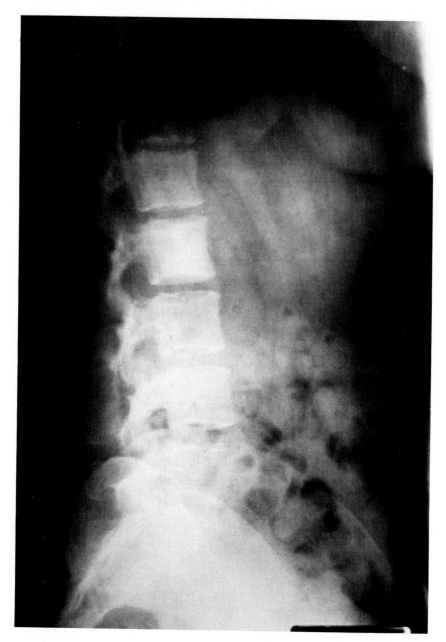

Figure 5-5. The ivory vertebrae of Hodgkin's disease.

Although most bone metastases are multiple, renal cell carcinoma and thyroid carcinoma have a propensity toward solitary metastases. Solitary bone metastases complicate renal cell carcinoma in 1–2% of cases; a vigorous surgical approach is indicated with such lesions, as a 25–30% five-year survival has been noted following surgical resection (25).

Several bones are more frequently involved by metastatic tumors than others. The spine and pelvis are the most common sites of involvement with metastatic disease. These are followed by the femur, skull, ribs, and humerus. Metastases distal to the elbows and knees are rare; metastases to the hand are so rare that only approximately 100 cases have been reported in the literature (26).

The most common symptom of bone metastases is pain in the affected area; occasionally such pain may be referred elsewhere. A not uncommon complication of bone metastases, and occasionally the first manifestation of primary and metastatic tumor, is that of a pathologic fracture (Fig. 5-6). The diagnosis of a malignant pathologic fracture should be considered in any older patient who sustains a fracture from a minor tension or stress.

Metastatic tumor in the spine may appear as a spinal compression; 90% of patients with spinal cord compression have an antecedent history of pain (27). The classic pain of spinal cord compression is a radicular pain that is described as "band- or viselike". In addition to pain, weakness, a sensory level, or signs and symptoms of bowel and bladder dysfunction may occur. Another symptom of bone metastases may be due to nerve involvement by an adjacent bony tumor; examples include sciatica due to lumbosacral metastases and cranial neuropathies due to metastases to the base of the skull.

The evaluation of patients with skeletal metastases begins with a history focusing on the character of the pain, associated nerve involvement, and factors precipitating the pain. The physical examination should key in on evidence of

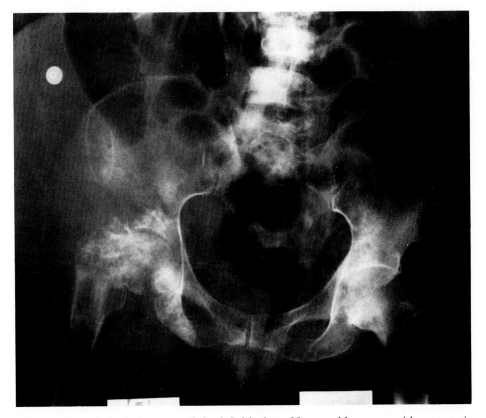

Figure 5-6. Pathologic fracture of the left hip in a 66-year-old woman with metastatic breast carcinoma. Both lytic and blastic lesions are present.

fractures, neurologic findings suggestive of spinal cord compression, and evidence of metastatic disease. Laboratory evaluation should include a CBC, platelet count, calcium test, alkaline phosphatase, liver function tests, and an acid phosphatase test. The acid phosphatase may be increased in primary and metastatic tumors to bone, including osteogenic sarcoma, myeloma, and prostatic carcinoma. The alkaline phosphatase is elevated in primary and metastatic tumors that are associated with osteoblastic activity or new bone formation; because multiple myeloma consists of purely lytic lesions, alkaline phosphatase is usually normal. If a fracture or bone healing occurs, alkaline phosphatase may be elevated in myeloma. If the clinical picture suggests myeloma, a serum and urine immunoelectrophoresis should be obtained. If prostate cancer is suspected or unexplained blastic lesions are seen in a male patient, an acid phosphatase determination should be obtained.

Radiographic studies are the most important diagnostic tools for the evaluation of skeletal metastases. The most sensitive detection technique is the radioisotope bone scan (28). Radionuclide bone scans can increase the yield of detection of areas of metastatic disease 30% over that of plain radiographs. Although several isotopes are employed, technetium-99-labeled pyrophosphate is most commonly used. The scanning techniques are based on the fact that the isotope is taken up by areas in which new bone is being formed. False negative studies may, therefore, occur with purely lytic lesions. Myeloma is a classic example of a disease giving a false negative bone scan in spite of extensive lytic lesions that are easily detected on plain radiographs. False positive bone scans are much more common. Degenerative arthritis and other arthritides are the most common causes of false positive scans. Other processes that may give a false positive reaction for malignancy include osteomyelitis, benign bone conditions such as hyperostosis frontalis, and overlying soft tissue diseases. One overlying soft tissue process that may yield a false positive bone scan is breast cancer, which may produce a pattern suggestive of underlying rib metastases.

Plain radiographs are also very useful in evaluating bony metastases, especially for examining specific areas of pain or suspected fracture. For neoplastic lesions to be detected on plain radiograph, a 50% increase or decrease in bone density is necessary. Tomography of the area in question may reveal metastases and is indicated when there is a high suspicion of neoplastic involvement in spite of normal plain films. In addition to painful areas, it is important to obtain x-ray films of weight-bearing and spinal areas that are positive on bone scan, even though asymptomatic. These areas should be scrutinized for large lytic lesions and areas of cortical involvement. Such areas in weight-bearing bones should be strongly considered for prophylactic surgical fixation to prevent subsequent fracture.

Plain films may also suggest the diagnosis. Blastic lesions may suggest prostate cancer; ivory vertebrae may suggest Hodgkin's disease. Plain films of the spine may help distinguish infectious and neoplastic processes. The earliest radiographic finding for spinal metastases is destruction of the pedicle. Metastases tend to involve the pedicles, spinous processes, and vertebral bodies; except in cases of vertebral collapse, there is preservation of the disc spaces. In infections, the disc space tends to be primarily involved with subsequent extention to adjacent bone (29).

Surgery and radiotherapy are the mainstays of therapy for tumors metastatic to bone. The choice of therapy depends on the location and extent of the lesion, the presence or absence of a pathologic fracture, the patient's overall medical condition, and the patient's estimated survival.

If a weight-bearing bone is involved by a pathologic fracture and the patient has an estimated survival of six weeks or more, surgical fixation is indicated (29). This situation is most commonly seen with femoral lesions. If the shaft is involved, placement of an intramedullary rod or pin is indicated. At the time of surgery, as much of the tumor as possible should be removed. Methylmethacrylate is frequently placed to give stability to the repaired bone and rod (30). Lesions of the femoral head and neck are best treated with insertion of a prosthesis. Acetabulum involvement with tumor or femoral head and neck lesions are best treated with total hip replacement (24). Before a patient undergoes surgery for a femoral lesion, radiographs of the humerus should be obtained. Lesions of the humerus that have a potential for fracture should be repaired as well, as the patient will not be able to use crutches to support his or her weight in ambulation. Patients with large lytic lesions of the femur or lesions involving the cortex should be considered for prophylactic surgical fixation if they have a life expectancy greater than one month and their general medical status permits (31).

Lesions of the proximal tibia are often treated with surgical fixation; other tibial lesions are treated with radiation. Humeral lesions in patients with reasonable life expectancy and performance status are treated with initial fixation and methylmethacrylate. Other patients may be treated with casting and subsequent irradiation. Patients with lesions in other nonweight-bearing bones can usually be safely managed by casting and radiation therapy.

In patients with spinal cord compression from bone metastases, decadron and radiation therapy are considered the treatment of choice in most centers. This followed a study of 235 patients with spinal cord compression secondary to malignancy treated at Memorial Sloan-Kettering Cancer Center; this study revealed that patients treated with radiation alone did as well as patients treated with laminectomy followed by radiation (32). The major criticism of this study is that it was nonrandomized. Patients in whom a tissue diagnosis of cancer has not been made and patients who do not respond to initial radiotherapy are treated with laminectomy.

Patients with bony involvement of the spine in whom there is no spinal cord compression are best treated with a brace for support and radiation therapy. Occasionally, painful lesions not responding to radiation are treated with laminectomy.

All patients with pathologic fractures that have been repaired, lesions that have been prophylactically fixed, and painful lesions in other sites should be irradiated. Even though the bone in question has been surgically stabilized, residual tumor should be sterilized by radiation to prevent further growth.

Radiation therapy should be directed to the smallest tumor volume possible to preserve bone marrow so that chemotherapy and further radiation therapy can be given if needed. Radiation therapy for bony metastases should be given in as short a time as possible so patients do not have to spend valuable time receiving therapy. Short-course, high-fraction therapy of 500 rads daily given over three to four days for a total of 1,500–2,000 rads has been shown to be as effective in palliation as 6,000 rads given over six weeks (33). Radiation generally palliates pain very well in a majority of patients, with a median duration of pain relief of six months.

In all patients with bone metastases, consideration should be given to systemic hormonal therapy or chemotherapy. Systemic hormone therapy with estrogens or orchiectomy can often provide dramatic relief of pain in prostatic cancer. Symptomatic relief may be immediate, with total pain alleviation occurring within hours of orchiectomy or the initiation of estrogens. The acid phosphatase level may also fall dramatically; it may normalize within a day in a hormone-sensitive patient. The acid phosphatase should be checked on the day before a hormone manipulation and on the fourth day after commencing therapy. In breast cancer, hormonal therapy or chemotherapy may be effective in halting the progression of disease and may cause regression and subsequent healing of bony lesions.

The skeletal system may occasionally be involved in the paraneoplastic syndromes associated with cancer; the two most important paraneoplastic syndromes related to the skeletal system are hypertrophic pulmonary osteoarthopathy and hypercalcemia. Arthritis is occasionally associated with malignancy as well.

Hypertrophic pulmonary osteoarthropathy consists of arthritis, clubbing of the fingers and toes, and periosteal new bone formation. The periosteal new bone formation, frequently associated with overlying swelling, most often involves the long bones; many other bones, including the ribs and facial bones, may be involved as well. The arthritis most often involves the wrists, ankles, and knees. Occasionally, autonomic dysfunction may be present.

Hypertrophic pulmonary osteoarthropathy typically complicates intrathoracic malignancies, especially bronchogenic carcinoma and occasionally, mesothelioma (34). Sometimes it may complicate nonmalignant conditions such as bronchiectasis and congenital heart disease. Clubbing of the fingers alone may be caused by a variety of disorders, including inflammatory bowel disease, cirrhosis, and a familial disorder known as pachydermoperiostosis; occasionally an "idiopathic" form of clubbing occurs. The bone scan in patients with hypertrophic pulmonary osteoarthropathy is usually positive in the areas of periosteal new bone formation and arthritis; plain radiographs of the long bones may show periosteal elevation (35).

The cause of hypertrophic pulmonary osteoarthropathy is unknown; ectopically produced mediators of bone growth, including growth hormone and somatostatin, have been postulated to mediate this syndrome (36). Treatment is directed at the underlying disorder; occasionally dramatic relief of the osteoarthropathy is noted with resection or remission of the primary disease. Osteoarthropathy may sometimes resolve within one day, as when dramatic chemotherapeutic responses occur in small cell lung cancer. Vagotomy has also been shown to relieve symptoms in some patients.

Hypercalcemia has been extensively discussed in another chapter. It may result from direct tumor invasion of bone, ectopic production of parathormone and prostaglandins, and production of osteoclast activating factor in multiple myeloma.

Rheumatoid arthritis may develop with malignancy; the simultaneous onset of breast cancer and rheumatoid arthritis has been noted by several investigators. The course of both diseases may parallel each other, with remissions and exacerbations of the arthritis coinciding with therapy-induced remissions and relapses of breast cancer. Infectious monoarticular arthritis, in which *Streptomyces bovis* is the offending organism, has been noted in patients with colonic carcinoma and may be the presenting manifestation of this neoplasm (37). In patients with this arthritis, a search for an occult colonic neoplasm is in order.

The therapy for cancer can affect the skeletal system. These complications are most frequently seen with responsive malignancies, such as Hodgkin's disease, non-Hodgkin's lymphomas, and head and neck cancer. In these neoplasms, treatment may result in long survival.

One of the leading therapeutic causes of bone complications is steroids. Steroids may cause osteoporosis if given over a prolonged period of time. Steroids as part of the MOPP combination have been reported to cause aseptic necrosis in patients treated for Hodgkin's disease.

Radiation therapy may cause a number of skeletal problems. Children treated for embryonal rhabdomyosarcoma, Ewing's sarcoma, and Hodgkin's disease may have arrested growth of the irradiated bone with resulting short stature or limb asymmetry (38). Careful attention to shielding the epiphyseal sites of bone growth in treatment planning is indicated. Large doses of radiation to bone may cause radio-osteonecrosis. This is most commonly seen in the mandible of patients receiving radiation for head and neck tumors. Osteonecrosis of the mandible occurs with severe pain, with or without associated edema; the involved bone may be exposed. Periodontal disease appears to predispose to this condition; prophylactic extractions in patients with poor dentition are recommended before beginning radiation therapy (39). Radiographs may show lytic areas with bone sequestration. Occasionally, surgical resection of the involved area of the mandible is needed to control severe pain.

Radiation may cause fractures of a previously irradiated bone several years after radiation has been completed. Transverse myelitis may complicate radiation therapy to vertebrae; to prevent this complication, shielding of the spinal cord and limiting the radiation dose to the spinal cord to less than 5,000 rads is in order. Finally, patients who have received prior radiotherapy to a portal overlying bone are at increased risk of developing osteogenic sarcomas and chondrosarcomas in bones lying within these areas of treatment.

Skeletal and rheumatologic problems have been noted to complicate the chemotherapy of cancer. Aseptic necrosis of the hips has been reported to complicate mithramycin therapy of testicular cancer (40). The aseptic necrosis is felt to be on an ischemic basis, complicating the veno-occlusive disease reported with mithramycin. Bleomycin therapy may also be complicated by vaso-occlusive phenomena, especially Raynaud's phenomenon.

REFERENCES

1. McKenna R, Schwinn C, Soong K, et al: Osteogenic sarcoma arising in Paget's disease. *Cancer* 17:42, 1964.
2. Kim J, Chu F, Woodard H, et al: Radiation induced soft tissue and bone sarcoma. *Radiology* 129:501, 1978.
3. Schimke R, Lowman J, Kowan G: Retinoblastoma and osteogenic sarcoma in siblings. *Cancer* 34:2077, 1974.

4. Dahlin D, Coventry M: Osteogenic sarcoma: A study of 600 cases. *J Bone Joint Surg* 49:101, 1967.

5. Dahlin D, Coventry M, Scanlon P: Ewing's sarcoma: A critical analysis of 165 cases. *J Bone Joint Surg* 43A:185, 1981.

6. Neifeld J, Michaelis L, Doppman J: Suspected pulmonary metastases: Correlation of chest x-ray, whole lung tomograms, and operative findings. *Cancer* 39:383, 1977.

7. Huvos A: *Bone Tumors: Diagnosis, Treatment and Prognosis.* Philadelphia, Saunders, 1979.

8. Ahuja S, Villacin A, Smith J, et al: Juxtacortical (parosteal) osteogenic sarcoma: Histologic grading and prognosis. *J Bone Joint Surg* 59:632, 1977.

9. Stout A: Discussion of the pathology and histiogenesis of Ewing's tumor of bone marrow. *Ann J Roent* 50:334, 1943.

10. Woodruff R, Malpas J, White F: Solitary plasmacytoma II: Solitary plasmacytoma of bone. *Cancer* 43:2344, 1979.

11. Morton D, Eilber F, Townsend C, et al: Limb salvage from a multidisciplinary treatment approach for skeletal and soft tissue sarcomas of the extremity. *Ann Surg* 184:268, 1976.

12. Graham-Pole J: Ewing's sarcoma: Treatment with high dose radiation and adjuvant chemotherapy. *Med Pediatr Oncol* 7:1, 1979.

13. Carter S, Frieman P: Osteogenic sarcoma: Treatment overview and some comments on interpretation of clinical trial data. *Cancer Treat Rep* 62:199, 1978.

14. Taylor W, Ivins J, Dahlin D, et al: Trends and variability in survival from osteosarcoma. *Mayo Clin Proc* 53:695, 1978.

15. Rosen G, Caparros B, Mosende C, et al: Curability of Ewing's sarcoma and consideration for future therapeutic trials. *Cancer* 41:888, 1978.

16. Gottlieb J, Baker L, O'Bryan R, et al: Adriamycin (NSC-123127) used alone and in combination for soft tissue and bony sarcomas. *Cancer Chemother Rep* 6:271, 1975.

17. Pinedo H, Kenis Y: Chemotherapy of advanced soft-tissue sarcomas in adults. *Cancer Treat Rev* 4:67, 1977.

18. Reimer R, Chabner B, Young R, et al: Lymphoma presenting in bone: Results of histopathology, staging and therapy. *Ann Intern Med* 87:50, 1977.

19. Alexanian R, Gehan E, Haut A, et al: Unmaintained remissions in multiple myeloma. *Blood* 51:1005, 1978.

20. Alexanian R, Salmon S, Bonnet J, et al: Combination therapy of multiple myeloma. *Cancer* 40:2765, 1977.

21. Case D, Lee B, Clarkson B: Improved survival time in multiple myeloma treated with melphalan, prednisone, cyclophosphamide, vincristine and BCNU: M-2 protocol. *Am J Med* 63:897, 1977.

22. Hendrickson F, Sheinkap M: Management of osseous metastases. *Semin Oncol* 2:399, 1975.

23. Lacher M: *Hodgkin's Disease.* New York, John Wiley & Sons, 1976.

24. Albright J, Gillespie T, Butaud T: Treatment of bone metastases. *Semin Oncol* 7:418, 1980.

25. de Kernion J: Natural history of metastatic renal cell carcinoma: A computer analysis. *J Urol* 120:148, 1978.

26. Basora J, Fery A: Metastatic malignancy of the hand. *J Bone Joint Surg* 40A:263, 1958.

27. Bruckman J, Bloomet W: Management of spinal cord compression. *Semin Oncol* 5:135, 1978.

28. McNeil B: Rationale for the use of bone scans in selected metastatic and primary bone tumors. *Semin Nucl Med* 8:336, 1978.

29. Parrish F, Murray J: Surgical treatment for secondary neoplastic fractures. *J Bone Joint Surg* 52A:665, 1970.

30. Harrington K, Sim F, Enis J, et al: Methylmethacrylate as an adjunct in internal fixation of pathological fractures. *J Bone Joint Surg* 58A:1047, 1976.

31. Ryan J, Rowe D, Salciccioli, G: Prophylactic internal fixation of the femur for neoplastic lesions. *J Bone Joint Surg* 58A:1071, 1976.

32. Gilbert R, Kim J, Posner J: Epidural spinal cord compression from metastatic tumor: Diagnosis and treatment. *Ann Neurol* 3:40, 1978.

33. Allen K, Johnson T, Hibbs, G: Effective bone palliation as related to various treatment regimens. *Cancer* 37:984, 1976.

34. Jao J, Barrow J, Krant M: Pulmonary hypertrophic osteoarthropathy, spider angiomata, and estrogen hypersecretion in neoplasia. *Ann Intern Med* 70:580, 1967.

35. Greenfield G, Schorsch H, Shkolnik A: The various roentgen appearances of pulmonary hypertrophic osteoarthropathy. *Am J Roentgenol Radium Ther Nucl Med* 101:927, 1967.

36. Rigammi A, Anderson E: Hypertrophic pulmonary osteoarthropathy: A clinical and biochemical study. *Br J Dis Chest* 68:193, 1974.

37. Hande K, Witebsky F, Brown M, et al: *Streptococcus bovis* septicemia and carcinoma of the colon. *Ann Intern Med* 91:560, 1979.

38. Probert J, Parker B, Kaplan H: Growth retardation in children after megavoltage irradiation of the spine. *Cancer* 32:634, 1973.

39. Regezzi J, Courtney R, Kerr, D: Dental management of patients irradiated for oral cancer. *Cancer* 38:994, 1976.

40. Margileth D, Smith F, Lane M: Sudden arterial occlusion associated with mithramycin therapy. *Cancer* 31:708, 1973.

6

Neurologic Complications of Cancer

Joseph Jankovic

Approximately 25% of patients with systemic cancer develop neurologic dysfunction at some time during the course of their illness. New advances in the treatment of cancer have greatly influenced the ultimate course of many malignant tumors. With prolongation of the natural history, the neurologic complications of malignant disease have been steadily gaining in importance. As outlined in Table 6-1, most of the neurologic complications are a result of direct metastatic involvement or are due to the secondary (nonmetastatic) effect of the cancer.

METASTATIC COMPLICATIONS OF CANCER

Intracranial Metastases

The most common neurologic complication of systemic cancer is due to metastatic parenchymal brain tumor or epidural spinal cord compression by metastases (1,2). Most of the intracranial metastases occur in persons between the ages of 40 and 60, with slightly higher frequency among males. There appears to be an inverse relationship between tendency for primary malignancy to metastasize to the brain and advancing age; thus in the elderly (over the age of 65), metastatic brain tumors are second in incidence after glioblastoma multiforme (3). Because of more effective treatment of systemic cancer, the incidence of intracranial metastases has been increasing. Metastatic brain tumor is the most frequent brain tumor in autopsy studies and accounts for about 50% of all brain tumors. In general, approximately 25% of cancer patients have brain metastases at the time of autopsy, but the incidence varies greatly with the type of tumor.

Certain neoplasms have special "affinity" for the brain. These include melanoma (Fig. 6-1), choriocarcinoma (Fig. 6-2), testicular carcinoma, lung and breast cancer, acute lymphoblastic leukemia, and non-Hodgkin's lymphoma. Lung and breast cancer account for about half of the primary tumor sites. Malignant melanoma, usually involving the brain gray matter, is found in over three-fourths

107

Table 6-1. Neurologic Complications of Cancer

Metastatic
  Intracranial metastases
  Metastases to the base of the skull
  Spinal cord metastases
  Meningeal carcinomatosis
  Metastases to peripheral nerves and roots
  CNS leukemia and reticulosis
Nonmetastatic
  Metabolic encephalopathy
  CNS infection
  Cerebrovascular disorders
  Complications of therapy
  Paraneoplastic ("remote") effects of cancer

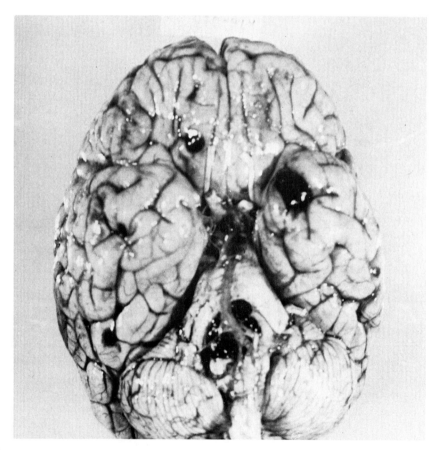

Figure 6-1. Metastatic melanoma: multiple nodules involving the inferior surface of the brain and meninges.

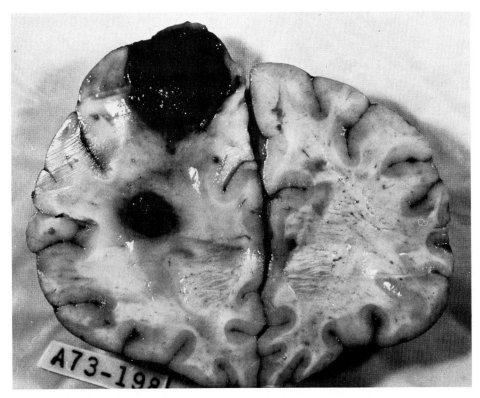

Figure 6-2. Metastatic choriocarcinoma: two tumors showing marked edema with central hemorrhagic necrosis.

of patients dying from this disease (4). Interestingly, melanomas, testicular carcinomas, choriocarcinomas (Fig. 6-3), and hypernephromas also have the greatest propensity toward intracranial hemorrhage (5,6). In contrast to the tumors listed above, other common systemic neoplasms only rarely spread to the brain. For example, ovary, pancreas, and uterine or cervical carcinomas rarely (in 5–10% of cases) involve the brain parenchyma. Prostate carcinoma may involve the dura or pituitary gland, but almost never involves the brain parenchyma. In approximately 20% of patients with brain metastases, the primary neoplasm is never found.

Pathologically, metastatic tumors are usually found in the middle cerebral artery distribution in the junction between gray and white matter. They are usually circumscribed lesions often with a necrotic center (Fig. 6-2) associated with considerable edema. Approximately 70% are supratentorial and 30% are infratentorial (7). Metastatic tumor is the most common cerebellar tumor of adults (Fig. 6-4) (8,9). Over half of the patients with brain metastases have multiple lesions at autopsy. Recently, a series of pituitary metastases was reported (10). In contrast to pituitary adenomas, the metastatic pituitary tumor occurred with diabetes insipidus and oculomotor palsies, but visual loss and anterior pituitary insufficiency, common in primary pituitary adenomas, were infrequently encountered in sellar metastases.

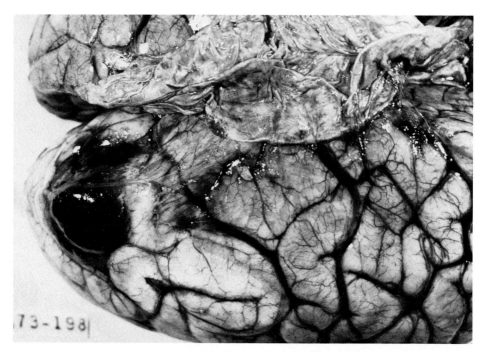

Figure 6-3. Metastatic choriocarcinoma: frontal lobe hemorrhagic necrotic tumor and secondary subarachnoid hemorrhage.

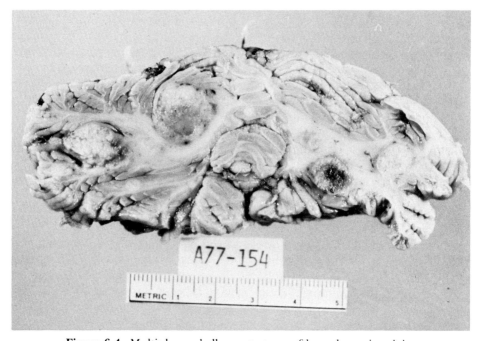

Figure 6-4. Multiple cerebellar metastases of bronchogenic origin.

110

The clinical presentation may be acute in onset in approximately half of the patients and gradual in onset in the other half. When metastatic tumor occurs acutely with sudden onset of focal weakness, it may simulate a stroke. Approximately two-thirds of patients with acute onset present with focal weakness and 15–20% of patients with metastatic tumor present with focal seizures that may remain focal or become secondarily generalized. Headache and mental disturbance are the two most common presentations in patients with gradual onset. The headache is mild, occurring usually on awakening.

Although the great majority of patients have extensive systemic involvement at the time of neurologic presentation, approximately 10% of these patients have neurologic problems as the first sign of systemic malignancy. The time interval between the diagnosis of primary tumor and the clinical manifestation varies with the tissue of origin, but has been estimated at approximately four months for lung cancer and three years for breast cancer (2).

When patients with known systemic cancer show neurologic problems suggestive of brain dysfunction, the differential diagnosis usually includes brain metastases, cerebral hemorrhage, infection, abscess, or metabolic encephalopathy. However, the possibility of an unrelated, including benign, process must always be considered. For example, patients with systemic cancer and neurologic presentation suggestive of intracranial neoplasm may have meningioma rather than metastatic tumor since there appears to be increased association between meningioma and extraneural malignancy, particularly breast cancer (11,12).

Computerized tomography (CT) of the brain is the diagnostic method of choice for intracerebral metastases (Fig. 6-5). It will detect tumors approximately 1 cm in diameter and larger. They are usually identified by an area of lucency representing edema surrounding the tumor. This area often demonstrates marked enhancement after administration of a contrast agent, although at times double concentration of the agent is required. The associated edema may produce a marked mass effect and may distort the surrounding structures causing ipsilateral ventricular compression, midline shift, and uncal or tonsillar herniation. Certain tumors, particularly melanomas and choriocarcinomas, may show increased density even before injection of contrast, presumably due to hemorrhage within the lesions (4). Angiography and pneumoencephalography are rarely required for diagnostic purposes. Skull x-ray films may reveal pineal shift, signs of increased intracranial pressure, and skull metastases. Lumbar puncture is potentially dangerous and should be performed only if associated bacterial or carcinomatous meningitis is suspected and CT scan has excluded large mass lesion. When cerebrospinal fluid (CSF) is available in patients with metastatic brain tumors, in addition to elevated CSF protein, certain specific assays may provide additional information. For example, human chorionic gonadotropin (HCG) and β-glucuronidase are often elevated in the cerebrospinal fluid of patients with intracranial metastases, particularly if the meninges are also involved (13,14). Rarely, biopsy is required for diagnostic purposes in patients without evidence of primary neoplasm.

Management of brain metastases is primarily directed toward reducing the mass effect of the tumor (15–17). In acute treatment, intravenous mannitol (2 g/kg 20% solution IV push) and dexamethasone (100 mg/day) often dramatically improve the clinical status because of their antiedema effect. Also, glycerol (1

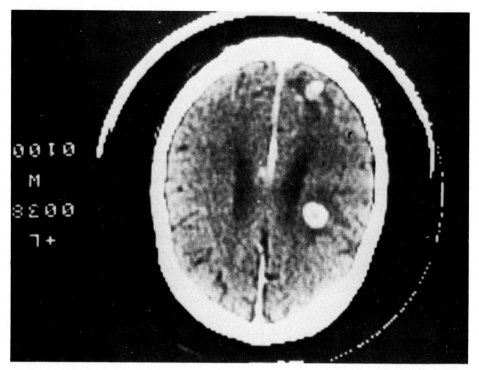

Figure 6-5. CT scan showing two cerebral metastases from bronchogenic carcinoma. There was a three-month history of right hand tremor and rapidly progressive right hemiparkinsonism.

g/kg orally every 4 hours) and hyperventilation are effective antiedema treatments. Because of the high incidence of seizures in patients with metastatic brain tumors (particularly melanoma), prophylactic treatment with anticonvulsants seems justified. Phenytoin may be started at a maintenance dose of 300–400 mg as a single daily dose. However, in patients who have had at least one seizure, a loading dose of 1,000 mg in 24 hours should be administered intravenously (at 50 mg/min) or orally. Blood levels must be carefully monitored and maintained at 10–20 μg/ml. Since glucocorticoids are epileptogenic, in patients receiving high-dose dexamethasone therapy prophylactic anticonvulsants are particularly recommended.

Radiotherapy to the brain using an equivalent of 3,000 rads over two to three weeks produces significant symptomatic relief in approximately 75% of patients with intracerebral metastases, although temporary exacerbation is often noted initially (18–20). Certain tumors, such as metastatic melanoma, are resistant to radiotherapy, while breast cancer, oat cell carcinoma of the lung, and testicular cancer respond quite favorably. In certain cases, especially with single metastatic lesions, surgical approach may be justified, and, recently, long-term survivors have been reported following surgical excision (2,21,22).

The prognosis for patients with metastatic cancer is quite poor after onset of symptoms related to brain metastases. Once the neurologic diagnosis is made, the median survival is approximately six months, depending on the histology of the primary tumor and the site of central nervous system (CNS) involvement. However, most patients die because of complications from the systemic cancer rather than from neurologic dysfunction due to brain metastases. One cannot overemphasize, however, that neurologic abnormality in a cancer patient may be totally unrelated to the underlying cancer or may represent a relatively and potentially curable benign process such as metabolic encephalopathy, infectious meningitis, and brain abscess.

Metastases to the Base of the Skull

Recently Greenberg et al. reviewed 43 patients in whom cancer metastasized to the base of the skull (23). They divided the patients into six groups according to the neurologic findings. These include (1) orbital syndrome (three patients), with diplopia, supraorbital pain, and numbness in V-1 distribution being the predominant symptoms; (2) parasellar syndrome (seven patients), with patients having ocular paresis with or without proptosis and unilateral frontal headache; (3) middle fossa syndrome (15 patients), with patients having numbness or pain in the face; (4) jugular foramen syndrome (nine patients), with hoarseness, dysphagia, and glossopharyngeal neuralgia being the most frequent complaints; (5) occipital condyle syndrome (nine patients), with unilateral twelfth cranial nerve paralysis and facial and upper cervical pain and eleventh nerve paralysis; and (6) atlantoaxial subluxation (14 patients), with symptoms being stiff neck, posterior cervical muscle spasm, and unilateral neck pain exacerbated by head turning, often associated with hyperreflexia in the lower extremities and extensor plantar response.

Some patients with metastases to the base of the skull have the "numb chin syndrome," which was recently also termed "mental neuropathy" because of involvement of the mental nerve or the inferior alveolar nerve. In half these patients the numb chin was the symptom of underlying malignancy. Of the 19 patients recently reported from Duke University, nine had lymphoreticular malignancy, three had breast cancer, and others had cancer of the lung and the prostate, multiple myeloma, melanoma, and rhabdomyosarcoma. Radiotherapy and chemotherapy improved symptoms in 16 of the 19 patients, but 84% died within 17 months of onset of symptoms of the neuropathy (24,25).

Radiographic studies in patients with base-of-the-skull metastases were positive in 85% of patients, with tomograms of the involved region providing the highest yield. In cases with atlantoaxial subluxation, lateral spine x-ray examination was the procedure of choice, showing lytic lesion of C-2 vertebral body in all 14 patients with this complication. Myelography was only infrequently necessary to document the extent of the epidural mass. Almost 90% of patients treated with radiotherapy had symptomatic improvement, but in patients with atlantoaxial subluxation, surgical stabilization was considered the treatment of choice.

Spinal Cord Metastases

In contrast to brain metastases, spinal cord complications are usually due to metastatic involvement of the surrounding bone, causing extramedullary epidural compression rather than intramedullary spinal cord lesion (26,27). Spinal metastases usually constitute true neurologic emergencies, and rapid diagnosis may facilitate effective treatment with prevention of irreversible neurologic damage. Approximately 90% of patients with epidural spinal cord compression have acute back pain as the most common early symptom. The pain is usually localized but may have a radicular character. Approximately 75% of patients complain of weakness at the time of diagnosis and 50% have a sensory loss and/or sphincter disturbance. Exquisite tenderness at the level of involvement is an important clue to the diagnosis.

Although plain x-ray films of the spine are abnormal in most cases, bone scans are more sensitive, but a myelogram is usually required for final confirmation. When a complete block is present on the myelogram, it is important to identify not only the lower extent of the lesion but also the rostral border. This often requires the instillation of a small amount of contrast material via cisternal or lateral cervical puncture. Recently, instead of pantopaque, water-soluble contrast media, such as metrizamide, combined with CT scan provide further refinement in the diagnosis of spinal metastases.

Since most of the spinal complications of metastatic cancer are due to involvement of the vertebral body, the incidence of the primary tumors reflects the tendency of these tumors to involve bone. Therefore lung, breast, prostate, and lymphoma followed by melanoma, myeloma, and renal cell carcinoma are the most common tumors producing spinal cord complications. In children sarcomas, neuroblastomas, and lymphomas are by far the most common primary tumors metastasizing to the spine. Intramedullary metastases are quite uncommon and usually induce sphincter disturbance early, whereas local pain and x-ray abnormalities are less common.

Differential diagnosis must include radiation myelopathy, paraneoplastic necrotizing myelitis, herniated intervertebral disc, and meningeal carcinomatosis with spinal cord involvement.

Acute treatment includes the use of steroids combined with radiation therapy, which usually reduces pain quite dramatically in most patients (27,28). Very high doses of dexamethasone have been recommended: 100 mg intravenously followed by 25 mg every 6 hours. Radiation therapy should be begun immediately once the cord compression is documented. The total dose should not exceed 3,900 rads in $2\frac{1}{2}$ weeks. Surgical decompression is only rarely necessary but should be considered if there is no evidence of primary disease, immediate radiation therapy is not available, or the tumor is resistant to radiotherapy. However, data comparing the effectiveness of surgical versus nonsurgical therapy are not available.

Leptomeningeal Metastasis (Tables 6-2 to 6-5)

Although the symptoms and signs of leptomeningeal metastasis may actually precede the diagnosis of primary neoplasm in more than 50% of patients, symptoms of meningeal infiltration follow within one year of the diagnosis of primary tumor. According to a recent retrospective study of 50 patients (29) with meningeal carcinomatosis, these initial symptoms included headache (38%); altered mental status (24%); radicular back pain (24%); parasthesias (10%); diplopia (8%); and other symptoms including nausea and vomiting, lightheadedness, gait ataxia, seizures, impaired hearing, and sphincter disturbance. Approximately

Table 6-2. Meningeal Carcinomatosis

	Reference	
	Olson (29)	Theodore (32)
Number of patients	50	33
Primary neoplasm (% of total)		
Breast	36	63
Lymphoma	26	0
Lung carcinoma	16	15
Melanoma	10	15
Pancreatic carcinoma	4	3
Liver	0	3
Unknown	4	0

three-fourths of patients have CSF pleocytosis in the form of mononuclear cells or even malignant cells (30). Repeated lumbar punctures are sometimes required to firmly establish the diagnosis. Low CSF sugar has also been reported in three-fourths of patients, and approximately half the patients have abnormal myelograms, usually revealing multiple nodular nerve root deficits.

The overall incidence of leptomeningeal metastasis appears to be increasing chiefly because of the longer survival of patients with systemic cancer and because of increasing awareness of this diagnosis (29,31,32). The overall incidence of leptomeningeal tumor is as high as 10% in the autopsied cancer cases. In the Memorial Sloan-Kettering Hospital series (29) carcinoma of the breast was the leading tumor, accounting for 36% of the cases, followed by lymphomas in 28%, carcinoma of the lung in 16%, malignant melanoma in 10%, and adenocarcinoma of the pancreas in 4%. In two out of the 50 cases no primary tumor could be identified. A recent study suggested that a correct diagnosis of leptomeningeal metastasis can be established by CT scan of the head in 56% of the cases (33).

Treatment of leptomeningeal metastasis consists of radiation therapy admin-

Table 6-3. Meningeal Carcinomatosis

		Reference	
	Initial	Olson (29) During Course	Theodore (32) During Course
Neurologic symptoms (% of total)			
Headache	38	50	39
Back pain	24	64	24
Altered mental status	24	52	54
Nausea and vomiting	12	36	12
Lightheadedness	12	22	—
Gait disorder	10	24	36
Seizures	8	26	12
Impaired vision	8	22	12
Diplopia	8	22	12

Table 6-4. Meningeal Carcinomatosis

	Olson (29)		Theodore (32)	
	Initial	During Course	Initial	During Course
Neurologic signs (% of total)				
Altered mental status	52	82	45	66
Visual field deficit	14	36	9	9
Papilledema	12	18	21	27
Ophthalmoparesis	46	70	39	51
Altered facial sensation	12	30	18	21
Facial weakness	42	44	30	48
Hearing loss	30	38	3	6
Bulbar palsy	24	40	30	45
Weakness	78	94	54	72
Sensory loss	50	62	33	39
Decreased reflexes	60	86	24	36
Extensor plantar	50	66	21	24
Meningeal irritation	16	34	33	45

istered to the focal area of involvement of the neuroaxis combined with intrathecal injection of methotrexate and cytosine arabinoside (34,35). If, in addition, cranial nerve signs are present, patients should receive whole brain irradiation. The spinal cord radiation rarely exceeds 3,000 rads in 15 treatments over 7 to 21 days. Radiation therapy is often combined with intrathecal chemotherapy using the Ommaya reservoir with cannula inserted in the right frontal horn of the lateral ventricle. This device allows for easy sampling of the cerebrospinal fluid and more uniform concentration of intrathecal chemotherapeutic agents. Although it is still too early to draw definite conclusions, it appears that the combination of radiation and intrathecal chemotherapy offers some hope for improvement of neurologic deficit and possibly prolonged survival. Using this combined approach in 45 patients with sufficient data to determine clinical outcome, the one-year survival for the entire group was 10%. In patients in whom the cause of death could be determined, half were directly related to

Table 6-5. Meningeal Carcinomatosis

	Olson (29)		Theodore (32)	
	First LP	All LPs	First LP	All LPs
CSF (% of total)				
Malignant cells	45	72	72	100
WBC > 4/cu mm^3	45	77	56	66
CSF protein > 45 mg/dl	74	91	72	79
CSF glucose < 50 mg/dl	40	77	54	60
CSF pressure > 150 mm H_2O	45	77	30	30
Abnormal Myelogram	7/18		2/5	

the meningeal involvement. More research is needed to develop techniques that lead to earlier diagnoses and more effective treatment.

Metastases to Peripheral Nerves and Roots

Brachial Plexopathy

Brachial plexus may be involved in several ways in patients with cancer, but the most likely causes are tumor infiltration and radiation injury (36). Patients with tumor infiltration usually have shoulder or arm pain (85%) that often precedes any neurologic deficit for several weeks. Only about 15% of patients complain of paresthesias, usually in the 4th through 5th digits. When weakness does occur, it is usually in the distribution of C7-T1 roots (70%). The proximal involvement in most patients is suggested by the presence of Horner's syndrome in more than half of them. In patients with lung cancer the presence of Horner's syndrome may suggest epidural extension, and a myelogram may be required. In contrast, patients with postradiation plexopathy only seldom present with pain (18%), although in most (65%) pain develops later. However, paresthesias, swelling of hand and arm, and proximal weakness in C5 to C7 root distribution were quite common in this group of patients. The radiation dose required to produce postradiation plexopathy is approximately 6,000 rads. The average latency from time of last radiation therapy to the onset of symptoms was 5.5 years, but the range was 3 months to 26 years.

Peripheral Nerve Involvement

Other than by spread from the surrounding carcinomatous tissue, peripheral nerves are rarely affected by systemic cancer. However, diffuse lymphocytic infiltration of peripheral and cranial nerves has been occasionally reported (37).

Central Nervous System Leukemia and Reticulosis (38–43)

Neurologic complications of leukemia are recognized clinically in 13% of adults with acute leukemia and in 25% of autopsied cases. Of the leukemias, the acute lymphocytic leukemia most frequently involves brain, spinal cord, and leptomeninges. With the use of newer chemotherapeutic agents, CNS relapse may occur in patients who have had a lasting remission. Therefore, the frequency of CNS involvement by leukemia has been increasing (40). In adult patients with acute lymphoblastic leukemia the CNS manifestations are usually related to increased intracranial pressure and cranial nerve palsies. In acute granulocytic leukemia, however, local signs such as root infiltration and cord compression appear to be more common. Intracranial hemorrhage, meningeal infiltration, and infection are also encountered in patients with leukemia. Whereas intracranial involvement is not uncommon in the leukemias, in patients with lymphoma and myeloma spinal cord involvement is more common (43). Although lymphoma may occur in the brain as a primary tumor, it usually produces neurologic complications by involving the epidural space and compressing the spinal cord and nerve roots. The overall incidence of spinal cord compression by epidural lymphoma is about 5%, with all lymphomas having similar incidence of spinal cord involvements (38). The thoracic and lumbar levels are most frequently involved, the cervical cord being involved in less than 20% of cases. The management of CNS leukemias and lymphomas consists of intrathecal injection of methotrexate and other chemotherapeutic agents and radiation therapy of the neuroaxis.

NONMETASTATIC NEUROLOGIC COMPLICATIONS OF CANCER

Metabolic Encephalopathy (44)

In hospitalized cancer patients the most common neurologic complication is metabolic encephalopathy. In fact, metabolic causes account for about 43% of cases of a confusional state (encephalopathy) in cancer patients. The other causes include effects of the underlying neoplasm (15%), such as metastasis, carcinomatous meningitis, and obstructive hydrocephalus; vascular causes (15%), such as disseminated intravascular coagulation, thrombotic or embolic infarction, and sagittal sinus thrombus; drugs (13%); and infections (8%). Metabolic encephalopathy associated with cancer is usually due to (1) liver failure; (2) hypercalcemia; (3) renal failure; (4) hypoxia/ischemia; (5) inappropriate ADH syndrome with hyponatremia; and (6) hyperosmolar state. These causes of encephalopathy must be excluded before the confusional and drowsy state of cancer patients can be attributed to brain metastases.

Infections of the Nervous System in Cancer Patients (45)

In cancer patients several defense mechanisms may be broken that predispose them to the development of infections and eventual involvement of the central nervous system. Lymphomas and leukemias are most frequently complicated by CNS infections, possibly because of association with immunologic deficiency. The third most common situation predisposing cancer patients to serious infection is following head and spine tumor surgery, possibly due to the destruction of the physical barriers that normally shield the brain and spinal cord from infection. In one large series the following organisms were identified as causes of meningitis in cancer patients: (1) Cryptococcus neoformans (28%); (2) Listeria monocytogenes (16%); (3) Pseudomonas aeruginosa (11%); (4) Staphylococcus aureus coagulase positive (11%); (5) Diplococcus pneumoniae (10%); (6) Escherichia coli (8%); and (7) anaerobic Streptococcus (5%). Other infections include abscess, herpes zoster, progressive multifocal leukoencephalopathy, and Toxoplasma gondii. Therefore, the usual distribution of organisms causing meningitis is not evident in cancer patients, and unusual forms of infection are the rule rather than the exception.

Cerebrovascular Disorders

Intravascular Coagulation (46–48)
Disseminated intravascular coagulation (DIC) is a nonspecific complication of a variety of medical conditions including cancer. Almost all patients have altered

mental status and many of them develop seizures, hemiparesis, cortical blindness, multifocal myoclonus, ataxia, and even epilepsia partialis continua. In most patients the neurologic symptoms are episodic in nature, but in some the neurologic disorder is rapidly progressive, often confused with a brain neoplasm. Leukemia and lymphoma are most frequently associated with DIC, but any form of cancer may be complicated by this order. The coagulation profile may be normal at onset, but all patients eventually develop thrombocytopenia and/or increased fibrinogen levels. At autopsy microvascular fibrin thrombi and multiple small infarcts and petechial hemorrhages are noted. In some patients subdural hematoma, subarachnoid hemorrhage, and arterial and venous fibrin thrombi have been well documented. Another complication of a "hypercoagulable state" associated with systemic malignancy is venous occlusion such as superior sagittal sinus thrombosis (49). Patients with this complication may present acutely with headache, seizures, hemiparesis, or lethargy or subacutely with progressive encephalopathy.

Nonbacterial (Marantic) Thrombotic Endocarditis (50)

In a survey of 18 patients with nonbacterial thrombotic endocarditis, five had stroke as the initial manifestation of cancer. Other patients had progressive encephalopathy or multifocal deficits. Therefore, this complication should always be considered in patients without obvious cause for embolic infarction. In patients in whom the primary carcinoma could be identified, adenocarcinoma of the lung, pancreas, prostate, and ovary accounted for the majority of the primary tumors.

Hyperviscosity Syndromes (39,51)

Hyperviscosity syndromes should also be considered in the differential diagnosis of cerebral vascular disease in a cancer patient. Patients with multiple myeloma and lymphomas are especially at risk for development of venous thrombosis or infarction as a result of increased production of proteins leading to blood hyperviscosity.

Complications of Anticancer Therapy

Complications of Chemotherapy (52,53)

Major advances have been made within the last decade in the chemotherapy of cancer. As a result of improved survival, many patients live long enough to develop further complications of the underlying cancer and neurologic toxicity from the chemotherapeutic agents. The latter can be divided into three major categories: (1) peripheral neuropathy; (2) encephalopathy; and (3) encephalomalacia.

Peripheral Neuropathy. The following drugs have been associated with peripheral neuropathy: vincristine, procarbazine, maytansine, hexamethylmelamine (HXM), 5-fluorouracil, 5-azacytidine, and cytosine arabinoside. Recently, *cis*-platinum has been associated mainly with ototoxicity, but mild peripheral neuropathy has also been reported.

Encephalopathy. Encephalopathic states have been produced by a variety of chemotherapeutic agents, particularly 5-fluorouracil, which also produces cerebellar degeneration related to the dose at each administration, rather than to the total cumulative dosage. The cerebellar syndrome is often accompanied by dementia and confusion as well as mild generalized weakness, rigidity, tremor, and parkinsonian features. In some patients even brain stem and pyramidal tract dysfunctions have been reported. Procarbazine also causes a confusional, delerious state, occasionally associated with ataxia and peripheral neuropathy. Other agents causing encephalopathy include asparaginase, mitotane (DDD), 5-azacytidine, and hexamethylmelamine.

Encephalomalacia. Necrotizing encephalopathy is most frequently due to methotrexate, especially if radiation therapy was previously employed as a prophylactic treatment. CT scan often reveals calcification in the brain, particularly in children. In addition to encephalopathy, some patients may actually develop focal neurologic symptoms such as hemiparesis and hemianopsia. Methotrexate may also cause meningeal irritation and myelopathy.

Complications of Radiotherapy

Radiation Myelopathy and Radiculopathy (54–57). Myelopathy may be transient, progressive, and arrested, and there may be anterior horn cell involvement or the patient may have disseminated demyelination. Although nerve cells are relatively radioresistant, the supporting tissue, consisting of glia and capillary endothelium, is much more susceptible to the effects of radiotherapy. Grossly, swelling of the spinal cord, demyelination, and tract degeneration may be noted. Microscopic evaluation reveals subendothelial edema, which results in vascular lumen narrowing, tissue ischemia, and infarction. It is not quite clear why symptoms are delayed, often for several months or years following the radiation therapy. It is, however, quite obvious that the dosage and the field of irradiation are the most important factors associated with radiation myelopathy. Thus, 3,500 rads in 17 days, considered by most as the usual dosage, is associated with 23% incidence of radiation myelopathy.

Radiation-induced Encephalopathy (58). Acute encephalopathy manifested by lethargy, decreased responsiveness, headaches, nausea and vomiting, behavioral changes and fever, as well as seizures and focal neurologic symptoms is usually due to radiation-induced cerebral edema. Approximately half the patients with an initial dose of 750 rads develop this acute encephalopathy. This is in contrast to only 15% incidence with an initial dose of 200 rads. Occasionally, pretreatment with steroids and lower initial dosage prevents the development of this potentially serious complication. Another form of encephalopathy is due to subacute demyelination. This is usually delayed by 10 to 13 weeks and usually follows radiotherapy to the head and neck regions. This disorder usually progresses to death or there may be complete spontaneous recovery in six to eight weeks. The pathology is quite similar to demyelination seen with multiple sclerosis.

Delayed Cerebral Radiation Necrosis (59). This condition is most frequently confused with recurrent brain tumor or brain abscess because it usually begins with a gradual onset of focal neurologic deficit suggesting a mass lesion (Fig. 6-6). CT scan often reveals an area of low density with mass effect with or without contrast enhancement in the surrounding white matter. Angiography usually reveals an avascular mass. The diagnosis is often confirmed by brain biopsy, which reveals necrosis and cavitation of white matter as well as glial proliferation and bizarre multinucleated astrocytes. The small vessels reveal fibrinoid necrosis, thrombus formation, and adventitial proliferation. Necrosis results from progressive ischemia as a result of the vascular changes, but other possible mechanisms include demyelination due to damage to the oligodendrogliocytes and autoimmune reaction directed against various central nervous system elements. Finally, cerebral atrophy may result months to years after radiation therapy to the whole brain. This is usually manifested clinically by progressive dementia and CT scan evidence of cerebral atrophy.

Cranial Neuropathy (60). The optic nerve is most frequently involved with radiotherapy to the head, particularly with radiation of the sinuses for nasal pharyngeal carcinoma. Again, latency of several years is not uncommon, and patients usually develop progressive painless loss of vision in one eye associated with optic nerve atrophy or may develop acute loss of vision due to central retinal artery thrombosis. The 12th, 8th, 10th, 11th, 5th, 6th, and other cranial nerves may also be involved as a result of radiotoxicity.

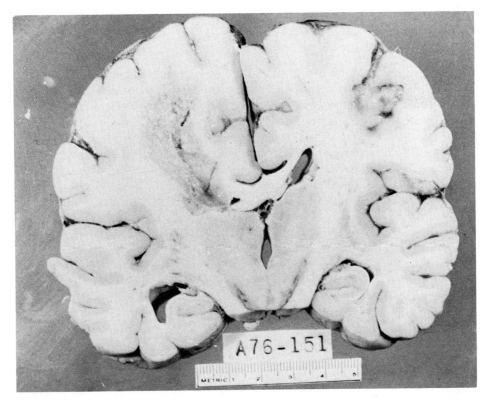

Figure 6-6. Metastasis of the breast, with postradiation necrosis producing mass effect.

Radiation-Induced Peripheral Neuropathy. Brachial plexopathy has been discussed in a previous section, "Metastases to the Peripheral Nerves and Roots (36,57).

Radiogenic Brain and Peripheral Nerve Tumors (61,62). Some patients have been reported to develop radiogenic brain tumors such as sarcomas, meningiomas, and, possibly, gliomas. This usually occurs following radiation therapy for pituitary tumors and primary CNS neoplasms. The interval between radiotherapy and the diagnosis of radiogenic brain tumor is usually several years. Furthermore, as a delayed effect of radiotherapy on peripheral nerves, painful neural tumors may develop and cause progressive neurologic dysfunction in the distribution of the affected nerve. Certain genetic factors (e.g., neurofibromatosis and specific susceptibility) play an important role in the pathogenesis of some of these peripheral nerve tumors.

Radiation-Induced Carotid Disease (63–65). Focal ulcerated narrowing and occlusion of internal carotid has been reported on angiography of some patients receiving radiotherapy to the head and neck region. The patients may present with a stroke and at autopsy have evidence of segmental vasculopathy with subintimal and medial fibrosis and disrupted internal elastic lamina.

Other Neurologic Complications of Radiotherapy. These include postradiation motor neuron syndrome (66) and peripheral neuropathy (67).

Paraneoplastic ("Remote") Effects of Cancer
(Tables 6-6 and 6-7)

In 1958 Brain and Henson introduced the term "carcinomatous neuromyopathy" to describe various neurologic syndromes that occur in patients with malignant tumors and that are not due to direct invasion or metastases (68). Subsequent reports emphasized the particularly high association of these paraneoplastic syndromes with cancer of the lung and ovary, where the incidence may be as high as 16%. The reported incidence of the paraneoplastic syndromes with other neoplasms is less than 6% (69). The importance of these paraneoplastic syndromes lies in the fact that they may precede the discovery of the primary carcinoma sometimes by several years and their recognition may lead to early diagnosis of otherwise occult carcinoma. Furthermore, they may be more disabling than the primary neoplasm.

Of the CNS paraneoplastic syndromes, dementia is the most frequent and may be a feature in as many as 40% of patients with remote effects of carcinoma (70,71). The mental changes may occur as an isolated neurologic abnormality or may be a part of a syndrome that also involves other portions of the central or peripheral nervous system. It may be a result of a metabolic derangement, viral infection (PML), or a nonspecific neuron degenerative process. In a few cases, the neuropathologic examination may reveal multifocal necrosis and perivascular lymphocytic infiltration, particularly in the region of hippocampal and amygdaloid nuclei. Corsellis et al. (72) have termed this condition "limbic encephalitis" and have pointed out the clinical and neuropathologic differences between this condition and herpes simplex encephalitis. Although in both con-

Table 6-6. Paraneoplastic "Remote" Effects of Neoplasm

Cerebral
  Encephalomyelitis (70–74)
  Dementia (70)
  Limbic encephalitis (72)
  Wernicke-Korsakoff syndrome (75)
Brainstem
  Encephalomyelitis (70–74,76)
  Central pontine myelinolysis (77,78)
  Midbrain encephalitis (79)
  Bulbar encephalitis (80)
Cerebellum
  Encephalomyelitis (70–74)
  Subacute cortical cerebellar degeneration (81–83)
  Opsoclonus-myoclonus-ataxia syndrome (84–87)
Spinal cord
  Necrotizing myelopathy (with or without vasculitis) (88–90)
  Subacute combined myelitis (73)
  Motor neuron disease (91–93)
Peripheral nerves, roots, and ganglia
  Sensorimotor polyneuropathy (94,95)
  Sensory neuropathy (102)
  Ganglioradiculitis (102,103)
  Radiculoneuropathy (105)
  Relapsing-remitting polyneuropathy (106)
  Mononeuritis (107)
Neuromuscular junction
  Myasthenia gravis (thymoma) (108)
  Myasthenic (Eaton-Lambert) syndrome (109,110)
Muscle
  Proximal myopathy (111,112)
  Dermatomyositis (113,114)
  Nonspecific degeneration (115)
  Myotonia (116)

ditions the medial temporal regions appear to be prominantly involved, the latter is more acute, produces more intensely necrotic reaction, and the characteristic intranuclear inclusion bodies are usually demonstrated. Previously Henson et al. (73) described inflammatory changes in the central nervous system of patients with carcinoma. Most of these patients harbored oat cell carcinoma of the bronchus (8 out of 10). In addition to limbic encephalitis, Henson et al. found evidence of bulbar encephalitis myelitis and ganglioradiculitis. Most of the patients had lesions in more than one of the four sites: 4 out of 10 had limbic encephalitis; 8 out of 10 had bulbar encephalitis; 3 out of 10 had myelitis; and 6 out of 10 had degeneration of the posterior root ganglia, posterior roots, and posterior columns. The neurologic complications were directly or indirectly responsible for 6 out of 10 deaths. Dorfman and Forno (74) described 30 patients with "paraneoplastic encephalomyelitis": 22 had dementia, 18 had cerebellar abnormalities, 15 had brainstem sign, 13 had spasticity, 16 had anterior horn cell

Table 6-7. Encephalomyelitis with Systemic Cancer: Review of Literature 1934–1981[a]

Neoplasm	
Lung	
Small Cell	31
Other	4
Ovary	4
Breast	4
Uterus	2
Stomach	2
Larynx	1
Lymphoma	5
Leukemia	1
Lesions	
Spinal cord	
Posterior root ganglia	
Brainstem	
Cerebellum	
Cerebral hemispheres	

[a]53 cases with autopsy: 26 women, 27 men. Mean age, 55.1 years (10–80).

involvement, and 15 had sensory abnormalities of the ganglioneuritis type. Pathologically, all patients had meningeal inflammation, and 10 patients had limbic encephalitis. In many patients several parts of the CNS had evidence of inflammation and degeneration. The average duration of illness was 10.5 months with a range of 2 to 24 months. Twenty-three of the 30 patients were found to have bronchogenic carcinoma (small cell or oat cell type). Pathologic changes consistent with Wernicke's encephalopathy have been described in patients with generalized invasion by a tumor of the lymphoid-hemopoietic systems (75).

The brainstem may be involved selectively or as a part of diffuse paraneoplastic inflammatory encephalomyelitis (76). Central pontine myelinolysis (CPM) is a neurologic syndrome characterized by rapidly evolving quadraparesis with pseudobulbar symptoms such as dysarthria and dysphagia, which may progress into a "locked-in" syndrome. Although demyelination of the pons is the most characteristic feature of this syndrome, other portions of the brain may also be affected. Thus, cerebral brain may also be affected. Thus, cerebral edema and pathologic changes of Wernicke's encephalopathy may accompany the more typical findings of CPM. Electrolyte imbalance, particularly hyponatremia, and alcohol abuse are most frequently associated with CPM, but occasional reference is made to association of CPM with remote neoplasms, particularly lymphoproliferation disease (77,78). Also midbrain (79) and bulbar (80) encephalitis have been reported as a remote effect of malignant neoplasm.

Approximately 3% of patients with nonmetastatic complications of cancer develop subacute cerebellar degeneration (81–82). The clinical picture of pancerebellar dysfunction with gait and limb ataxia and dysarthria evolves over a period of weeks or months, and approximately half the patients have associated dementia and some have nystagmus or opsoclonus. In seven out of 17 cases reported by Croft and Wilkinson (83) clinical features of cerebellar degeneration preceded the diagnosis of carcinoma by three to 93 months. Carcinoma of the lung, ovary, and breast accounted for almost all cases. However, even the lymphoproliferative disorders may be associated with cerebellar degeneration (83). In some cases, there was CSF pleocytosis and an increase in CSF protein. On pathologic examination the most prominent finding was diffuse loss of Purkinje cells throughout the cerebellum. Frequently, meningeal and perivascular lymphocytic infiltration was present. Some degenerative change may also be observed in the brainstem, basal ganglia, and the spinal cord.

In 1962 Kinsbourne described six cases of a new disorder he termed "myoclonic encephalopathy of infants" (84). Subsequently, a number of similar cases were described using various terminology, including "dancing eyes, dancing feet syndrome." In almost half the children a neuroblastoma can be identified (85). Clinically, these young children have cerebellar ataxia, myoclonus of limbs, and trunk and ocular dyskinesias. Opsoclonus consists of involuntary, rapid, chaotic, multidirectional, but conjugate eye movements. Occasionally, evidence of increased catecholamine excretion is found, but this is not consistent. Although some children may remit spontaneously, most require removal of the neuroblastoma and treatment with ACTH or prednisone. In contrast to the subacute cerebellar degeneration described before, in the syndromes of opsoclonus, ataxia, and myoclonus no definite cerebellar pathology could be demonstrated. Besides neuroblastoma, opsoclonus has also been described in association with bronchogenic carcinoma and carcinoma of the breast, uterus, and heart (86). The important site of pathology in the pathogenesis of opsoclonus has been suggested to be the cerebellum; however, brainstem encephalitis has also been described in association with opsoclonus. A recent report of "opsoclonic cerebellopathy" responsive to thiamine therapy links this interesting disorder to some nutritional deficiency (87).

The spinal cord may be involved in several pathologic processes. Mancall and Rosales (88) described an acute or subacute necrotizing myelopathy in two cases of their own and nine other cases from the literature. The characteristic clinical features included rapid onset of flaccid paraplegia and loss of sensation, reflexes, and sphincter control below the level of the lesion. Pathologically there was marked noninflammatory necrosis affecting the white and gray matter. The spinal cord may also be involved by a subacute myelitis involving chiefly the anterior horn cells. This form of myelitis is usually a part of the encephalomyelitis syndrome described by Henson et al. (73,89). Severe acute vasculitis was noted in a case of necrotizing myelopathy associated with Hodgkin's disease (90).

Motor neuron disease is another form of spinal cord involvement in patients with cancer. Brain et al. (91) described 11 patients, five of whom had neurologic complaints three months to five years before the occult carcinoma was diagnosed. Five patients had weakness in the upper limbs, two had symptoms in the lower limbs; one patient presented with bulbar palsy and three other patients presented with generalized weakness. Weakness and wasting in the arms or hands was present in all patients and was less frequent in the lower limbs. All patients demonstrated fasciculations. The reflexes were either exaggerated or diminished. Neoplasm of the lung and the breast were again most frequent. The neuropathologic features of two patients examined were similar to those of classical motor neuron disease. Interestingly, when compared clinically, the motor neuron disease associated with cancer appears to have a more benign course than the classical motor neuron disease. Some of the patients in the carcinoma series reached a plateau or actually improved following resection of the carcinoma. Therefore, atypical cases of motor neuron disease should be investigated for the possibility of an occult neoplasm (91–93).

Disorders of the peripheral nerves account for one of the most frequent remote complications of neoplasm. In a recent study of 195 patients with malignancies at various sites, muscle weakness and wasting was observed in 22% (generalized 14%, proximal 7%) (94). Neuropathic sensory symptoms were present in 15%, although objective sensory abnormalities were present in only 7%. Muscle weakness as a predominant symptom was reported by only 7 patients (3.5%). Of the patients with muscle wasting 86% had an abnormal electromyograph (EMG) and 35% had abnormal nerve conduction velocities (NCVs). The overall incidence of EMG and NCV abnormalities was 32% and 26%, respectively. Of the clinically normal patients 35% were found to have abnormal electrophysiologic studies. The various clinical and electrophysiologic abnormalities were noted in carcinoma of the lung (48–64%), ovary (46–64%), testes (42–58%), penis, stomach, and oral cavity, in that order.

Croft et al. (95) divided the carcinomatous peripheral sensorimotor neuropathies into three types. Type A (10 patients) neuropathy is a relatively mild, symmetrical sensory neuropathy that often occurs late in the course of a neoplastic illness. Type B (15 patients) is a more acute or subacute and more severe sensorimotor neuropathy, which may present early in the course often before the diagnosis of a neoplasm is made. This type of neuropathy may rapidly progress to a severe paralysis. Type C (8 patients) represents a group of peripheral neuropathies clinically similar to type B, but with a remitting and occasionally relapsing course. In the entire series 16 out of 33 patients had carcinoma of the lung, 4 out of 33 had carcinoma of the breast, and 4 out of 33 had carcinoma of the stomach. Other carcinomas and the lymphoreticular malignancies have been reported in association with Guillain-Barré syndrome and other peripheral neuropathies (96–101). Demyelination, axonal changes, and vasculitis (101) have been described on pathologic examination of the peripheral nerves.

In 1948 Denny-Brown described two patients with severe proprioceptive ataxia and sensory loss. Both patients had brochogenic carcinoma and coincidental polymyositis (102). Horwich et al. (103) described seven patients with subacute sensory neuropathy and reviewed 29 previously reported cases. Pathologic examination revealed inflammation and degeneration of dorsal root ganglia and secondary degeneration of the posterior root and posterior columns. In 24 of 29 patients the neurologic symptoms preceded the diagnosis of neoplasm by 1 to 46 months (mean of 14 months in men and 11 months in women). Carcinoma of the lung was found in 24 of 29 patients (17 of 24 with oat cell variety). Clinical features include subacute onset of pain, parathesias, dysesthesias, and numbness with proprioceptive ataxia. In addition, severe sensory loss and distal muscle wasting and loss of reflexes are found on the neurologic examination. Ocular abnormalities include nystagmus, diplopia, anisocoria, irregular pupils, and depressed light reaction. The CSF analysis usually demonstrates elevated protein and mild pleocytosis. Recently, clinically indistinguishable progressive sensory neuropathy has been reported in patients without obvious carcinoma (104). Myelopathy and radiculoneuropathy may occasionally be combined in association with lymphoproliferative disease (105). Also remitting polyneuropathy (106) and mononeuritis (107) have been rarely reported as remote effects of underlying malignancy.

The "neuromuscular disorder" group accounted for 65% of the patients with "carcinomatous neuromyopathy." In these neuromuscular groups of disorders, a definite peripheral neuropathy was found in 19% and definite myopathy, myasthenic syndrome, or myasthenia gravis was found in 16%. Myasthenia gravis (MG) is associated with a tumor of the thymus in approximately 10% of the cases, and in 4% of the myasthenic patients a malignant thymoma is found (108). However, MG has been described in association with other neoplasms, particularly oat cell carcinoma of the lungs, although most authors believe that the incidence of neoplasm other than thymoma is the same in the myasthenia gravis group as in the general population. The myasthenic syndrome of Eaton and Lambert is clinically characterized by a male preponderance, proximal weakness, fatigability, dysphagia, dry mouth, stiffness, areflexia, and increased sensitivity to curare or curarelike drugs (e.g., "mycin" antibiotics). On repetitive stimulation following the initial transient decrement, there is an increase in amplitude indicating facilitation of transmission. Although the myasthenic syndrome has been reported without associated neoplasm, in most cases the suspected neoplasm will be found, usually in the chest (109–112). In contrast to MG, in the myasthenic syndrome the defect in neuromuscular transmission is presynaptic and is associated with decreased amounts of acetylcholine released from the presynaptic nerve ending. This is manifested clinically by proximal weakness and muscle wasting with loss of reflexes.

A recent review of the literature contends that the incidence of malignancy in dermatomyositis is five to seven times that of the general population (113). The most frequent sites of neoplasm are breast, lung, ovary, stomach, uterus, and colon (113,114). Proximal weakness with nonspecific degeneration of the muscle (115) and myotonia (116) and other neuromuscular complications of cancer have also been described in association with malignancy (117).

REFERENCES

1. Posner JB, Chernik NL: Intracranial metastasis from systemic cancer. *Adv Neurol* 19:575, 1978.
2. Black P: Brain metastasis: Current status and recommended guidelines for management. *Neurosurgery* 5:617, 1979.
3. Tomita T, Raimond, AJ: Brain tumors in the elderly. *JAMA* 246:53, 1981.
4. Enzmann DR, Kramer R, Norman D, Pollock J: Malignant melanoma metastatic to the central nervous system. *Radiology* 127:177, 1978.
5. Little JR, Dial B, Belanger G, Carpenter S: Brain hemorrhage from intracranial tumor. *Stroke* 10:283, 1979.
6. Mandybur TI: Intracranial hemorrhage caused by metastatic tumors. *Neurology* 27:650, 1977.
7. Weiss HD, Richardson EP: Solitary brainstem metastasis. *Neurology* 28:562, 1978.
8. Amici R, Avanzini G, Pacin L: Cerebellar tumors, in *Monograms in Neural Sciences*, vol 4. Basel, S. Karger, 1976, p 36.

9. Gilman S, Bloedel JR, Lechtenberg R: Disorders of the cerebellum, in *Contemporary Neurology Series*, vol 21. Philadelphia, F.A. Davis, 1981, p 352.

10. Max MB, Deck MDF, Rottenberg DA: Pituitary metastasis: Incidence in cancer patients and clinical differentiation from pituitary adenoma. *Neurology* 31:998, 1981.

11. Schoenberg BS, Christine BW, Whisenant JP: Nervous system neoplasms and primary malignancies of other sites: The unique association between meningiomas and breast cancer. *Neurology* 25:705, 1975.

12. Bellur S, Chandra V, McDonald LW: Association of meningiomas with extraneural primary malignancy. *Neurology* 29:1165, 1979.

13. Shuttleworth E, Allen N: CSF B-glucuronidase assay in the diagnosis of neoplastic meningitis. Arch Neurol 37:684, 1980.

14. Schold SC, Wasserstrom WR, Fleisher M, et al: Cerebrospinal fluid biochemical markers of central nervous system metastasis. *Ann Neurol* 8:597, 1980.

15. Weinstein JD, Toy JF, Jaffee ME, Goldberg HI: The effect of dexamethasone on brain edema in patients with metastatic brain tumors. *Neurology* 23:121, 1973.

16. Gutin PH: Corticosteroid therapy in patients with cerebral tumors: Benefits, mechanisms, problems, practicalities. *Semin Oncol* 2:49, 1975.

17. Markesbery WR, Brook WH, Glipta G, Young AB: Treatment for patients with cerebral metastasis. *Arch Neurol* 35:754, 1978.

18. Cairncross JG, Chernik NL, Posner JB: Sterilization of cerebral metastases by radiation therapy *Neurology* 29:1195, 1979.

19. Cairncross JG, Kim JH, Posner JB: Radiation therapy for brain metastases. *Ann Neurol* 7:529, 1980.

20. Cox JD, Stanley K, Petrovich Z, et al: Cranial irradiation in cancer of the lung of all cell types. *JAMA* 245:469, 1981.

21. White KT, Fleming TR, Laws ER: Single metastasis to the brain: Surgical treatment in 122 consecutive patients. *Mayo Clinic Proc* 56:424, 1981.

22. Mosberg WH: Twelve-year "cure" of lung cancer with metastasis to the brain. *JAMA* 235:2745, 1976.

23. Greenberg HS, Deck MDF, Vikram B, et al: Metastasis to the base of the skull: Clinical findings in 43 patients. *Neurology* 31:530, 1981.

24. Massey EW, Schold SC, Moore J: Mental neuropathy from systemic cancer. *Neurology* 31:1277, 1981.

25. Dugan TM, Bermat JL, O'Donnel JF: Lymphoma initially appearing with chin numbness. *Arch Neurol* 37:327, 1980.

26. Gilbert RW, Kim JH, Posner JB: Epidural spinal cord compression from metastatic tumor: Diagnosis and treatment. *Ann Neurol* 3:40, 1978.

27. Black P: Spinal metastasis: Current status and recommended guidelines for management. *Neurosurgery* 5:726, 1979.

28. Greenberg HS, Kim JH, Posner JB: Epidural spinal cord compression from metastatic tumor: Results with a new treatment protocol. *Ann Neurol* 8:361, 1980.

29. Olson ME, Chernik NL, Posner JB: Infiltration of the leptomeninges by systemic cancer: A clinical and pathologic study. *Arch Neurol* 30:122, 1976.

30. Glass JP, Melamed M, Chernik NL, Posner JB: Malignant cells in cerebrospinal fluid (CSF): The meaning of a positive CSF cytology. *Neurology* 29:1369, 1979.

31. Little JR, Dale AJD, Okazaki H: Meningeal carcinomatosis: Clinical manifestations. *Arch Neurol* 30:138, 1974.

32. Theodore WH, Gendelman S: Meningeal carcinomatosis. *Arch Neurol* 38:696, 1981.

33. Ascherl GF, Hilal SK, Brisman R: Computed tomography of disseminated meningeal and ependymal malignant neoplasms. *Neurology* 31:567, 1981.

34. Glass JP, Shapiro WR, Posner JB: Treatment of leptomeningeal metastases. *Neurology* 28:350, 1978.

35. Hasegawa H, Allen JC, Mehta BM, et al: Enhancement of CNS penetration of methotrexate by hyperosmolar intracarotid mannitol or carcinomatosis meningitis. *Neurology* 29:1280, 1979.

36. Kori SH, Foley KM, Posner JB: Brachial plexus lesions in patients with cancer: 100 cases. *Neurology* 31:45, 1981.

37. Guberman A, Rosenbaum H, Braciale T, Schlaepfer WW: Human neurolymphomatosis. *J Neurol Sci* 36:1, 1978.

38. Portlock CS: Lymphomatous involvement of the central nervous system, in Whitehouse JMA, Kay HEM (eds): *CNS Complications of Malignant Disease.* Baltimore, University Park Press, 1979, p 113.

39. Davies-Jones GAB, Preston FE, Timperley WR: Neurological complications, in *Clinical Haematology.* Oxford, Blackwell Scientific Publications, 1980, p 36.

40. Dawson DM, Rosenthal DS, Moloney WC: Neurological complications of acute leukemia in adults: Changing rate. *Ann Intern Med* 79:541, 1973.

41. Ballard JD, Towfighi J, Brennan RW, et al: Neurologic complications of acute myelomonoblastic leukemia of four year's duration. *Neurology* 28:174, 1978.

42. Bunn PA, Schein PS, Banks PM, DeVita VT: Central nervous system complications in patients with diffuse histiocytic and undifferentiated lymphoma: Leukemia revisited. *Blood* 47:3, 1976.

43. Currie S, Henson RA: Neurological syndromes in the reticuloses. *Brain* 94:307, 1971.

44. Posner JB: Neurological complications of systemic cancer. *Med Clin North Am* 55:625, 1971.

45. Chernik NL, Armstrong D, Posner JB: Central nervous system infections in patients with cancer. *Medicine* 52:563, 1973.

46. Collins RC, Al-Mondhiry H, Chernik NL, Posner JB: Neurologic manifestations of intravascular coagulation in patients with cancer: A clinicopathologic analysis of 12 cases. *Neurology* 25:795, 1975.

47. Reagan TJ, Okazaki H: The thrombotic syndrome associated with carcinoma: A clinical and neuropathologic study. *Arch Neurol* 31:390, 1974.

48. Chernik NL, Loewenson RB, Posner JB, Resch JA: Cerebral atherosclerosis and stroke in cancer patients. *Neurology* 28:350, 1978.

49. Sigsbee B, Deck MDF, Posner JB, Resch JA: Nonmetastatic superior sagittal sinus thrombosis complicating systemic cancer. *Neurology* 29:139, 1979.

50. Kooiker JC, Maclean JM, Sumi S: Cerebral embolism, marantic endocarditis, and cancer. *Arch Neurol* 33:260, 1976.

51. Azzarelli B, Itani A-L, Catanzaro PT: Cerebral phlebothrombosis: A complication of lymphoma. *Arch Neurol* 37:126, 1980.

52. Weiss HD, Walker MD, Wiernik PH: Neurotoxicity of commonly used antineoplastic agents. *New Engl J Med* 75:127, 1974.

53. Allen JC: The effects of cancer therapy on the nervous system. *J Pediatr* 93:903, 1978.

54. Kramer S, Lee KF: Complications of radiation therapy: The central nervous system. *Semin Roentgenol* 9:75, 1974.

55. Godwin-Austen RB, Howell DA, Worthington B: Observations on radiation myelopathy. *Brain* 98:557, 1975.

56. Sundaresan N, Gutierrez FA, Larsen MB: Radiation myelopathy in children. *Ann Neurol* 4:47, 1978.

57. Ashenhurst EM, Quartey GRC, Starreveld A: Lumbosacral radiculopathy induced by radiation. *Can J Neurol Sci* 4:259, 1977.

58. Rottenberg DA, Horten B, Kim JH, Posner JB: Progressive white matter destruction following irradiation of an extracranial neoplasm. *Ann Neurol* 8:76, 1980.

59. Rottenberg DA, Chernik NL, Deck MDF, Ellis F, Posner JB: Cerebral necrosis following radiotherapy of extracranial neoplasms. *Ann Neurol* 1:339, 1977.

60. Berger PS, Bataini JP: Radiation-induced cranial nerve palsy. *Cancer* 40:152, 1977.

61. Averback P: Mixed intracranial sarcomas: Rare forms and a new association with previous radiation therapy. *Ann Neurol* 4:229, 1978.

62. Foley KM, Woodruff JM, Ellis FT, Posner JB: Radiation-induced malignant and atypical peripheral nerve tumors. *Ann Neurol* 7:311, 1980.

63. Nardelli E, Fiaschi A, Ferrari G: Delayed cerebrovascular consequences of radiation to the neck: A clinico-pathological study of a case. *Arch Neurol* 35:538, 1978.

64. Painter MJ, Chutorian AM, Hilal S: Cerebrovasculopathy following irradiation in childhood. *Neurology* 25:189, 1975.

65. Silverberg GD, Britt RH, Goffinet DR: Radiation-induced carotid artery disease. *Cancer* 41:130, 1978.

66. Sadowsky CH, Sachs E, Ochoa J: Postradiation motor neuron syndrome. *Arch Neurol* 33:786, 1976.

67. Stoll BA, Andrews JT: Radiation-induced peripheral neuropathy. *Br Med J* 1:834, 1966.

68. Brain WR, Henson RA: Neurological syndromes associated with carcinoma: The carcinomatous neuromyopathies. *Lancet* 2:971, 1958.

69. Croft PB, Wilkinson M: The incidence of carcinomatous neuromyopathy in patients with various types of carcinoma. *Brain* 88:427, 1965.

70. Henson RA, Urich H: Remote effects of malignant disease: Certain intracranial disorders, in Vinken PJ, Bruyn GG (eds): *Handbook of Clinical Neurology*, vol 38. Amsterdam, North Holland Publishing Company, 1979, p 625.

71. Shapiro WR: Remote effects of neoplasm on the central nervous system: Encephalopathy. *Adv Neurol* 15:101, 1976.

72. Corsellis JAN, Goldberg GJ, Norton AR: "Limbic encephalitis" and its association with carcinoma. *Brain* 91:481, 1968.

73. Henson RA, Hoffman HL, Urich H: Encephalomyelitis with carcinoma. *Brain* 88:449, 1965.

74. Dorfman LJ, Forno LS: Paraneoplastic encephalomyelitis. *Acta Neurol Scand* 48:556, 1972.

75. De Reuck JL, Sieben GJ, Sieben-Praet MR: Wernicke's encephalopathy in patients with tumors of the lymphoid-hemopoietic systems. *Arch Neurol* 37:388, 1980.

76. Halperin JJ, Richardson EP, Ellis J, et al: Paraneoplastic encephalomyelitis and neuropathy. *Arch Neurol* 38:773, 1981.

77. Messert B, Orrison WW, Hawkins MJ, Quaglieri CE: Central pontine myelinolysis. Considerations on etiology, diagnosis, and treatment. *Neurology* 29:147, 1979.

78. Tomlinson BK, Pierides AM, Bradley WG: Central pontine myelinolysis. *Q J Med* 45:374, 1976.

79. Reddy RV, Vakii ST: Midbrain encephalitis as a remote effect of a malignant neoplasm. *Arch Neurol* 38:781, 1981.

80. McGill T: Carcinomatous encephalomyelitis with auditory and vestibular manifestations. *Ann Otol* 85:120, 1976.

81. Brain WR, Wilkinson M: Subacute cerebellar degeneration associated with neoplasms. *Brain* 88:465, 1965.

82. Brazis PW, Biller J, Fine M, et al: Cerebellar degeneration with Hodgkin's disease: Computed tomographic correlation and literature review. *Arch Neurol* 38:253, 1981.

83. Croft PB, Wilkinson M: The course and prognosis in some types of carcinomatous neuromyopathy. *Brain* 92:1, 1969.

84. Kinsbourne M: Myoclonic encephalopathy of infants. *J Neurol Neurosurg Psychiatry* 25:271, 1962.

85. Brandt S, Carlsen N, Glenting P, Helwea-Larsen J: Encephalopathia myoclonica infantilis (Kinsbourne) and neuroblastoma in children: A report of three cases. *Dev Med Child Neurol* 16:286, 1974.

86. Bellur SH: Opsoclonus: Its clinical value. *Neurology* 25:502, 1975.

87. Nausieda PA, Tanner CM, Weiner WJ: Opsolenic cerebellopathy: A paraneoplastic syndrome responsive to thiamine. *Arch Neurol* 38:780, 1981.

88. Mancall EL, Rosales RK: Necrotizing myelopathy associated with visceral carcinoma. *Brain* 87:639, 1965.

89. Sieben GM, DeReuck JL, DeBruyne JC, Vander Eecken HM: Subacute necrotic myelopathy: Its appearance eight years after cure of breast carcinoma. *Arch Neurol* 38:775, 1981.

90. Lester EP, Feld E, Kinzie JJ, Wollmann R: Necrotizing myelopathy complicating Hodgkin's disease. *Arch Neurol* 36:583, 1979.

91. Brain WR, Croft PB, Wilkinson M: Motor neuron disease as a manifestation of neoplasm. *Brain* 88:479, 1965.

92. Buchanan DS, Malamud N: Motor neuron disease with renal cell carcinoma and postoperative neurologic remission: A clinicopathologic report. *Neurology* 23:891, 1973.

93. Schold SC, Choe ES, Somasundaram M, Posner JB: Subacute motor neuropathy: A remote effect of lymphoma. *Ann Neurol* 5:271, 1979.

94. Paul T, Katiyar BC, Misra S, Pant GC: Carcinomatous neuromuscular syndromes: A clinical and quantitative electrophysiological study. *Brain* 101:53, 1978.

95. Croft PB, Urich H, Wilkinson M: Peripheral neuropathy of sensorimotor type associated with malignant disease. *Brain* 90:31, 1967.

96. Dyck PJ, Kiely JM: Differential diagnosis of neuropathy associated with cancer. *Adv Neurol* 15:149, 1976.

97. Read D, Warlow C: Peripheral neuropathy and solitary plasmacytoma. *J Neurol Neurosurg Psychiatry* 41:177, 1978.

98. Hildebrand J, Coers C: The neuromuscular function in patients with malignant tumors: Electromyographic and histiological study. *Brain* 90:67, 1967.

99. Trojaborg W, Frantzen E, Andersen I: Peripheral neuropathy and myopathy associated with carcinoma of the lung. *Brain* 92:71, 1969.

100. Barron SA, Heffner RR: Weakness in malignancy: Evidence for a remote effect of tumor on distal axons. *Ann Neurol* 4:268, 1978.

101. Johnson PC, Rolak LA, Hamilton RH, Laguna JF: Paraneoplastic vasculitis of nerve: A remote effect of cancer. *Ann Neurol* 5:437, 1979.

102. Denny-Brown DE: Primary sensory neuropathy with muscular changes associated with cancer. *J Neurol Neurosurg Psychiatry* 11:73, 1948.

103. Horwich MS, Cho L, Porro RJ, Posner JB: Subacute sensory neuropathy: A remote effect of carcinoma. *Ann Neurol* 2:7, 1977.

104. Kaufman MD, Hopkins LC, Hurwitz BJ: Progressive sensory neuropathy in patients without carcinoma: A disorder with distinctive clinical and electrophysiological findings. *Ann Neurol* 9:237, 1981.

105. Peress NS, Su PC, Turner I: Combined myelopathy and radiculoneuropathy with malignant lymphoproliferative disease. *Arch Neurol* 36:311, 1979.

106. Patten JR: Remittent peripheral neuropathy and cerebellar degeneration complicating lymphosarcoma. *Neurology* 21:189, 1971.

107. Rubinstein MK: Mononeuritis in association with malignancy. *Bull Los Angeles Neurol Soc* 31:157, 1966.

108. Goldman AJ, Herrmann C, Keesey JC, et al: Myasthenia gravis and invasive thymoma: A 20 year experience. *Neurology* 25:1021, 1975.

109. Kennedy WR, Jimenez-Pabon E: The myasthenic syndrome associated with small cell carcinoma of the lung (Eaton-Lambert syndrome). *Neurology* 18:757, 1968.

110. Lauritzen M, Smith T, Fischer-Hansen B, et al: Eaton-Lambert syndrome and malignant thymoma. *Neurology* 30:634, 1980.

111. Hawley RJ, Cohen MH, Salni N, Armbrust-Macher VW: The carcinomatous neuromyopathy of oat cell lung cancer. *Ann Neurol* 7:65, 1980.

112. Tervainen H, Larsen A: Some features of the neuromuscular complications of pulmonary carcinoma. *Ann Neurol* 2:495, 1977.

113. Barnes BE: Dermatomyositis and malignancy: A review of the literature. *Ann Intern Med* 84:68, 1976.

114. Rowland LP, Clark C, Olarte M: Therapy for dermatomyositis and polymyositis. *Adv Neurol* 17:63, 1977.

115. Brownell B, Hughes JT: Degeneration of muscle in association with carcinoma of the bronchus. *J Neurol Neurosurg Psychiatry* 38:363, 1975.

116. Humphrey JC: Myotonia associated with small cell carcinoma of the lung. *Arch Neurol* 33:375, 1976.

117. Engel WK, Askanas V: Remote effects of focal cancer on the neuromuscular system. *Adv Neurol* 15:119, 1976.

7
Cutaneous Manifestations of Malignant Disease

Andrew Rudolph and James Callen

A number of cutaneous signs can be associated with internal malignancy (1–9). These signs may be nonspecific—acquired dermatoses—or specific—malignant infiltration into the skin (metastatic disease). Occasionally, the first manifestation of an internal malignancy is the occurrence of skin lesions. Although these acquired skin lesions are not common, their recognition may be vital for the early diagnosis of internal malignancy.

A causal relationship between a skin disorder and internal malignancy may be suggested if the following criteria are met: (*1*) The conditions begin at the same time; (*2*) the conditions follow a parallel course; (*3*) a specific tumor occurs with the dermatosis; (*4*) the dermatosis is uncommon; and (*5*) the incidence of association is high.

A number of cutaneous signs, syndromes, or skin lesions that have been associated with internal malignancy follow; these are listed in alphabetical order.

ACANTHOSIS NIGRICANS

Acanthosis nigricans exists in two forms: that associated with internal malignancy and that occurring in a variety of situations unrelated to internal malignancy (10). The clinical picture in these two forms is identical except that in the type associated with internal malignancy other signs of the malignancy may be present. In addition to internal malignancy, acanthosis nigricans may be associated with endocrine disease, the most common being Cushing's syndrome; may be familial, associated with a positive family history; or may occur without history of malignancy, endocrinopathy, or a positive family history. The term applied to the latter is benign acanthosis nigricans. Pseudo-acanthosis nigricans indicates acanthosis nigricans occurring in obese people.

Acanthosis nigricans can occur in any age group; however, it is more frequently associated with internal malignancy in persons over the age of 30 (11). Benign acanthosis nigricans is more common in women; however, in malignant acanthosis the sexes are equally affected. Acanthosis nigricans associated with internal malignancy is uncommon; its exact incidence is unknown. The cause of malignant acanthosis nigricans is unknown, but most authors believe the tumor secretes a substance that is responsible for the skin changes (12–15). This theory is supported by the disappearance of acanthosis nigricans with tumor treatment and reappearance with tumor regrowth or metastases (16).

The characteristic feature of acanthosis nigricans is the presence of hyperpigmented velvety thickening of the skin folds, especially at the nape and sides of the neck (Fig. 7-1), the axillae, and the groin. Any intertriginous surface may be involved, however, as well as such areas as the umbilicus, nipples, elbows, knees, thighs, and knuckles. Occasionally, the oral mucosa will have thickened papillomatous changes without hyperpigmentation. The palms and soles may show hyperkeratotic changes (17). Verrucous or papillary lesions may appear with the hyperpigmentation. Skin lesions of acanthosis nigricans are clinically identical whether internal malignancy, endocrinopathy, or obesity is present or not. No malignant changes are present in the skin lesions. Itching may occur but is usually not a prominent symptom. Hyperpigmentation of the skin in the intertriginous areas is often the first change noted. The hyperpigmentation varies from brown to black and represents melanin deposition in the skin. As the acanthosis nigricans becomes more prominent, velvety, verrucous, or papillomatous lesions may develop. Occasionally, acanthosis nigricans may become generalized (18).

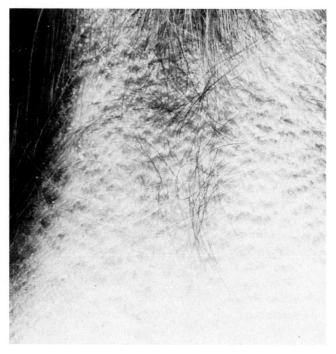

Figure 7-1. Acanthosis nigricans: posterior neck.

Acanthosis nigricans may develop during childhood, at puberty, or later in life. It may precede the development of a malignancy; however, it may also follow the appearance of the malignancy or both may develop simultaneously. Curth et al. (11) found that in 61% of all cases the dermatoses and malignancy appeared concomitantly, in 17% the dermatoses preceded tumor by up to 16 years, and in 22% the dermatoses followed the tumor by up to $4\frac{1}{2}$ years. Other clinical features of internal malignancy, for example, weight loss, cachexia, or specific symptoms related to the tumor, may be associated with malignant acanthosis nigricans. Patients with malignant acanthosis nigricans are rarely obese. Cancers associated with acanthosis nigricans have been reported to occur in many sites. Curth et al. (11) observed that intra-abdominal neoplasia was present in 91% of the patients examined. In addition, these authors suggest that nearly all the cancers are adenocarcinomas. Brown and Winkelmann (19) found that 13 of 17 patients had adenocarcinomas, one had squamous cell carcinoma of the cervix, and three had lymphoma. Malignancies in sites outside the abdomen, such as testicle, lung, and hypopharynx, have also been reported.

The appearance of acanthosis nigricans and internal malignancy appears to be an ominous sign. The tumors associated with acanthosis nigricans are highly malignant. In the series of Brown and Winkelmann (19) death occurred in all but two patients in less than one year. Exceptions to this, however, have been noted in the recent literature, particularly when tumor resection was possible (16).

In summary, acanthosis nigricans is a highly characteristic dermatosis that can be diagnosed clinically by the presence of hyperpigmented velvety skin involving the intertriginous areas. It appears to be a significant marker of internal malignancy in adults who are not obese. The malignancies are often, but not always, abdominal, and although many are adenocarcinomas, squamous carcinomas and lymphomas have also been reported. The dermatosis may be progressive and often suggests a rapid and fatal outcome.

ACQUIRED ICHTHYOSIS

Ichthyosis is a scaly dermatosis that is usually inherited and usually appears at birth or early in life. Occasionally, the disease first develops during adulthood, and then the term *acquired ichthyosis* is used. Acquired ichthyosis has a clinical appearance similar to that of ichthyosis vulgaris (Fig. 7-2). The scales usually are rhomboidal and often have free edges. The extremities are most commonly involved. Similar lesions may occur in hypothyroidism or severe xerotic eczema, and these conditions must be carefully ruled out. The appearance of acquired ichthyosis has been associated with concomitant internal malignancy, usually a lymphomatous process such as Hodgkin's disease (20,21). However, acquired ichthyosis is rarely, if ever, the initial manifestation of the malignancy, and its course may not follow that of the malignancy. While Hodgkin's disease is the usual type of malignancy associated with acquired ichthyosis, solid tumors have been reported to occur with acquired ichthyosis (22,23).

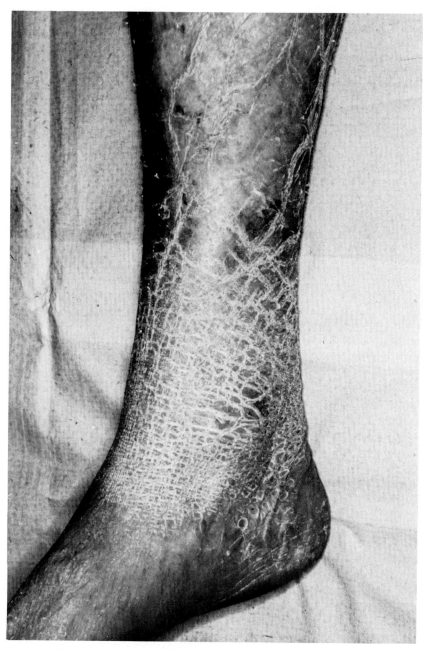

Figure 7-2. Acquired ichthyosis in a patient with lymphoma.

BOWEN'S DISEASE

Bowen's disease is a form of squamous cell carcinoma of the skin, characterized by epidermal dysplasia (24). Invasion of the dermis may occur late in the course of the disease. Sun exposure undoubtedly plays a role in the development of many lesions of Bowen's disease. Bowen's disease may also be related to arsenic ingestion.

Clinically, Bowen's disease has an appearance similar to that of eczema. The lesion is usually flat but may become hyperkeratotic or verrucose (warty). Nodular or crusted areas may also develop within the lesions. The borders of the lesion are often undulating or irregular (Fig. 7-3). Bowen's disease should be suspected in any patient with a nonhealing patch of eczema or psoriasiform dermatitis, particularly if nodularity, crusting, or erosion are present. Bowen's disease may occur on any area of the body, but in ⅔ of the cases exposed skin surfaces are involved.

The relationship between Bowen's disease and internal malignancy is surrounded by controversy. In 1959 Graham and Helwig (25) first reported the occurrence of internal malignancy with Bowen's disease. In 35 patients with the disease, 28 (80%) had visceral malignancy. Thirty-three patients with Bowen's disease, five of whom had internal malignancy, were described in 1969 by Epstein (26). Subsequent reports have suggested the incidence of internal malignancy occurring with Bowen's disease to be between 15 and 30% (27–30). Patients with Bowen's disease occurring on an unexposed area may have an increased incidence of internal malignancy, whereas patients with lesions on exposed surfaces may have a lesser incidence of internal malignancy (27). However, Callen and

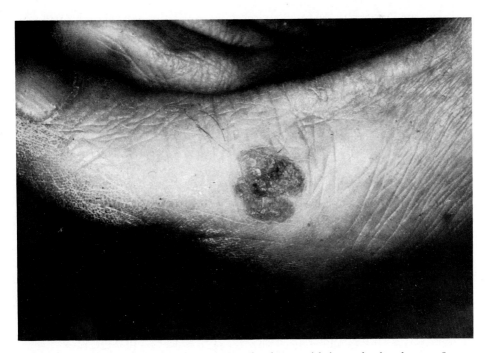

Figure 7-3. Bowen's disease: hyperkeratotic plaque with irregular borders on foot.

Headington were unable to confirm this predilection (31). In contrast, Anderson et al. (32) reported no significant difference in the incidence of internal malignancy with Bowen's disease compared to a matched group in the general population.

The type of the internal malignancies seen with Bowen's disease varies from study to study. No one site or type of lesion appears to predominate. While patients with Bowen's disease may have a disposition to internal malignancy, this disposition may not be manifest until many years after appearance of the skin lesions. Thus, extensive evaluation for malignancy beyond a complete history, physical examination, and routine laboratory testing is probably not warranted in patients with Bowen's disease.

BULLOUS DERMATOSES

The bullous dermatoses have been associated with internal malignancy. Controversy continues regarding the relationship of bullous pemphigoid, a chronic subepidermal bullous dermatosis (Fig. 7-4), and internal malignancy. A well-controlled study at Mayo Clinic has shown that the occurrence of malignancy is perhaps no more than an age-related coincidence (33). However, Hodge et al. (34) and others (35) have suggested that malignancy was more common in bullous pemphigoid patients with negative immunofluorescence.

Pemphigus, a group of chronic bullous diseases characterized by intraepidermal blister formation, has been associated with malignancy, particularly thymoma (36,37). Myasthenia gravis often occurs in these patients also (38). The relation of pemphigus to other malignancies seems coincidental (39).

Dermatitis herpetiformis is an intensely pruritic subepidermal blistering disease in which small, tense vesicles, symmetrically grouped in clusters, are distributed over the extensor surfaces of the body (Fig. 7-5). Dermatitis herpetiformis may be more frequently associated with intestinal lymphoma than expected (40). This may relate to the presence of gluten sensitive enteropathy in these patients, rather than being a function of the cutaneous disease (3). This association, however, requires further documentation.

CARCINOID SYNDROME

Carcinoid syndrome may include such features as episodic facial flushing, diarrhea or other gastrointestinal complaints, respiratory distress, valvular heart disease, and a carcinoid tumor, usually with metastases (41). The flushing associated with carcinoid syndrome usually begins with acute, bright red erythema of the cheeks, neck, and upper chest. A dusky, cyanotic hue may follow the erythema. Telangiectasias eventually develop in the flushed area, and a permanent cyanotic hue may develop after years of flushing, producing a plethoric appearance. Skin lesions resembling pellegra may occur (41). Carcinoids may be found in the appendix and small intestine. Bronchial adenomas of the carcinoid type can also produce the syndrome (42); however, the duration of flushing in these patients may last hours rather than the usual 10 to 30 minutes and may be associated with fever, sweating, lacrimation, anxiety, and disorientation.

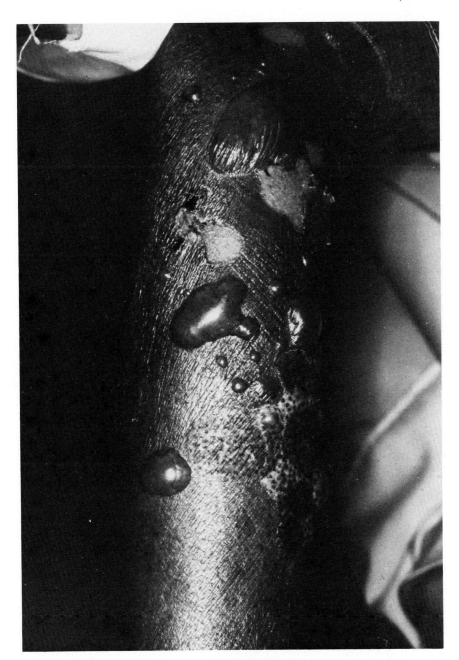

Figure 7-4. Bullous pemphigoid: tense bullae on a noninflammatory base.

DERMATOMYOSITIS

Dermatomyositis is the term used for the presence of characteristic cutaneous lesions with inflammatory muscle disease characterized by proximal, symmetric, and progressive weakness. Dermatomyositis may occur at any age, but most cases occur in adults between the ages of 30 and 60. Dermatomyositis appears to be mediated through immunologic mechanisms, but the exact etiologic factors are

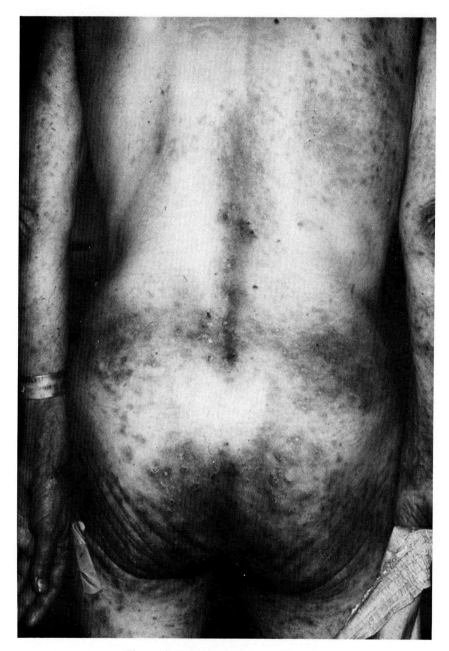

Figure 7-5. Dermatitis herpetiformis.

unknown. Neoplasms may be associated with dermatomyositis, but the exact pathogenesis of this relationship is also not fully understood.

Characteristic cutaneous features of dermatomyositis are heliotrope rash and Gottron's papules (Fig. 7-6) (43,44). The heliotrope rash consists of an edematous, dusky, violaceous to erythematous discoloration of the eyelids. Gottron's papules are slightly elevated, erythematous to violaceous papules that occur most

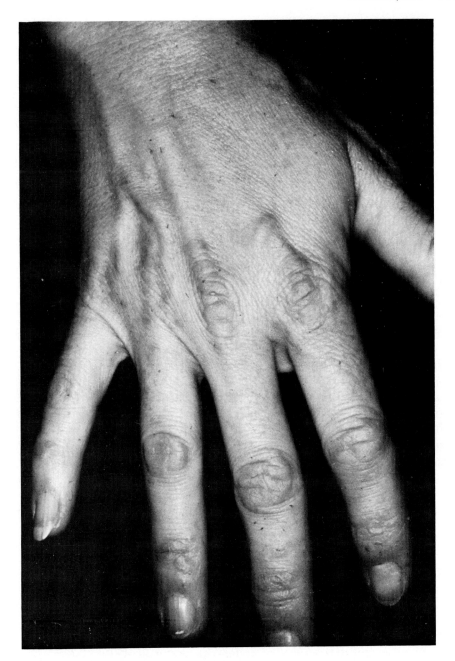

Figure 7-6. Gottron's papules of dermatomyositis.

commonly over the knuckles. However, they may also be present over the elbows, knees, and ankles. Other cutaneous findings of dermatomyositis include photosensitivity, malar erythema, periungual telangiectasias, and poikiloderma (45). Poikiloderma is the term applied to the combination of hypo- and hyperpigmentation, telangiectasia, and mild atrophy of the skin.

Reports of the association of dermatomyositis and malignancy are common

(43,46–50), and the incidence of malignancy in adults with dermatomyositis is significant, approaching 25%. However, when malignancy occurs it may precede, occur with, or follow the onset of dermatomyositis. Carcinoma may involve almost any organ, but the genitourinary tract, colon, breast, and lungs are among the most common sites. While it is obligatory to look for cancer in adults with dermatomyositis, the value of an extensive search for malignancy in an otherwise asymptomatic patient with dermatomyositis is controversial. A recent review of the literature by Callen has indicated that in evaluation of a "routine" patient with dermatomyositis, a complete history, physical examination, and routine laboratory tests, including a chest x-ray examination, should be sufficient (43,51). In patients with atypical symptoms, in patients who have failed to respond to conventional therapy, or in patients with a history of previous malignancy, a more extensive evaluation should be conducted.

ERYTHEMA GYRATUM REPENS AND ERYTHEMA ANNULARE CENTRIFUGUM

Erythema gyratum repens is a bizarre cutaneous eruption consisting of characteristic, persistent, erythematous lesions that form gyrate, serpiginous bands (Fig. 7-7). These bands of erythema have a slightly raised border with a fine collarette of scale. They migrate very slowly across the skin surface producing a pattern resembling "grains in wood." Pruritus is common and may be severe.

Erythema gyratum repens has been associated with internal malignancy in almost all cases (52–56), but no one cell type has been consistently reported. The eruption may precede, occur concurrently, or follow the appearance of the malignancy. Successful treatment of the malignancy has led to resolution of the eruption in many reported cases; recurrence of the tumor can cause reappearance of the eruption. The pathogenesis of erythema gyratum repens is not known, although the finding of granular deposits of IgG in the lesions has suggested that the dermatosis is immunologically mediated. Erythema gyratum repens appears to have a significant association with internal malignancy, and its presence in a patient should trigger an extensive search for an underlying neoplasm.

Lesions of erythema annulare centrifugum begin as papules that enlarge peripherally to form erythematous annular lesions; these may coalesce to form polygyrate lesions (Fig. 7-8). Characteristically, the advancing borders are palpable, and scaling is present along their inner edges.

Erythema annulare centrifugum appears to be a hypersensitivity phenomenon that may be due to a variety of causes, including neoplasia. Since erythema annulare centrifugum has only occasionally been associated with internal malignancy (57–59), extensive search for malignant tumor does not seem warranted in patients with this condition.

EXFOLIATIVE DERMATITIS

In exfoliative dermatitis, the skin is erythematous and scaly. Edema, weeping, and desquamation of the skin may occur. Pruritus is usually pronounced. Ex-

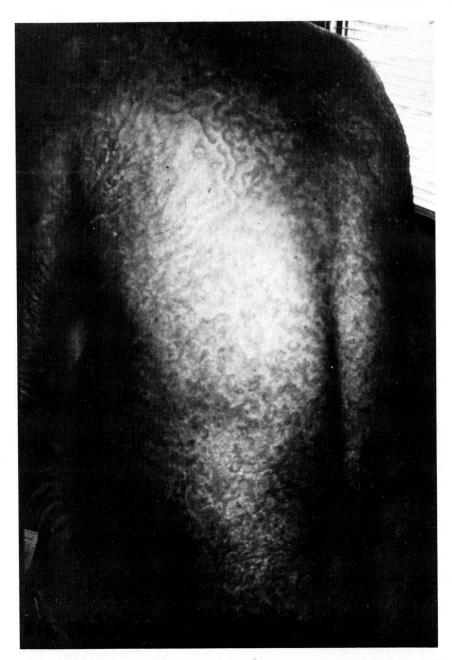

Figure 7-7. Erythema gyratum repens in a patient with squamous cell carcinoma of the lung.

coriation and lichenification of the skin may be present. Scalp and body hair may be lost. Fever, generalized lymphadenopathy, and hepatosplenomegaly may also be present. Exfoliative dermatitis is a cutaneous reaction pattern that may be the manifestation of a number of diseases. Common causes of exfoliative dermatitis are a preexisting cutaneous disease or a drug eruption. However,

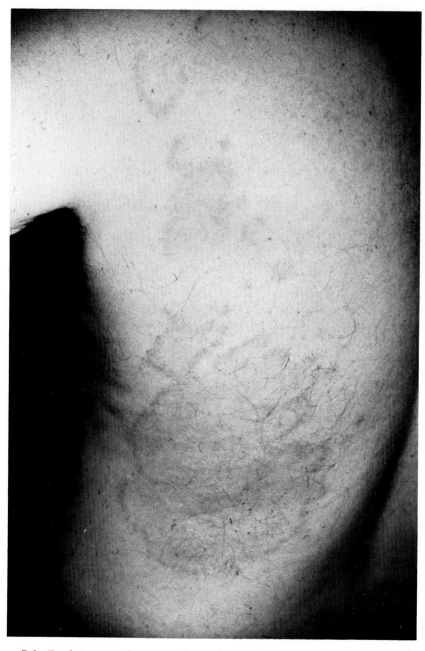

Figure 7-8. Erythema annulare centrifugum in a patient occurring following irradiation of a malignant thymoma.

malignancies such as lymphoma, leukemia, carcinoma, adenocarcinoma, and mycosis fungoides may also be causes. Exfoliative dermatitis may precede or develop at the time of the appearance of the leukemia, lymphoma, or carcinoma.

GARDNER'S SYNDROME

In Gardner's syndrome a variety of cutaneous lesions and bony abnormalities are associated with precancerous adenomatous polyps of the colon and rectum (60,61). The potential for malignant change of these polyps approaches 100% if the patient lives long enough. According to one review, 53% of patients over 20 who had the syndrome also had carcinoma of the colon (62). Other gastro-intestinal carcinomas have also been reported in patients with Gardner's syndrome (63).

The skin lesions preceding the development of the colonic polyps are most commonly epidermoid cysts of the face and scalp. Fibromas, desmoid tumors, and fibrosarcomas may also develop (62). Osteomas are the most common bone lesions. The diagnosis of this syndrome obligates the patient to colectomy and close follow-up.

GLUCAGONOMA SYNDROME (NECROLYTIC MIGRATORY ERYTHEMA)

The glucagonoma syndrome comprises a specific group of symptoms that includes a characteristic rash associated with a glucagon-secreting tumor of the pancreas (64). Numerous recent case reports have drawn attention to this important marker of internal malignancy (64–77). Symptoms usually develop in middle age. Signs of the syndrome include anorexia, weakness, and weight loss. A normocytic, normochromic anemia suggestive of chronic disease may be present, and the erythrocyte sedimentation rate often is elevated. Glucose intolerance, biochemically and occasionally clinically, is present in nearly all patients with glucagon-secreting tumors. The cutaneous eruption (necrolytic migratory erythema) is helpful in diagnosing the syndrome.

Initial skin lesions of glucagonoma are often patches of erythema that are angular, annular, or irregular in outline. Circinate and polycyclic lesions may develop. Flaccid vesicles and bullae are often present within the erythematous patches; these quickly break to leave eroded, crusted surfaces. The active margins of the lesions may demonstrate a collarette of scale, vesicles, or bullae. These changes are due to edema and epidermal cell death that results in cleavage of the upper third of the epidermis. Central healing with hyperpigmentation may occur. Characteristically, the lesions of necrolytic migratory erythema occur centrally on the body with the perineum, buttocks, groin, and lower abdomen most commonly affected, but the proximal extremities and perioral areas of the face may also be involved. An angular cheilitis, vaginitis, and perianal dermatitis may be present. Painful glossitis is a major feature of the syndrome, with the tongue appearing red, shiny, and smooth. The presence of these cutaneous lesions and systemic symptoms should suggest the existence of a glucagon-secreting tumor.

Although the tumor may occur in any region of the pancreas, the tail is the most common site. In about half of the cases, metastatic disease, usually localized to the liver, is present. However, there have been reports of lymph node involvement and the occurrence of bony metastases. Elevated glucagon levels are helpful in establishing a diagnosis and dictate a search for the tumor.

Skin lesions and systemic symptoms usually are reversed with surgical removal of the tumor. In addition chemotherapy may also cause resolution of the dermatitis (77).

HERPES ZOSTER

Herpes zoster is an acute cutaneous eruption caused by a recurrence of herpesvirus varicellae infection. Clinically, the eruption consists of grouped, edematous papules or vesicles on an erythematous base, arranged in a bandlike distribution following one of the dermatomes (Fig. 7-9). At times, a generalized eruption may occur, usually in patients with underlying disorders known to alter the immune state (78). In these patients, pneumonitis can occur and may be fatal. Pain of variable severity may precede the eruption, occur coincidentally with the eruption, or follow the eruption. The majority of patients with herpes zoster are otherwise healthy. However, herpes zoster may be secondary to or precipitated by a number of conditions, including malignancy. In this regard, herpes zoster frequently complicates Hodgkin's disease, lymphosarcoma, and leukemia. Thus, because there is more than a chance association between herpes zoster and malignant disease, particularly the lymphomas and leukemias, it would be judicious to consider an underlying lymphoma or leukemia in adults with herpes zoster, especially if it is disseminated.

HYPERTRICHOSIS LANUGINOSA ACQUISITA (MALIGNANT DOWN)

Hypertrichosis lanuginosa is a rare entity characterized by excessive generalized growth of lanugo hair (Fig. 7-10) (79). Lanugo hair refers to fine, soft hair in contrast to coarse, terminal hair. Hypertrichosis lanuginosa usually is inherited as a simple dominant trait, occurring at birth or during the first year of life. In all patients, other causes of languo hair, such as endocrinopathies, mucopolysaccharidosis, and porphyria cutanea tarda, should be ruled out. Patients with the malignant down usually have an accompanying glossitis. In cases acquired late in life, the occurrence of an internal malignancy is almost certain (80–82). Acquired hypertrichosis lanuginosa has antedated the appearance of tumor in most reported cases and, therefore, provides a skin sign that should not be disregarded. The type of malignancy is not uniform (81–84). Bladder carcinoma, mammary carcinoma, and carcinoma of the lung have been reported. When malignancy is not found, frequent reevaluation of these patients is warranted (81, 84).

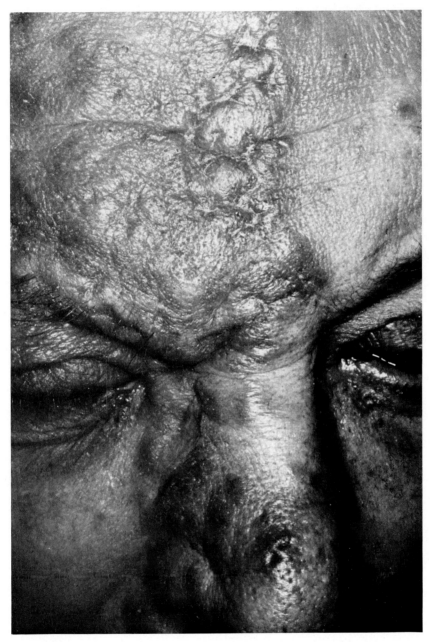

Figure 7-9. Herpes zoster occurring in a patient with chronic lymphocytic leukemia (ophthalmic branch of trigeminal nerve).

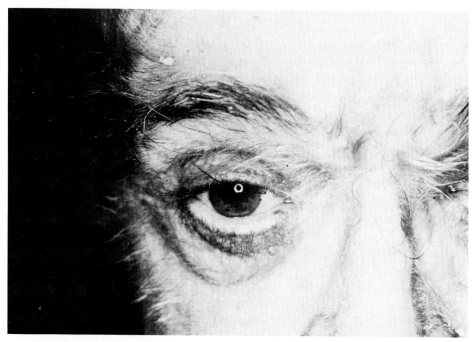

Figure 7-10. Hypertrichosis lanuginosa in a patient with squamous cell carcinoma of the lung.

MIGRATORY THROMBOPHLEBITIS (TROUSSEAU'S SYNDROME)

While superficial thrombophlebitis is a common medical problem, that which cannot be readily explained by ordinary causes may be a manifestation of cancer. Migratory thrombophlebitis, or Trousseau's syndrome, is frequently associated with pancreatic carcinoma; it reportedly can occur with other malignancies as well (85). The migratory recurrent thrombophlebitis is believed to be caused by chronic low-grade disseminated intravascular coagulopathy. The veins of the neck, chest, abdomen, pelvis, and lower extremities may be involved; different areas may be involved sequentially or simultaneously. The veins appear as palpable, tender cords.

MULTICENTRIC RETICULOHISTIOCYTOSIS

Multicentric reticulohistiocytosis is a rare disorder characterized by polyarthritis and nodular skin lesions (86). The skin lesions are small, flesh-colored to purplish brown nodules appearing on the scalp, ears, face, extremities, trunk, and mucous membranes. Arthritis involving the joints of the extremities occurs in more than 50% of patients with this disorder. The arthritis may be destructive and mutilating, resulting in severe deformities of the fingers. Catterall and White (87) in a review of the literature found that 27% of reported cases were associated with internal malignancy. In all but one case the malignant lesion was a carcinoma (87). Thus, patients with multicentric reticulohistiocytosis should be carefully evaluated for internal malignancy.

MULTIPLE HAMARTOMA SYNDROME (COWDEN'S DISEASE)

The multiple hamartoma syndrome (Cowden's disease) has been associated with internal malignancy, particularly of the thyroid and breast (88–93). In addition, cancers of the lung and colon have also been reported. Cowden's disease is inherited as an autosomal dominant trait with varible expressivity (88). A number of cutaneous lesions are found, including warty, keratotic papules of the dorsa of the hands and flat-topped (lichenoid) papules of the ear, neck, and central portion of the face (Fig. 7-11). These papular lesions also are present on the mucous membranes involving the gingiva and palate; they may coalesce, forming a cobblestone appearance. Punctate keratoses of the hands and feet may also be present. Patients and family members with Cowden's disease should be carefully and frequently evaluated for malignancy.

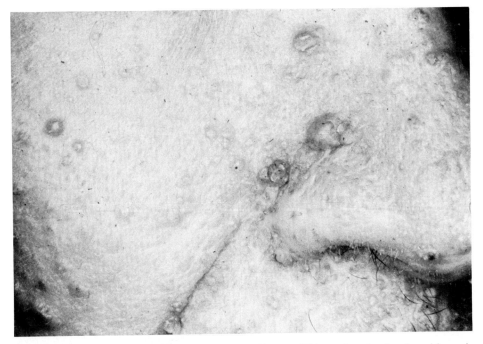

Figure 7-11. Trichofolliculomas in Cowden's disease. This patient had a thyroid carcinoma as well as bilateral breast carcinomas.

NEUROFIBROMATOSIS

Neurofibromatosis is a familial disorder consisting of cutaneous neurofibromas, cutaneous pigmentary changes, tumors of the peripheral nerves and the central nervous system, and bony abnormalities. Cutaneous lesions of neurofibromatosis include several types of tumors such as superficial, fusiform, and plexiform neurofibromas. Axillary freckling (small pigmented macules in the axillae) may occur (94). Café-au-lait spots (yellowish to brown macules) varying in size and configuration usually occur on nonexposed areas of the skin. The presence of six or more café-au-lait spots larger than 1.5 cm in diameter is presumptive evidence of the disease (95). Malignant transformation of the neurofibromas to neurosarcomas may occur (96). An increased incidence of melanoma, thyroid carcinoma, and breast cancer has also been reported in patients with neurofibromatosis. Neurofibromatosis has also been associated with leukemia, especially in children (97).

PAGET'S DISEASE

Paget's disease represents involvement of the epidermis with adenocarcinomatous cells. The lesions may occur on the breasts (mammary Paget's) or in the anogenital area, lower abdominal wall, upper thighs, or axilla (extramammary Paget's disease). Clinically, Paget's disease has an eczematous appearance (Fig. 7-12). The lesion is often erythematous and may show crusting or weeping. Its

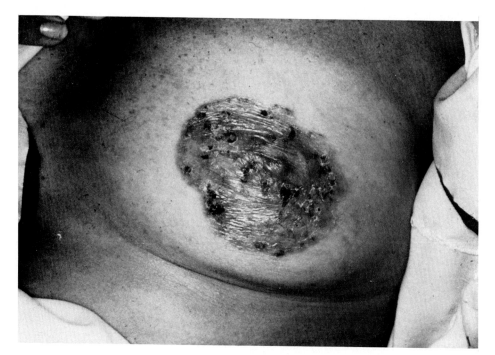

Figure 7-12. Paget's disease on breast with underlying ductal adenocarcinoma.

border is often sharply marginated. Paget's disease of the breasts is typically unilateral, involving the nipple or areola or both. Itching, burning, or tenderness of the lesion may occur. Extramammary Paget's disease usually appears as infiltrated whitish plaques that are occasionally eczematoid, crusting, scaling, papillomatous, or ulcerated. The disease usually appears in persons over age 50, with women being more commonly affected than men. Paget's disease of the breast and extramammary locations are identical histologically (98,99). The epidermis contains numerous large, round cells with clear cytoplasm (Paget's cells). The clear cytoplasm of these cells is due to accumulation of mucopolysaccharides.

Paget's disease of the breast should be suspected whenever a middle-aged or older patient has eczematoid involvement of the nipple and areola. Extramammary Paget's disease should be suspected in patients with chronic, sharply demarcated eczematoid plaques in the anogenital region. Mammary Paget's disease is indicative of an underlying ductal adenocarcinoma of the breast (99). Metastatic disease is found in the axillary nodes of $\frac{2}{3}$ of patients with a palpable mass in the breast and $\frac{1}{3}$ without a palpable mass (99). Extramammary Paget's disease is associated with underlying malignancy in more than 50% of cases (98,100). The malignancy may be of eccrine, apocrine, or adenoid origin. Metastases to both local lymphatics and wide-spread metastases have been reported at the time of diagnosis. The prognosis appears to be worse when adenocarcinoma is present (101).

PEUTZ-JEGHERS SYNDROME

Peutz-Jeghers syndrome is an inherited autosomal dominant disorder characterized by melanotic macules on the oral mucosa, lips, and oral skin combined with hamartomatous gastrointestinal polyps (102,103). Usually these hamartomatous polyps are benign in nature. However, multiple recent reports have described malignant transformation of the polyps (104–108). In addition colonic carcinoma may be more common in these patients (102). The skin lesions consist of melanotic asymptomatic macules and appear in childhood and adolescence. Usually patients appear for evaluation of abdominal pain or gastrointestinal hemorrhage, but any unusual symptoms or signs must be closely followed.

PUNCTATE PALMAR KERATOSES, TYLOSIS, AND ARSENICAL KERATOSES

Punctate keratoses are discrete, yellow to brown, hyperkeratotic papules occurring on the palmar surfaces of the hands and occasionally on the plantar surfaces of the feet (Fig. 7-13). The lesions often have a central plug that is lost, leaving a shallow depressed crater. Although numerous, the lesions do not coalesce and are usually asymptomatic. Clinical differentiation from arsenical keratoses or verruca is often impossible. The disorder may be familial, being inherited in a dominant manner, or acquired.

Acquired punctate keratoses have at times been associated with internal malignancy. Dobson et al. (109) reported that punctate keratoses were seen four

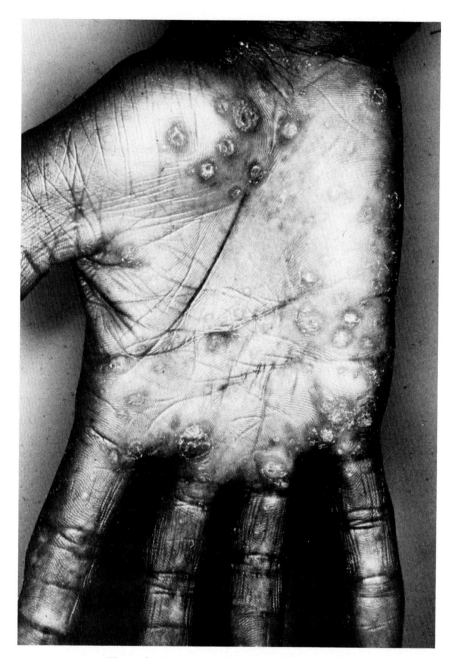

Figure 7-13. Punctate keratoses of the palms.

to five times more frequently in cancer patients than in a controlled group. However, other studies have failed to confirm this relationship (110,111). Therefore, the association of internal malignancy with acquired punctate keratoses remains questionable.

Tylosis palmaris et plantaris is the occurrence of palmar and plantar hyper-keratosis with esophageal carcinoma (112,113). The palmar and plantar hyper-keratosis is usually bilateral and symmetrical. Most reported cases are familial but sporadic cases have also been reported.

Pentavalent arsenic ingestion has also been associated with the development of discrete punctate keratotic lesions on the palms and soles and with the appearance of multiple basal cell carcinomas and Bowen's disease. However, the incidence of internal malignancy and the association of arsenic ingestion remain controversial. In one report of 27 cases of long-term arsenic ingestion, 10 patients had multiple skin cancers as well as visceral malignancy (114). The latency period seemed to range from 15 to 30 years following arsenic ingestion. On the other hand, Yeh et al. (115), examined a population exposed to arsenic in their drinking water and concluded that while there was an increased incidence of skin cancer, there was no significant increase in internal malignancy. Similarly, others have found no increased incidence of internal malignancy with arsenic ingestion (116). Jackson and Grainge (117) recently reviewed the literature for the relationship of inorganic arsenic ingestion and malignancy and found malignancies in 58 of 916 cases. Although the relationship of arsenic ingestion and internal malignancy is unproved, unexplained symptoms in patients with arsenical keratosis should be evaluated (117,118).

PYODERMA GANGRENOSUM

Pyoderma gangrenosum is characterized by necrotic ulceration with over-hanging borders (119). The pathogenesis of pyoderma gangrenosum is unknown. It is a rare entity most often seen in adults; women are slightly more frequently affected than men. Clinically, the lesions may appear on any area of the body, including the mucous membranes. Characteristically, the lesions develop rapidly, beginning as a red plaque or pustule that spreads concentrically with necrosis and ulceration of its central portion (Fig. 7-14). In time a typical lesion, consisting of a necrotic ulcer with an elevated overhanging border surrounded by a violaceous area, develops. The ulceration may enlarge rapidly and progressively.

Pyoderma gangrenosum has been associated with lymphoreticular malignancies, including myeloma, myelofibrosis, leukemia, and lymphoma (120–136). Pyoderma gangrenosum has also been associated with other disorders, such as ulcerative colitis, regional enteritis, and polyarthritis (possibly rheumatoid arthritis) (136, 137).

SIGN OF LESER-TRÉLAT

The sign of Leser-Trélat is rare; several recent reports have reemphasized its association with internal malignancy (138–142). However, as with many other symptoms of internal malignancy, this sign has been a subject of controversy. Seborrheic keratoses are common in older patients as is internal malignancy; therefore, the simultaneous occurrence of both may only be coincidental. No consistent tumor type has been reported with the sign of Leser-Trélat. Most

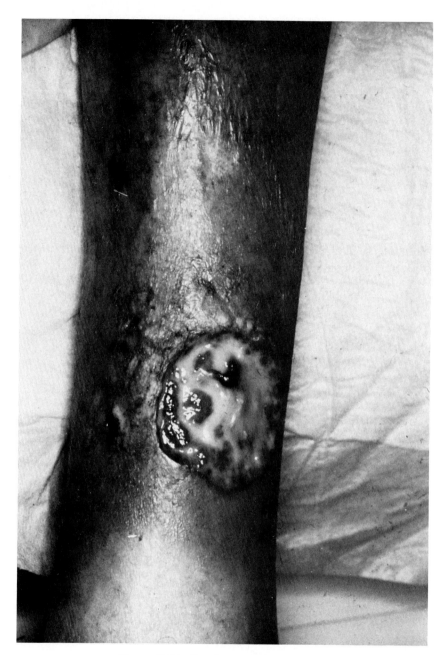

Figure 7-14. Pyoderma gangrenosum.

recently, the sign of Leser-Trélat has been associated with squamous cell carcinoma of the lung, Sézary syndrome, lymphoma, and mycosis fungoides (140–146). The presence of multiple seborrheic keratoses alone is not sufficient to warrant thorough evaluation. However, the rapid appearance of multiple new lesions and/or rapid increase in their size or the development of pruritus should lead to suspicion of internal malignancy.

TORRE'S SYNDROME

In Torre's syndrome, multiple cutaneous sebaceous gland tumors are associated with carcinoma, primarily of the gastrointestinal tract (147). The syndrome may be inherited as an autosomal dominant trait with high penetrance (148). Most of the sebaceous gland tumors are adenomas, but carcinomas have also been reported. The sebaceous gland neoplasms are multiple and 70% are noted on the trunk (149). The visceral carcinomas are primarily of the colon, but many patients have had multiple cancers involving other areas of the gastrointestinal tract as well as other organ systems (150).

REFERENCES

1. Curth HO: Skin lesions and internal carcinoma, in Andrade R, et al (eds): *Cancer of the Skin.* Philadelphia, Saunders, 1978, p 1308.
2. Shelley WB: Cutaneous signs of internal malignancy. *Minn Med* 57:773, 1974.
3. Callen JP: Skin signs of internal malignancy, in J. P. Callen (ed) *Cutaneous Aspects of Internal Disease.* Chicago, Yearbook Medical Publishers, 1981, p 207.
4. Braverman IB: *Skin Signs of Systemic Disease.* Philadelphia, Saunders, 1981, p 3.
5. Kierland RR: Cutaneous signs of internal malignancy. *South Med J* 65:563, 1972.
6. Moschella SL: Cutaneous manifestations of internal malignancy. *Med Clin North Am* 59:471, 1975.
7. Stone SP: Cutaneous clues to cancer. *Am Fam Physician* 12:82, 1975.
8. Samitz MH: Clinical significance of skin lesions in the diagnosis of gastrointestinal malignancies. *Cutis* 19:649, 657, 1977.
9. Perry HO: Less common skin markers of visceral neoplasms. *Int J Dermatol* 15:19, 1976.
10. Schwartz RA: Acanthosis nigricans, florid cutaneous papillomatosis and the sign of Leser-Trélat. *Cutis* 28:319, 1981.
11. Curth HO, Hilberg AW, Machacek GF: The site and histology of the cancer associated with malignant acanthosis nigricans. *Cancer* 15:364, 1962.
12. Hage E, Hage J: Malignant acanthosis nigricans: A para-endocrine syndrome? *Acta Derm Venereol* 57:169, 1977.
13. Mikhail GR, Fachnie DM, Drukker BH, et al: Generalized malignant acanthosis nigricans. *Arch Dermatol* 115:201, 1979.
14. Reid JH, Pierson DL, Rodman OG: Malignant acanthosis nigricans universalis. *J Assoc Milit Dermatol* 4:10, 1979.
15. Safai B, Grant JM, Kurtz R, et al: Cutaneous manifestations of internal malignancies (1): Acanthosis nigricans. *Int J Dermatol* 17:312, 1978.
16. Möller H, Eriksson S, Holen O, et al: Complete reversibility of paraneoplastic acanthosis nigricans after operation. *Acta Med Scand* 203:245, 1978.
17. Breathnach SM, Wells GC: Acanthosis palmaris: tripe palms: A distinctive pattern of palmar keratoderma frequently associated with internal malignancy. *Clin Exp Dermatol* 5:181, 1980.
18. Andreev VC, Boyanov L, Tsankov N: Generalized acanthosis nigricans. *Dermatologica* 163:19, 1981.
19. Brown J, Winkelmann RK: Acanthosis nigricans: A study of 90 cases. *Medicine* 47:33, 1968.
20. Sneddon IB: Acquired ichthyosis in Hodgkin's disease. *Br Med J* 1:763, 1955.
21. Van Dijk E: Ichthyosiform atrophy of the skin with internal malignant disease. *Dermatologica* 127:413, 1963.

22. Reiches AJ: Acquired ichthysosis: Report of a case associated with breast cancer. *Urol Cutan Rev* 54:160, 1950.

23. Flint GL, Flam M, Soter NA: Acquired ichthyosis: A sign of nonlymphoproliferative malignant disorders. *Arch Dermatol* 111:1446, 1975.

24. Bowen JT: Precancerous dermatosis: A study of two cases of chronic atypical epithelial proliferation. *J Cutan Dis* 30:241, 1912.

25. Graham JH, Helwig EB: Bowen's disease and its relationship to systemic cancer. *Arch Dermatol* 8:33, 1959.

26. Epstein E: Association of Bowen's disease with visceral cancer. *Arch Dematol* 82:349, 1960.

27. Peterka ES, Lynch FW, Goltz RW: An association between Bowen's disease and internal cancer. *Arch Dermatol* 84:623, 1961.

28. Graham JH, Helwig EB: Bowen's disease and its relationship to systemic cancer. *Arch Dermatol* 83:738, 1961.

29. Hugo NE, Conway H: Bowen's disease: Its malignant potential and relationship to systemic cancer. *Plast Reconstr Surg* 39:190, 1967.

30. Goldman AL: Lung cancer in Bowen's disease. *Am Rev Res Dis* 108:1205, 1973.

31. Callen JP, Headington J: Bowen's and non-Bowen's squamous intra-epidermal neoplasia of the skin: Relationship to internal malignancy. *Arch Dermatol* 116:422, 1980.

32. Anderson SLC, Nielsen A, Reymann F: Relationship between Bowen's disease and internal malignant tumors. *Arch Dermatol* 108:367, 1973.

33. Stone SP, Schroeter AL: Bullous pemphigoid and associated malignant neoplasms. *Arch Dermatol* 111:991, 1975.

34. Hodge L, Marsden RA, Black MM, et al: Bullous pemphigoid: The frequency of mucosal involvement and concurrent malignancy related to indirect immunofluorescence findings. *Br J Dermatol* 105:65, 1981.

35. Greer KE, Beacham BE, Askew PC Jr.: Benign mucous membrane pemphigoid in association with internal malignancy. *Cutis* 25:183, 1980.

36. Krain LS, Bierman SM: Pemphigus vulgaris and internal malignancy. *Cancer* 33:1091, 1974.

37. Krain LS: The association of pemphigus with thymoma or malignancy: A critical review. *Br J Dermatol* 90:397, 1974.

38. Maize JC, Dobson RL, Provost TT: Pemphigus and myasthenia gravis. *Arch Dermatol* 111:1334, 1975.

39. Callen JP: Internal disorders associated with bullous disease of the skin: A critical review. *J Am Acad Dermatol* 3:107, 1980.

40. Fowler JM, Thomas DJB: Lymphoma in dermatitis herpetiformis. *Br Med J* 2:757, 1976.

41. Sjoerdsma A, Weissbach H, Udenfriend S: Clinical, physiologic and biochemical study of patients with malignant carcinoid (argentaffinoma). *Am J Med* 20:520, 1956.

42. Melmon KL, Sjoerdsma A, Mason DT: Distinctive clinical and therapeutic aspects of the syndrome associated with bronchial carcinoid tumors. *Am J Med* 39:568, 1965.

43. Callen JP, Hyla JF, Bole GG, et al: The relationship of dermatomyositis and polymyositis to internal malignancy. *Arch Dermatol* 116:295, 1980.

44. Winkelmann RK: Dermatomyositis in childhood. *J Cont Ed Dermatol* 18:13, 1979.

45. Samitz MH: Cuticular change in dermatomyositis: A clinical sign. *Arch Dermatol* 110:866, 1974.

46. Williams RC Jr.: Dermatomyositis and malignancy: A review of the literature. *Ann Intern Med* 50:1174, 1959.

47. Curtis AC, Blaylock HC, Harrell ER: Malignant lesions associated with dermatomyositis. *JAMA* 150:844, 1952.

48. Arundell FD, Wilkinson RD, Haserick JR: Dermatomyositis and malignant neoplasm in adults: A survey of twenty years experience. *Arch Dermatol* 82:772, 1960.

49. Talbott JH: Acute dermatomyositis-polymyositis and malignancy. *Semin Arthritis Rheum* 6:305, 1977.

50. Barnes BE: Dermatomyositis and malignancy: A review of the literature. *Ann Intern Med* 84:68, 1976.

51. Callen JP: The vlaue of malignancy evaluation in patients with dermatomyositis. *J Am Acad Dermatol* 6:253, 1982.

52. Skolnick M, Mainman ER: Erythema gyratum repens with metastatic adenocarcinoma. *Arch Dermatol* 111:227, 1975.

53. Summerly R: The figurate erythemas and neoplasia. *Br J Dermatol* 76:370, 1964.

54. Willia WF: The gyrate erythemas. *Int J Dermatol* 17:698, 1978.

55. Gammel JA: Erythema gyratum repens: Skin manifestations in patients with carcinoma of the breast. *Arch Dermatol Syph* 66:494, 1952.

56. Leavell UW Jr, Winternitz WW, Black JH: Erythema gyratum repens and undifferentiated carcinoma. *Arch Dermatol* 95:69, 1967.

57. Leimert JT, Corder MP, Skibba CA, et al: Erythema annulare centrifugum and Hodgkin's disease: Association with disease activity. *Arch Intern Med* 139:486, 1979.

58. Lazar P: Cancer, erythema annulare centrifugum, autoimmunity. *Arch Dermatol* 87:246, 1963.

59. White JW, Perry HO: Erythema perstans. *Br J Dermatol* 81:641, 1969.

60. Gardner EJ, Richards RC: Multiple cutaneous and subcutaneous lesions occurring simultaneously with hereditary polyposis and osteomatosis. *Am J Hum Genet* 5:139, 1953.

61. Watne AL, Johnson JG, Change CH: The challenge of Gardner's syndrome. *CA* 19:266, 1969.

62. Weary PE, Linthicum A, Cawley EP, et al: Gardner's syndrome: A family group study and review. *Arch Dermatol* 90:20, 1964.

63. Jones TR, Nance FC: Periampullary malignancy in Gardner's syndrome. *Am Surg* 185:565, 1977.

64. Lewis AE: The glucagonoma syndrome. *Int J Dermatol* 18:17, 1979.

65. Church RE, Crane WAJ: A cutaneous syndrome associated with islet-cell carcinoma of the pancreas. *Br J Dermatol* 79:284, 1967.

66. Amon RB, Swenson KH, Hanifin JM, et al: The glucagonoma syndrome (necrolytic migratory erythema) and zinc. *N Engl J Med* 295:962, 1976.

67. Tasman-Jones C, Kay RG: Zinc deficiency and skin lesions. *N Engl J Med* 293:830, 1975.

68. Wilkinson DS: Necrolytic migratory erythema with carcinoma of the pancreas. *Trans St Johns Hosp Dermatol Soc* 59:244, 1973.

69. Mallinson CN, Bloom SR, Warin AP, et al: A glucagonoma syndrome. *Lancet* 2:1, 1974.

70. Sweet RD: A dermatosis specifically associated with a tumor of pancreatic alpha cells. *Br J Dermatol* 90:301, 1974.

71. Kahan RS, Perez-Figaredo RA, Neimanis A: Necrolytic migratory erythema: Distnctive dermatosis of the glucagonoma syndrome. *Arch Dermatol* 113:792, 1977.

72. Pedersen NB, Jonsson L, Holst JJ: Necrolytic migratory erythema and glucagon cell tumor of the pancreas: The glucagonoma syndrome: Report of two cases. *Acta Derm Venereol* 56:391, 1976.

73. Binnick AN, Spencer SK, Dennison WL Jr, et al: Glucagonoma syndrome: Report of two cases and literature review. *Arch Dermatol* 113:749, 1977.

74. Headington JT: Glucagonoma syndrome. *Challenges Dermatol* 1:20, 1979.

75. Swenson KH, Amon RB, Hanifin JM: The glucagonoma syndrome: A distinctive cutaneous marker of systemic disease. *Arch Dermatol* 114:224, 1978.

76. Broder LE, Carter SK: Pancreatic islet cell carcinoma II: Results of therapy with streptozotocin in 52 patients. *Ann Intern Med* 79:108, 1973.

77. Marynick SP, Fagadau WR, Duncan LA: Malignant glucagonoma syndrome: Response to chemotherapy. *Ann Intern Med* 93:453, 1980.

78. Mazur MH, Dolin R: Herpes zoster at the NIH: A 20 year experience. *Am J Med* 65:738, 1978.

79. Fretzin DF: Malignant Down. *Arch Dermatol* 95:294, 1967.

80. Hegedus SI, Schorr WF: Acquired hypertrichosis languinosa and malignancy: A clinical review and histopathologic evaluation with special attention to the "mantle" hair of pinkus. *Arch Dermatol* 106:84, 1972.

81. Goodfellow A, Calvert H, Bohn G: Hypertrichosis languinosa acquisita. *Br J Dermatol* 103:431, 1980.

82. Gonzalez JJ, Ungaro PC, Hooper JW, et al: Acquired hypertrichosis lanuginosa: Rare manifestation of urinary bladder carcinoma. *Arch Intern Med* 140:969, 1980.

83. McLean DI, Macaulay JC: Hypertrichosis lanuginosa acquisita associated with pancreatic carcinoma. *Br J Dermatol* 96:313, 1977.

84. Wadskov S, Bro-Jorgensen A, Sondergaard J: Acquired hypertrichosis lanuginosa: A skin marker of internal malignancy. *Arch Dermatol* 112:1442, 1976.

85. Sack GH Jr, Levin J, Bell WR: Trousseau's syndrome and other manifestations of chronic disseminated coagulopathy in patients with neoplasms: Clinical, pathophysiologic and therapeutic features. *Medicine* 56:1, 1977.

86. Goltz RW, Laymon CW: Multicentric reticulohistiocytosis of the skin and synovia: Reticulohistiocytoma or ganglioneuroma. *Arch Dermatol Syph* 69:717, 1954.

87. Catterall MD, White JE: Multicentric reticulohistiocytosis and malignant disease. *Br J Dermatol* 98:221, 1978.

88. Weary PE, Gorlin RJ, Gentry WC Jr, et al: Multiple hamartoma syndrome (Cowden's disease). *Arch Dermatol* 106:682, 1972.

89. Thyresson HN, Doyle JA: Cowden's disease (multiple hamartoma syndrome). *Mayo Clin Proc* 56:179, 1981.

90. Wade TR, Kopf AW: Cowden's disease: A case report and review of the literature. *J Dermatol Surg Oncol* 4:459, 1978.

91. Weinstock JV, Kawanishi H: Gastrointestinal polyposis with orocutaneous hamartomas (Cowden's disease). *Gastroenterology* 74:890, 1978.

92. Brownstein MH, Wolf M, Bikowski JB: Cowden's disease: A cutaneous marker of breast cancer. *Cancer* 41:2393, 1978.

93. Burnett JW, Goldner R, Calton GJ: Cowden's disease: Report of two additional cases. *Br J Dermatol* 93:329, 1975.

94. Crowe FW, Schull WJ: Diagnostic importance of café-au-lait spot in neurofibromatosis. *Arch Intern Med* 91:758, 1953.

95. Crowe FW: Axillary freckling as a diagnostic aid in neurofibromatosis. *Ann Intern Med* 61:1142, 1964.

96. D'Agostino AN, Soule EH, Miller RH: Sarcomas of the peripheral nerves and somatic soft tissues associated with multiple neurofibromatosis (von Recklinghausen's disease). *Cancer* 16:1015, 1963.

97. Bader JL, Miller RW: Neurofibromatosis and childhood leukemia. *J Pediatr* 92:925, 1978.

98. Helwig EB, Graham JH: Anogenital (extramammary) Paget's disease: A clinicopathological study. *Cancer* 16:387, 1963.

99. Ashikari R, Park K, Huvos AG, et al: Paget's disease of the breast. *Cancer* 26:680, 1970.

100. Yoell JH, Price WG: Paget's disease of the perianal skin with associated adenocarcinoma. *Arch Dermatol* 82:986, 1960.

101. Murrell TW Jr, McMullan FH: Extramammary Paget's disease: A report of two cases. *Arch Dermatol* 85:600, 1962.

102. Utsunomiya J, Gocho H, Miyanaga T, et al: Peutz-Jeghers syndrome: Its natural course and management. *Johns Hopkins Med J* 136:71, 1975.

103. Bartholomew LG, Dahlin DC, Waugh JM: Intestinal polyposis associated with mucocutaneous melanin pigmentation (Peutz-Jeghers syndrome): A review of literature and report of six cases with special reference to pathologic findings. *Gastroenterology* 32:434, 1957.

104. Matuchansky C, Babin P, Coutrot S, et al: Peutz-Jeghers syndrome with metastasizing carcinoma arising from a jejunal hamartoma. *Gastroenterology* 77:1311, 1979.

105. Reid JD: Duodenal carcinoma in the Peutz-Jeghers syndrome: Report of a case. *Cancer* 18:970, 1965.

106. Cochet B, Carrel J, Desbaillets L, et al: Peutz-Jeghers syndrome associated with gastrointestinal carcinoma. *Gut* 20:169, 1979.

107. Hsu SD, Zaharopoulos P, May JT, et al: Peutz-Jeghers syndrome with intestinal carcinoma: Report of the association in one family. *Cancer* 44:1527, 1979.

108. Lin JI, Caracta PF, Lindner A, et al: Peutz-Jeghers polyposis with metastasizing duodenal carcinoma. *South Med J* 70:882, 1977.

109. Dobson RL, Young MR, Pinto JS: Palmar keratoses and cancer. *Arch Dermatol* 92:553, 1965.

110. Bean SF, Foxley EG, Fusaro RM: Palmar keratoses and internal malignancy. A negative study. *Arch Dermatol* 97:528, 1968.

111. Stolman LP, Kopf AW, Garfinkel L: Are palmar keratoses a sign of internal malignancy? *Arch Dermatol* 101:52, 1970.

112. Parnell DD, Johnson SA: Tylosis palmaris et plantaris: Its occurrence with internal malignancy. *Arch Dermatol* 100:7, 1969.

113. Woscoff A, Abulafia J, Lacentre EC, et al: Queratodermal plantar con carcinoma de pulmon. *Med Cutan Ano* 5:125, 1970.

114. Sommers SC, McManus RG: Multiple arsenical cancers of skin and internal organs. *Cancer* 6:347, 1953.

115. Yeh S, How SW, Lin CS: Arsenical cancer of skin: Histologic study with special reference to Bowen's disease. *Cancer* 21:312, 1968.

116. Reymann R, Möller R, Nielsen A: Relationship between arsenic intake and internal malignant neoplasms. *Arch Dermatol* 114:378, 1978.

117. Jackson R, Grainge JW: Arsenic and cancer. *Can Med Assoc J* 113:396, 1975.

118. Spoor HJ: Arsenic and skin cancer: Cocarcinogenicity. *Cutis* 18:631, 1976.

119. Callen JP, Taylor WB: Pyoderma gangrenosum: A literature review. *Cutis* 21:61, 1978.

120. Cream JJ: Pyoderma gangrenosum with a monoclonal IgM red cell agglomerating factor. *Br J Dermatol* 84:223, 1971.

121. Jablonska S, Stachow A, Dabrowska H: Rapports entre la pyodermite gangreneuse et le myelome. *Ann Dermatol Syph* 94:121, 1967.

122. Thivolet J, Perrot H, Hermier-Abgrall CR: Phagedenisma et dysglobulinemice G. *Ital Derm Sif* 44:148, 1969.

123. Sluis I: Two cases of pyoderma (ecthyma) gangrenosum associated with the presence of an abnormal serum protein (beta-2-paraproteins): With a review of the literature. *Dermatologica* 132:409, 1966.

124. Thompson DM, Main RA, Beck JS, et al: Studies on a patient with leukocytoclastic vasculitis "pyoderma gangrenosum" and paraproteinaemia. *Br J Dermatol* 88:117, 1973.

125. Callen JP, Dubin HV, Gehrke CF: Recurrent pyoderma gangrenosum and agnogenic myeloid metaplasia. *Arch Dermatol* 113:1585, 1977.

126. Perry HO, Brunsting LA: Pyoderma gangrenosum: A clinical study of nineteen cases. *Arch Dermatol* 75:380, 1957.

127. Perry HO, Winkelmann RK: Bullous pyoderma gangrenosum and leukemia. *Arch Dermatol* 106:901, 1972.

128. Goldin D: Pyoderma gangrenosum with chronic myeloid leukemia. *Proc R Soc Med* 67:1239, 1974.

129. Pye RJ, Choundhury C: Bullous pyoderma as a presentation of acute leukemia. *Clin Exp Dermatol* 2:33, 1977.

130. Shore RN: Pyoderma gangrenosum, defective neutrophil chemotaxis and leukemia. *Arch Dermatol* 112:1792, 1976.

131. Tay CH: Pyoderma gangrenosum and leukemia. *Arch Dermatol* 108:580, 1973.

132. Lewis SJ, Poh-Fitzpatrick MB, Walther RR: Atypical pyoderma gangrenosum with leukemia. *JAMA* 239:935, 1978.

133. Walther RR, Poh-Fitzpatrick MB: Malignant pyoderma. *Cutis* 22:316, 1978.

134. Mahood JM, Sneddon IB: Pyoderma gangrenosum complicating non-Hodgkin's lymphoma. *Br J Dermatol* 102:223, 1980.

135. Perry HO: Pyoderma gangrenosum. *South Med J* 62:899, 1969.

136. Lazarus GS, Goldsmith LA, Rocklin RE, et al: Pyoderma gangrenosum, altered delayed hypersensitivity and polyarthritis. *Arch Dermatol* 105:46, 1972.

137. Stolman LP, Rosenthal D, Yaworsky R, et al: Pyoderma gangrenosum and rheumatoid arthritis. *Arch Dermatol* 111:1020, 1975.

138. Ronchese F: Keratosis, cancer and "the sign of Leser-Trélat." *Cancer* 18:1003, 1965.

139. Liddell K, White JE, Caldwell IW: Seborrheic keratoses and carcinoma of the large bowel: Three cases exhibiting the sign of Leser-Trélat. *Br J Dermatol* 92:449, 1975.

140. Dantzig PL: Sign of Leser-Trélat. *Arch Dermatol* 108:700, 1973.

141. Safai B, Grant JM, Good RA: Cutaneous manifestation of internal malignancies (II): The sign of Leser-Trélat. *Int J Dermatol* 17:494, 1978.

142. Doll DC, McCagh MF, Welton WA: Sign of Leser-Trélat. *JAMA* 238:236, 1977.

143. Wagner RF Jr, Wagner KD: Malignant neoplasms and the Leser-Trélat sign. *Arch Dermatol* 117:598, 1981.

144. Halevy S, Halevy J, Feuerman EJ: The sign of Leser-Trélat in association with lymphocytic lymphoma. *Dermatologica* 161:183, 1980.

145. Sperry K, Wall J: Adenocarcinoma of the stomach with eruptive seborrheic keratoses. *Cancer* 45:2434, 1980.

146. Kechijian P, Sadick NS, Mariglio J, et al: Cytarabine-induced inflammation in the seborrheic keratoses of Leser-Trélat. *Ann Intern Med* 91:868, 1979.

147. Torre D: Multiple sebaceous tumors. *Arch Dermatol* 98:549, 1968.

148. Anderson DE: Familial cancer and cancer families. *Semin Oncol* 5:11, 1978.

149. Rulon DB, Helwig EB: Multiple sebaceous neoplasms of the skin: An association with multiple visceral carcinomas, especially of the colon. *Am J Clin Pathol* 60:745, 1973.

150. Lynch HT, Lynch PM, Pester J, et al: The cancer family syndrome: Rare cutaneous phenotypic linkage of Torre's syndrome. *Arch Intern Med* 141:607, 1981.

8
Disorders
of Erythrocytes

Edward C. Lynch

Anemia is among the most common manifestations of malignant disease. In some patients diagnostic evaluation of an anemia results in the discovery of an occult neoplasm. In other patients anemia does not appear until late in the course of the illness. The mechanisms of anemia in patients with malignancies are quite varied (Table 8-1) but are similar, in general, to the causes of anemia in persons who have no malignancy. A thorough diagnostic study to define the mechanism of anemia is important in all patients with an anemia. In many cases the possibility of malignancy must be considered along with various nonneoplastic disorders. Rational treatment of an anemia cannot be initiated until the mechanism of the anemia is understood.

BLOOD LOSS

Acute blood loss from the gastrointestinal, urinary, or female genital systems may be of sufficient degree to cause anemia. Cancers of the stomach, colon, uterus, bladder, and kidney may abruptly bleed, leading to the sudden appearance of anemia. Bleeding from other organs is rarely severe enough to cause anemia due to acute blood loss. However, unexplained hemorrhage from any organ deserves prompt evaluation. Certainly unexplained bleeding is a common manifestation of neoplasms.

IRON DEFICIENCY ANEMIA

In the vast majority of instances of iron deficiency anemia in adults in the United States, chronic loss of blood is responsible for the lack of iron. Excessive menstrual loss of blood is a frequent cause of iron deficiency in younger women. In postmenopausal women and adult men the source of the chronic blood loss is usually the gastrointestinal tract, although occasionally it is the genitourinary tract. Blood loss from the gastrointestinal tract, sufficient to cause anemia, may be totally inapparent to the patient. Additionally, tests of the stools for occult

Table 8-1. Mechanisms of Anemia in Malignant Disease

Blood loss
Iron deficiency
Anemia of chronic disorders
Myelophthisis
  Hematologic and lymphatic malignancies
  Metastatic cancer
  Myelofibrosis
Erythroid hypoplasia
Aplastic anemia
Megaloblastic erythropoiesis
  Vitamin B_{12} deficiency
  Folic acid deficiency
  Erythroleukemia
  Antimetabolite chemotherapy
Sideroblastic erythropoiesis
Autoimmune hemolytic
  Warm antibodies
  Cold antibodies
Microangiopathic hemolytic
Paroxysmal nocturnal hemoglobinuria
Hypersplenism
Erythrophagocytosis
Dilutional "anemia"

blood may be negative at times because the blood loss is intermittent. The occurrence of iron deficiency in an adult without evidence of urinary blood loss or unusual menstrual loss most likely is due to gastrointestinal blood loss even when tests of the stool for blood are negative. Aside from chronic bleeding, other causes of iron deficiency are pregnancies, chronic hemoglobinuria, impaired absorption of iron related to gastrectomy, and dietary deficiency of iron. Insufficient intake of iron occurs in infants on deficient diets, occasionally in growing children, and in adult food fadists. Relative dietary deficiency of iron contributes to the iron deficient state of women with substantial menstrual loss and in pregnant women.

Characteristically, the anemia of iron deficiency is hypochromic microcytic (Fig. 8-1). However, when the anemia is mild the red blood cell indices may be normochromic normocytic. The finding of a decreased value of the serum iron coupled with an elevated level of the serum iron-binding capacity is ordinarily sufficient for confirmation of the diagnosis of iron deficiency. Bone marrow stores of iron, estimated by Prussian blue staining of a marrow aspirate, are depleted in persons with iron deficiency anemia. Because the level of serum ferritin accurately reflects the status of iron storage, it is not necessary to perform a marrow aspirate to quantitate iron stores.

Iron deficiency must be distinguished from other causes of a hypochromic microcytic anemia, such as thalassemia minor, lead poisoning, and some cases of sideroblastic anemia. Usually the finding of the typical values of the serum iron and iron-binding capacity is sufficient for diagnosis. The anemia of chronic disorders may, however, at times be difficult to discriminate from iron deficiency.

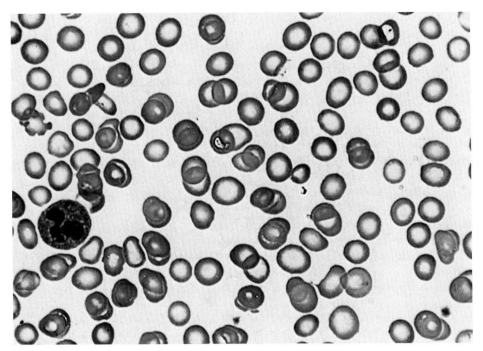

Figure 8-1. Peripheral blood film demonstrating hypochromic microcytic erythrocytes in a patient with iron deficiency anemia. (Magnification $800\times$.)

Although usually the red cell indices are normochromic normocytic in the anemia of chronic disorders, occasionally the indices and review of the peripheral blood film disclose a hypochromic and/or microcytic anemia. Additionally, the value of the serum iron is regularly decreased in the anemia of chronic disorders. However, in contrast to iron deficiency, the serum iron-binding capacity is usually decreased and values of the serum ferritin are normal or high, indicative of an abundance of storage iron.

The responsibilities of the physician do not end with the discovery that an anemia is due to deficiency of iron and the administration of iron therapy. Thorough radiographic examinations of the esophagus, stomach, small bowel, and colon should be obtained in (1) patients who have occult blood in their stools, or (2) patients with iron deficiency in whom no blood loss has been found and in whom there is no reasonable explanation of the iron deficiency. Approximately 10% of adults with iron deficiency due to occult gastrointestinal blood loss have malignancies. The most common sites are the stomach and the cecum. In these adults, gastroscopy and colonoscopy are often advisable if radiographic studies fail to reveal a gastrointestinal lesion responsible for the blood loss.

ANEMIA OF CHRONIC DISORDERS

The anemia of chronic disorders occurs secondary to three general types of disease: (1) malignancies; (2) infections and chronic inflammatory conditions;

and (3) collagen disorders, particularly rheumatoid arthritis and systemic lupus erythematosus. When a malignancy is responsible for the anemia, the neoplasm is frequently disseminated rather than limited to its primary site.

The anemia is moderate in severity, with hemoglobin values varying between 7 and 11 g/dl. Usually the anemia is normochromic normocytic, but occasionally it is hypochromic microcytic. The hypochromia and microcytosis are rarely as striking as that seen in iron deficiency. The anemia of chronic disorders is an example of relative bone marrow failure. Reticulocyte counts are within the normal range, indicating that there is no increase in marrow erythroid activity in response to the anemia. The marrow is less responsive than normal to erythropoietin. Mild shortening of red cell life span is commonly found by ^{51}Cr-erythrocyte survival studies.

Values of the serum iron and serum iron-binding capacity are decreased. Iron stores in histiocytes, estimated by measuring serum ferritin or by marrow aspirate, are normal or increased. The amount of iron in normoblasts, judged by Prussian blue stain of marrow aspirates, is reduced. The decreased level of serum iron is due to impaired release of iron from histiocytes to circulating transferrin. Normally iron derived from the histiocytic breakdown of senescent red cells is returned promptly to the plasma, but this process is blocked in the anemia of chronic disorders. The mechanism of the decreased serum iron-binding capacity has not been firmly established. One hypothesis is excessive binding of transferrin to the surface of iron-laden histiocytes.

The diagnosis of the anemia of chronic disorders is clinically established with reasonable certainty if values of the serum iron and iron-binding capacity are reduced and the serum ferritin level is normal or increased. In the absence of clinical evidence of an inflammatory condition or a collagen disorder, establishment of the anemia of chronic disorders as the mechanism of an anemia dictates a thorough diagnostic search for an occult malignancy. Particular attention should be given to the possibilities of lymphoma and malignancies of the kidney, pancreas, stomach, lung, and breast. Occasionally a marrow aspirate will disclose metastatic tumor. However, in patients with malignancies, there is no correlation of the development of the anemia of chronic disorders with the presence of marrow metastases. The anemia is unresponsive to iron therapy and will improve only if the underlying disease (malignancy, infection, or collagen disease) is brought under control.

Case 1

A 65-year-old woman was referred for hematologic consultation because of an anemia. Twenty-six months previously the patient had undergone right radical mastectomy for adenocarcinoma. Resected axillary lymph nodes showed no evidence histologically of metastatic carcinoma. She received radiotherapy postoperatively. She thereafter felt well until about six months before her consultation visit when she noted the appearance of fatigue with mild exertion. A few weeks later she saw a physician, who found the hematocrit value to be 30%. Treatment with iron orally did not result in improvement in her anemia. She had not experienced fever or loss of weight.

Physical examination revealed a very obese woman with mild pallor. There were no findings indicative of local recurrence of her breast cancer. A mass, thought to be the liver, was felt in the right upper quadrant of the abdomen. The mass extended 7 cm beneath the right costal margin. The spleen was not palpable. Except for a rectocele, pelvic and rectal examinations were normal.

The hemoglobin value was 9.4 g/dl, hematocrit 30%, reticulocyte count 1.5%, platelet count 720,000/mm^3, and total leukocyte count 9,400/mm^3, with a normal differential count. Examination of the peripheral blood film showed normochromic normocytic erythrocytes. Urinalysis gave normal results. A stool specimen was negative for occult blood. Roentgenograms of the chest were normal. Serum iron was 15 μg/dl, serum iron-binding capacity 249 μg/dl, and serum ferritin 93 ng/ml.

At this point the diagnostic impression was the anemia of chronic disorders. The most likely underlying cause was considered to be metastatic breast cancer to organs such as liver and bone. Bone marrow aspirate and biopsy disclosed a normocellular specimen with orderly granulopoiesis and erythropoiesis, increased megakaryocytes, and abundant histiocytic iron, but absent erythroblast iron judged by Prussian blue stain. No tumor cells were seen. A radionuclide bone scan was negative. Radioisotopic scan of the liver and spleen revealed these organs to be normal in size without "cold" defects. At this point in pursuit of the cause of the anemia of chronic disorders, a search for a primary malignancy arising in an abdominal organ was initiated. Contrast radiographic studies of the upper gastrointestinal tract, small bowel, and colon were all normal. However, an intravenous pyelogram with nephrotomograms disclosed a large space-occupying lesion of the right kidney, explaining the abdominal mass felt by physical examination. Selective right renal arteriogram yielded findings indicative of carcinoma (Fig. 8-2). A hypernephroma was removed by right nephrectomy. Invasion of the renal vein was found, but no distant metastases were observed.

Comment
This case illustrates the necessity of vigorous diagnostic evaluation searching for an underlying cause of an anemia of chronic disorders.

MYELOPHTHISIC ANEMIA

A myelophthisic anemia arises because of an infiltrative process in the bone marrow. The basic disease may be a primary malignancy of the marrow, metastatic neoplasm to the marrow, myelofibrosis, or a benign inflammatory process such as a granulomatous infection. The anemia is commonly accompanied by granulocytopenia and thrombocytopenia. The depression in blood cell counts results from displacement of marrow precursor cells by the infiltrative process. The anemia is normochromic normocytic with reticulocyte counts normal or low. Examination of the peripheral blood film reveals considerable morphologic abnormality of the red cells with various poikilocytes, such as teardrop erythrocytes, elliptocytes, and schizocytes, evident. Frequently, the so-called leukoerythroblastic picture of the peripheral blood is observed. This term refers to

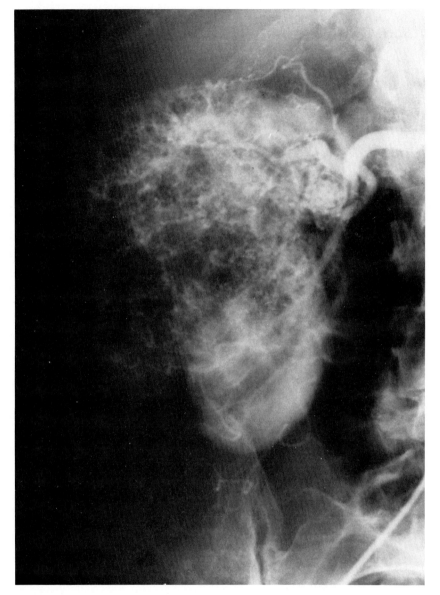

Figure 8-2. Selective right renal arteriogram (Case 1) showing a carcinoma of the upper pole of the right kidney.

the presence of small to moderate numbers of circulating normoblasts and immature granulocytes.

The most frequent mechanism of anemia (and pancytopenia) in patients with acute leukemia is myelophthisis. Usually circulating blast cells are found. However, some patients have pancytopenia without blast cells evident in the peripheral blood. The anemia in patients with multiple myeloma is commonly related to reduction in erythroid precursors due to proliferation of the myeloma cells.

In lymphocytic or histiocytic lymphoma, anemia may result from marrow infiltration by the neoplastic cells. Involvement of the marrow by lymphoma is sometimes more easily detected by biopsy of the marrow than by aspirate (1). Bilateral posterior iliac spine marrow biopsies increase significantly the yield of positive samples compared to a biopsy of one iliac spine (2). Improvement of a myelophthisic anemia or pancytopenia due to a hematologic malignancy depends on control of the malignancy with chemotherapy.

Approximately 10% of patients with Hodgkin's disease have involvement of the bone marrow demonstrable by biopsy (3) and thus are classified as stage IV. With intensive combination chemotherapy with MOPP, 13 of 18 patients with Hodgkin's disease accompanied by marrow involvement treated at the National Cancer Institute achieved complete remission (3).

The three solid tumors most commonly leading to myelophthisic anemia due to marrow metastases are carcinomas of the prostate, breast, and lung. However, many other neoplasms occasionally involve the marrow resulting in myelophthisic anemia. Tumor cells may be recognized by examination of aspirates of marrow with Wright's or Giemsa stain. Usually the tumor cells occur in clumps. The histologic pattern of a metastatic tumor may be discerned by examination of a needle biopsy of marrow stained with hematoxylin and eosin. Examination of biopsies is more reliable than aspirates in the diagnosis of carcinoma metastatic to the marrow. In about one-half of patients with oat cell carcinoma of the lung, bone marrow involvement is demonstrable at the time of initial presentation (1,4). Determination of the bone marrow acid phosphatase level is helpful in the diagnosis of metastatic prostatic carcinoma. Elevation of this enzyme in a marrow aspirate is probably the earliest evidence of medullary metastases of prostatic cancer (5).

Case 2

A 63-year-old woman was seen in hematologic consultation because of pancytopenia. Three months previously she had seen her physician complaining of low grade fever, malaise, and a weight loss of 15 pounds. Bronchoscopy, performed after a right hilar mass was observed on chest roentgenograms, established the diagnosis of oat cell carcinoma. At that time peripheral blood counts, bone marrow aspirate and biopsy, and radioisotopic scans of the liver, brain, and bones were all normal. Radiation treatment to the right hilum resulted in disappearance of the mass. However, about two and one half months after discovery of the carcinoma, pain in the right hip and right shoulder, weakness, and fever appeared. A radioisotopic bone scan was again negative. Her hemoglobin level was 7.0 g/dl, hematocrit 22%, reticulocyte count 1.1%, platelet count 49,000/mm^3, and total leukocyte count 2,900/mm^3, with a differential count of 77 segmented neutrophils, 3 bands, 4 metamyelocytes, 1 myelocyte, 2 eosinophils, 3 basophils, 5 monocytes, and 5 lymphocytes. Three normoblasts per 100 leukocytes were seen. Examination of the peripheral blood film revealed teardrop erythrocytes and elliptocytes. Bone marrow aspirate disclosed most of the cells to be anaplastic carcinoma cells (Fig. 8-3).

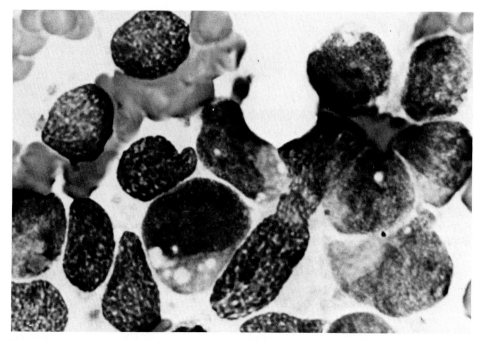

Figure 8-3. Bone marrow aspirate in Case 2 disclosed small, undifferentiated carcinoma cells, a few of which had characteristics of oat cells. (Magnification 1,250×.)

Comment

In the evaluation of the pancytopenia in this patient with a prior history of an undifferentiated carcinoma, the peripheral blood findings of teardrop eryth-rocytes, elliptocytes, immature granulocytes, and normoblasts all suggested a myelophthisic process. This was confirmed by finding tumor cells in the marrow aspirate.

Fibrosis of the bone marrow is most commonly due to the idiopathic myelo-proliferative disorder, myelofibrosis. Patients with this disease usually have ex-tramedullary hematopoiesis in the spleen and liver, that is, myeloid metaplasia. The majority of cases of myelofibrosis occur without an antecedent hematologic disorder. However, in some patients myelofibrosis occurs during the course of other hematologic diseases, specifically polycythemia vera, chronic myeloid leu-kemia, and essential thrombocythemia. Approximately 25% of patients with idiopathic myelofibrosis enter a terminal phase of the illness characterized by proliferation of blast cells and the clinical picture of acute leukemia.

Several malignant diseases may be associated with extensive fibrosis of the marrow, detected by biopsy. In patients with Hodgkin's disease involving the marrow, fibrosis almost always accompanies other histologic features of the dis-ease. Leukemic reticuloendotheliosis, or "hairy-cell leukemia," is a disorder in which the marrow is infiltrated with "hairy" leukemic cells and, additionally, usually has increased fibrous tissue (6). Rarely, multiple myeloma has been as-sociated with myelofibrosis and myeloid metaplasia (7). Occasionally, extensive fibrosis is found on examination of a marrow biopsy involved by metastatic cancer, such as carcinoma of the breast, stomach, or prostate (8). In such cases myeloid metaplasia of the spleen and liver is commonly present.

Case 3

A 53-year-old woman was referred for hematologic consultation because of severe anemia. Two years previously she had been treated for infiltrating lobular carcinoma of the right breast with preoperative radiotherapy and radical mastectomy. Ten of 25 lymph nodes were positive for metastatic cancer. When we saw the patient, the spleen was palpable 3 cm below the left costal margin. Hematocrit value was 19%, reticulocyte count 6.1%, platelet count 150,000/mm^3, and total leukocyte count 5,500/mm^3, with a differential count of 62 segmented neutrophils, 1 band, 4 metamyelocytes, 6 myelocytes, 2 promyelocytes, 1 myeloblast, 1 basophil, 1 eosinophil, 3 monocytes, and 19 lymphocytes. Examination of a peripheral blood film disclosed many teardrop erythrocytes and elliptocytes (Fig. 8-4) and 12 normoblasts per 100 leukocytes. No marrow cells could be aspirated, but a needle biopsy of posterior iliac spine marrow revealed myelofibrosis with metastatic tumor cells (Fig. 8-5). A ferrokinetic study with external scanning indicated splenic erythropoiesis.

The patient was one year postmenopausal. She was treated with radiation to

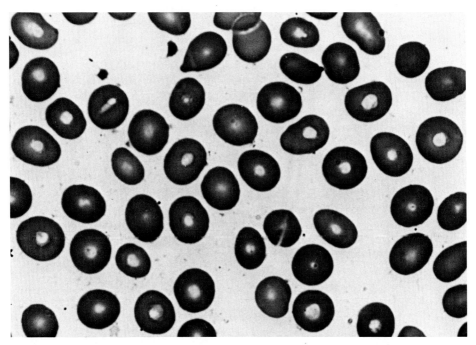

Figure 8-4. Examination of the peripheral blood film in Case 3 revealed teardrop red cells and elliptocytes, a finding commonly seen in patients with myelophthisic anemia. (Magnification 1,250×.)

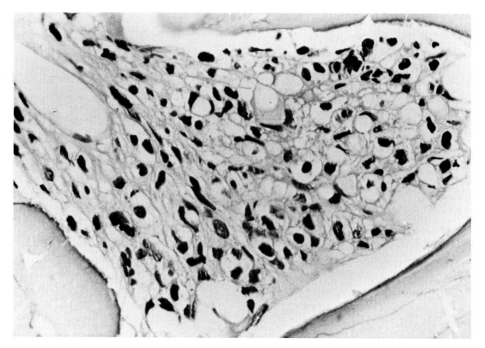

Figure 8-5. Bone marrow biopsy (Case 3) showing fibrosis and metastatic carcinoma cells. (Magnification 525×.)

the ovaries and fluoxymesterone 30 mg daily. Marked hematologic improvement occurred. Three months after initiation of androgen therapy, her hematocrit value was 44% with a platelet count of 390,000/mm³. However, five months later anemia recurred with the hematocrit value 17% and the platelet count 70,000/mm³. The spleen was palpable 8 cm below the left costal margin. In spite of the administration of corticosteroids, thiotepa, and transfusions, severe anemia and thrombocytopenia persisted and splenomegaly increased. Radiochromium red blood cell survival ($t\frac{1}{2}$) was quite short, with a value of 12 days. Splenectomy was performed. Histologic sections disclosed extensive extramedullary hematopoiesis. Before the splenectomy, hematocrit was 14%, reticulocyte count 17.8%, and platelet count 47,000/mm³. Two weeks after splenectomy, the hematocrit stabilized at 30% with a platelet count of 153,000/mm³. She did well for about six weeks. Then severe anemia and thrombocytopenia recurred. She died two months later as a result of extensive metastatic carcinoma in the liver and bone marrow.

Comment
In most instances myelofibrosis occurs as an idiopathic myeloproliferative disorder. However, occasionally metastatic carcinoma can be responsible for myelofibrosis and a myelophthisic anemia. In such patients extramedullary hematopoiesis may appear in the spleen and liver. In the patient described above enlargement of the spleen reached such proportions that hypersplenism became a contributing mechanism to her anemia and thrombocytopenia.

ERYTHROID HYPOPLASIA

Anemia due to erythroid hypoplasia of the bone marrow is uncommon. Affected patients have a normochromic normocytic anemia with reticulocytopenia. Leukocyte and platelet counts are usually normal. The diagnosis of erythroid hypoplasia is established by demonstration of reduced or absent erythroid precursors in a marrow aspirate. Causes of erythroid hypoplasia include both neoplastic and nonneoplastic disorders (Table 8-2). Because the hypoplasia is commonly very severe, the disorder is often termed *pure red cell aplasia*.

Congenital erythroid hypoplasia, the Diamond-Blackfan syndrome, is an uncommon disorder in which severe anemia appears in early childhood. Usually leukocyte and platelet counts are normal. Associated congenital abnormalities are common and include in some cases strabismus, exophthalmos, webbed neck, double ureters with hydronephrosis, and, particularly, bony abnormalities of the fingers. Remissions of the anemia may occur spontaneously or with corticosteroid therapy. Hemosiderosis due to transfusions is a major complicating feature of the disease. In three reported patients death has resulted from malignancies—acute myeloblastic leukemia, acute lymphoblastic leukemia, and hepatocellular carcinoma (9,10).

Most cases of acquired erythroid hypoplasia in adults in the United States belong to the pure red cell aplasia group. Approximately 50% of such patients have a thymoma. Viewed from the reverse standpoint, about 7% of patients with thymomas have pure red cell aplasia. Histologically in patients with pure red cell aplasia, the thymoma is usually encapsulated, noninvasive, and composed mainly of spindle cells. The thymoma shows histologic evidence of malignancy in 15% of cases. About two-thirds of affected patients are women. In some patients the red cell aplasia is not pure, there being either leukopenia or thrombocytopenia or both. The likely mechanism of the erythroid aplasia is immune

Table 8-2. Classification of Erythroid Hypoplasia

Congenital
  Diamond-Blackfan syndrome
Acquired "pure red cell aplasia"
  With thymoma
  No thymoma
Hematologic malignancies
  Acute leukemia
  Chronic leukemia
  Multiple myeloma
  Hodgkin's disease
"Aplastic crisis" in chronic hemolytic disorders
Drugs
  Diphenylhydantoin
  Chloramphenicol
  Cephalothin
  Chlorpropamide
  Sulfonamides
Riboflavin deficiency

destruction of erythroid precursors. Antibodies, cytotoxic for erythroblasts, have been demonstrated in the immunoglobulin G fraction of plasma of several patients with pure red cell aplasia (11). In one patient with panhypoplasia of the marrow, an inhibitor of erythropoietin was found (12). Hypogammaglobulinemia is present in 18% of patients with thymoma and pure red cell aplasia (13). In addition, myasthenia gravis occurs in about 15% of affected patients. Occasionally, immunologic abnormalities, such as antinuclear antibodies, a positive direct Coombs' reaction, positive cold agglutinin test, or a false-positive test for syphilis, have been found.

When a thymoma is present, thymectomy results in remission of the anemia in approximately 25–30% of patients with pure red cell aplasia. Because the disorder is apparently immunologically mediated, cortiocosteroids and immunosuppressive agents such as cyclophosphamide have been used in treatment, with beneficial results in some patients. Splenectomy occasionally causes improvement in the anemia. In patients in whom the anemia is responsive to thymectomy or to immunosuppressive therapy the serum inhibitor of erythropoiesis may no longer be demonstrable (14).

Case 4

A 64-year-old salesman was referred for hematologic consultation concerning an anemia. Five weeks previously he had noted the appearance of pallor and weakness. Two weeks later he saw his family physician, who found the hemoglobin level to be 7.5 g/dl. He received transfusions of five units of blood during the two weeks before consultation. Ten years previously he was found to have myasthenia gravis; symptoms were subsequently fairly well controlled with medications.

Physical examination disclosed moderate ptosis of the left eyelid, slight ptosis of the right eyelid, bilateral facial weakness, and easy fatigue of the muscles in all extremities. No enlargement of lymph nodes, liver, or spleen was found.

His hemoglobin value was 11.4 g/dl (history of recent transfusions), hematocrit 32%, reticulocyte count 0.0%, platelet count 391,000/mm^3, and total leukocyte count 7,700/mm^3, with a normal differential count. Examination of a peripheral blood film disclosed normochromic normocytic erythrocytes with no morphologic abnormalities. Bone marrow aspirate revealed normal megakaryocytes and granulopoiesis but no erythroid precursors. No incorporation of radioiron into new erythrocytes was found by a ferrokinetic study. Urinary erythropoietin level was elevated. Serum protein electrophoresis disclosed a value of 2.0 g/dl for the gammaglobulin. Roentgenograms of the chest showed a large anterior mediastinal mass (Fig. 8-6). At this point the most likely hematologic diagnosis was considered to be erythroid aplasia related to a thymoma.

Thoracotomy was performed. An anterior mediastinal mass was encountered. The mass could not be resected because it extended into the superior vena cava and into the strap muscles. Histologic sections of a biopsy of the mass revealed a thymoma, predominantly of the spindle cell type (Fig. 8-7). Radiation, amounting to 4,000 rads, was directed at the tumor mass. For a period of four days during the course of radiation therapy the reticulocyte count rose, to a maximum of 1.8%, then fell to zero. The patient's myasthenia gravis was much improved

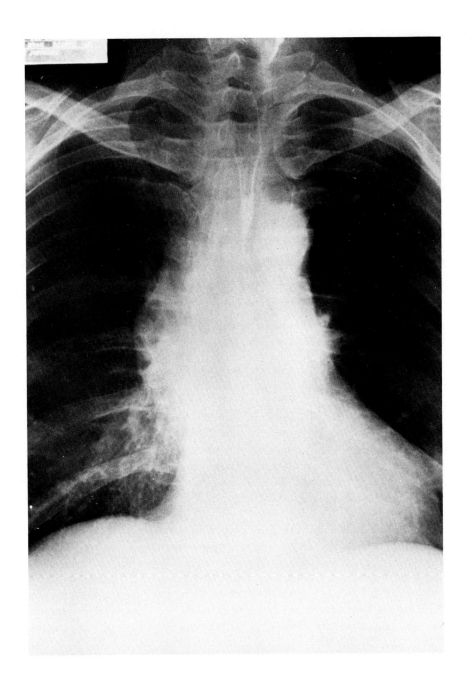

Figure 8-6. Roentgenogram of the chest demonstrated a mediastinal mass in Case 4. The lateral radiographic projection showed the mass to be in the anterior mediastinum.

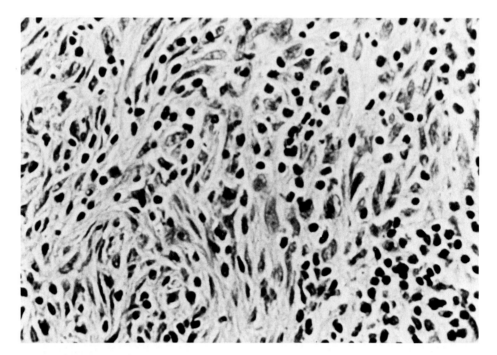

Figure 8-7. Biopsy of an anterior mediastinal mass in Case 4 established the diagnosis of thymoma of the spindle-cell type. (Magnification 525×.)

after the radiotherapy, but the anemia was not benefited. With subsequent treatment with prednisone and fluoxymesterone for several months, no reticulocytes were ever found and severe anemia persisted.

Comment

In this patient erythroid aplasia and myasthenia gravis were associated with a thymoma of the spindle cell type. Leukopenia, thrombocytopenia, and hypo-gammaglobulinemia were not present. Radiotherapy directed at the thymoma resulted in improvement in the myasthenia gravis but not in the erythroid aplasia.

In seven reported patients with pure red cell aplasia, acute leukemia appeared as a terminal event (15). Other hematologic malignancies that rarely may be associated with pure red cell aplasia are chronic lymphocytic leukemia (16), chronic myelogenous leukemia (17), multiple myeloma (18), and Hodgkin's disease (19).

Seven patients with pure red cell aplasia have been reported in whom carcinoma later appeared (20). The interval between the onset of the anemia and the discovery of the carcinoma varied from six weeks to three years. The causal relationship between the two disorders is uncertain.

APLASTIC ANEMIA

Patients with aplastic anemia ordinarily have pancytopenia (anemia, granulocytopenia, and thrombocytopenia). Morphologically the erythrocytes are normochromic and normocytic with little or no anisocytosis or poikilocytosis. Reticulocytopenia is present. Marrow aspirate and biopsy are needed to differentiate aplastic anemia from other causes of pancytopenia. Examination of the aspirate discloses hypocellularity with spicules consisting mainly of fat cells rather than hematopoietic cells. Prussian blue stain reveals abundant iron in the marrow particles. Biopsy of the marrow is necessary to confirm the diagnosis of aplastic anemia because hypocellular aspirates may be found in other disorders, particularly in patients with infiltrative diseases of the marrow. In patients with aplastic anemia, the marrow biopsy shows a paucity of hematopoietic cells and an abundance of fat cells.

Values of the serum iron are generally greater than normal in patients with aplastic anemia, while values of the serum iron-binding capacity are less than normal. Thus, the percentage saturation of the serum iron-binding protein is substantially above normal and may approach 100% when there is severe erythroid hypoplasia. Ferrokinetic studies show low to normal values for plasma iron turnover with much reduced incorporation of the radioiron into new erythrocytes.

It is commonly difficult to pinpoint the underlying cause of aplastic anemia, and, thus, in large clinical studies substantial percentages of cases are classified as "idiopathic" (Table 8-3). So-called idiopathic aplastic anemia is sometimes followed by acute leukemia. Sixty-three such cases have been reported (15).

Fanconi's anemia is an uncommon congenital hypoplastic anemia with pancytopenia that becomes evident in the first few years of life. Associated nonhematologic abnormalities are common and include renal and splenic hypoplasia, microcephaly, mental retardation, and hypoplasia of the thumb or radius. Chromosomal studies of marrow cells are generally abnormal, with findings such as chromosomal breakages, chromatid exchanges, and chromosomal gaps. From the standpoint of neoplasia, it is significant that there is a high incidence of transformation of this congenital hypoplastic anemia to acute leukemia, either myeloblastic or myelomonocytic (15,21). In addition, there may be a predisposition in Fanconi's anemia to the development of squamous cell carcinomas and hepatocellular carcinoma (22,23).

Exposure to certain drugs represents the most commonly discovered underlying cause of acquired aplastic anemia. By a wide margin chloramphenicol has been the most frequently cited causative therapeutic agent. Other drugs in which the relationship with aplastic anemia seems established are phenylbutazone, gold salts, sulfonamides, sulfonylurea compounds, quinacrine, and certain anticonvulsants (phenantoin and diphenylhydrantoin). Fortunately, the incidence of aplastic anemia in persons taking these drugs is quite low. Occasionally persons with aplastic anemia due to chloramphenicol or to phenylbutazone later develop

Table 8-3. Classification of Aplastic Anemia

Idiopathic acquired
Congenital (Fanconi's syndrome)
Drugs and chemicals
Irradiation
Viral hepatitis
Paroxysmal nocturnal hemoglobinuria
Miscellaneous

acute leukemia (24–26). The temporal relationship of leukemia to chloramphenicol therapy usually consists of protracted marrow hypoplasia followed by acute myeloblastic leukemia (24,25). Pierre (15) in 1974 found in a search of the medical literature 27 cases of acute leukemia attributed to chloramphenicol and 27 cases of acute leukemia (24 acute nonlymphoblastic) in which phenylbutazone was implicated as a causative agent.

The most commonly reported chemical agent to be associated with the development of pancytopenia is benzene. The relationship of benzene to bone marrow dysfunction was well established by studies in American industry 40 years ago. With subsequent lowered exposure to benzene, the frequency of cases in industrial workers declined. The marrow aspirate may be either hypocellular or hyperplastic in affected persons. In patients sustaining pancytopenia related to benzene, there is clearly an increased incidence of the subsequent development of acute leukemia, usually myeloblastic in type (27). Pierre (15), in his review of the medical literature, collected 105 cases of acute leukemia thought to be secondary to exposure to benzene.

Ionizing irradiation is another example of an agent that may cause both aplastic anemia and acute leukemia. The increased incidence of acute myeloblastic leukemia in patients with Hodgkin's disease may be related, in part, to radiation therapy (28). The addition of chemotherapy to radiation therapy substantially increases the likelihood of acute leukemia (29).

Among other causes of aplastic anemia, mostly rare, are viral hepatitis, systemic lupus erythematosus, congenital immunodeficiency disorders in children, and paroxysmal nocturnal hemoglobinuria (PNH). Patients with PNH may occasionally during the course of their illness sustain aplastic anemia. Additionally, patients who initially have aplastic anemia may have the PNH defect of their erythrocytes demonstrable by sucrose hemolysis or acid hemolysis tests.

MEGALOBLASTIC ANEMIA

The megaloblastic anemias are generally due to deficiency of either vitamin B_{12} or folic acid. Other causes include erythroleukemia, an uncommon form of acute leukemia, and the therapeutic administration of certain drugs, largely antineoplastic agents, which inhibit nucleic acid synthesis in hematopoietic cells. Megaloblastic anemias are macrocytic, judged both by red cell indices and by examination of peripheral blood films. There is marked anisocytosis, with microcytes as well as macrocytes seen. Small numbers of nucleated erythrocytes with megaloblastic nuclear features may be found in the peripheral blood and provide a valuable clue to the mechanism of the anemia. The reticulocyte count is not elevated, indicating that marrow dysfunction is responsible for the anemia. Granulocytopenia is frequent, with hypersegmented neutrophils observed microscopically. Thrombocytopenia likewise is very common. A greater than normal percentage of the platelets are large.

The bone marrow aspirate shows hyperplasia of erythroid, granulocytic, and megakaryocytic elements. Megaloblastic erythropoiesis is the prominent diagnostic feature. Erythroid precursors have nuclei that are larger and have more finely dispersed chromatin than one would expect for a particular stage of development. While nuclear maturation is delayed, cytoplasmic development of erythroid precursors proceeds more or less normally (so-called nuclear-cytoplasmic asynchrony). Granulopoiesis is characterized both by similar changes in the nuclear chromatin and a propensity for the midmyeloid cells, that is, myelocytes and metamyelocytes, to be unusually large. Prussian blue stains disclose abundant iron in both histiocytes and erythroid precursors.

"Ineffective erythropoiesis" is the term used to designate the mechanism of anemia in the megaloblastic anemias. Erythroid precursors are plentiful in the marrow, but output of new erythrocytes is inappropriately low judged by the reticulocyte count. Ferrokinetic studies reveal increased plasma iron turnover indicative of increased *total* erythropoiesis but much reduced incorporation of radioiron into new erythrocytes, because of *ineffective erythropoiesis*. This disparity between total erythropoiesis and effective erythropoiesis is attributable to ineffective erythropoiesis.

Approximately 75% of patients with megaloblastic anemia due to vitamin B_{12} deficiency have subacute combined system disease and/or peripheral neuropathy. Folic acid deficiency does not result in these pathologic changes. Combined system disease refers to degeneration of the posterior and lateral columns of the spinal cord. Patients deficient in vitamin B_{12} complicated by neurologic deficit complain of parathesias of the feet and hands and distal weakness. On examination diminished vibratory sensation and proprioception distally in the extremities, weakness, and, commonly, a positive Babinski reaction are found. More severe neurologic abnormalities due to vitamin B_{12} deficiency include ataxia, optic atrophy, and organic psychosis.

Once the physician has established the presence of a megaloblastic anemia, the next step is to distinguish vitamin B_{12} deficiency from folic acid deficiency. In most instances this is accomplished by measurement of serum levels of vitamin B_{12} and folic acid and the red cell folate content. Alternatively, the response to specific therapy, judged by serial values of hemoglobin, hematocrit, and percentage of reticulocytes, may be used. To avoid nonspecific responses to treatment, small doses of vitamin B_{12} (1–5 µg IM daily) or folic acid (50–200 µg daily) must be used.

The causes of vitamin B_{12} deficiency are numerous (Table 8-4). Dietary deficiency is rare in the United States. Pernicious anemia is characterized by gastric atrophy, achlorhydria, and deficiency of production of intrinsic factor by the stomach. Intrinsic factor is necessary for the absorption of vitamin B_{12} in the ileum. The Schilling tests (stages I and II) are used to establish pernicious anemia as the cause of vitamin B_{12} deficiency in a particular patient. In the stage I Schilling test in pernicious anemia, cobalt radiolabeled vitamin B_{12} administered orally is poorly absorbed and thus little radioactivity is excreted in the urine. Less than 7% of the orally administered radiolabel is found in the urine in 24 hours and, in fact, commonly less than 2% is identified in the urine. Intrinsic factor is administered with the radiolabeled vitamin B_{12} in the stage II Schilling test. In patients with pernicious anemia the vitamin B_{12} is absorbed normally in the presence of intrinsic factor and more than 7% of the isotope is found in the urine. In persons with disorders of the ileum, poor absorption of vitamin B_{12} is found in both stages of the Schilling test. The procedure for the Schilling test involves intramuscular administration of 1,000 µg of unlabeled vitamin B_{12} in

Table 8-4. Classification of Vitamin B_{12} Deficiency

Stage I Schilling test normal
    Dietary deficiency of vitamin B_{12}
Stage I Schilling test abnormal, stage II normal
    Pernicious anemia
    Gastrectomy
Stage I and stage II Schilling tests abnormal
    Sprue, celiac disease
    Intestinal infiltrative diseases
    Crohn's disease
    Ileal resection or bypass
    Drug-related malabsorption
    Bacterial overgrowth
    Fish tapeworm infestation
    Chronic pancreatic insufficiency

order to flush out labeled absorbed vitamin B_{12} into the urine. Thus, all patients given a Shilling test receive a therapeutic dose of vitamin B_{12}.

There are two main relationships of vitamin B_{12} deficiency to malignancies. One is carcinoma of the stomach and the other is lymphoma of the small bowel. Carcinoma of the stomach, like pernicious anemia, is frequently associated with gastric atrophy and achlorhydria. Rarely, pernicious anemia and carcinoma of the stomach coexist at the time of initial presentation of a patient (30). More frequent is the appearance of carcinoma of the stomach several years after the diagnosis and treatment of pernicious anemia. At the Boston City Hospital approximately 10% of patients with pernicious anemia developed cancer of the stomach on an average of 6.6 years after the appearance of the anemia (30). Among 2,115 autopsies performed on patients with pernicious anemia, Chanarin (31) found the incidence of carcinoma of the stomach to be 5.2%. Gastric carcinoma is distinctly more likely to occur in patients with pernicious anemia who have blood group A (32). In addition to carcinoma of the stomach, there may be a relationship between pernicious anemia and gastric carcinoid, a rare tumor. Five such cases have been reported (33). Lymphomas extensively involving the ileum may prevent adequate absorption of vitamin B_{12} and provoke the deficiency state. Such cases, however, are rare.

Case 5

A 79-year-old woman was referred for evaluation of an anemia. Three months previously, she was hospitalized in her community hospital with weakness. She was told that she was "anemic and low on protein." She thereafter took iron and protein supplements, but weakness and the anemia persisted. Anorexia and ankle edema appeared. She denied weight loss, fever, abdominal pain, diarrhea, and melena.

The past history was of interest in that the patient was given a diagnosis of pernicious anemia 45 years previously by her father, who was a physician. Her anemia responded to liver shots for many years. During the past 20 years, she had taken an intramuscular injection of vitamin B_{12} every other day. A recent stage I Schilling test had shown less than 1% excretion of the radioisotope.

Physical examination revealed general debility and moderate pallor but no jaundice. A mass, thought to be the spleen, was felt in the left upper quadrant of the abdomen extending 4 cm below the left costal margin. The liver was not enlarged. There was no ascites, but two plus edema of the ankles was detected bilaterally. Deep tendon reflexes were two plus positive at the knees but absent at the ankles. Proprioception and vibratory sensations were good.

Her hemoglobin value was 8.7 g/dl, hematocrit 28%, red blood cell count 3.58 million/mm^3, reticulocyte count 1.4%, platelet count 700,000/mm^3, and total leukocyte count 24,800/mm^3, with a differential count of 87 segmented neutrophils, 4 bands, 1 eosinophil, 4 monocytes, and 4 lymphocytes. Examination of a peripheral blood film showed a mildly hypochromic, microcytic erythrocyte population. Leukocyte alkaline phosphatase score was 143 (control score 84). Serum iron level was 10 μg/dl with a serum iron-binding capacity of 153 μg/dl. Bone marrow aspirate revealed orderly granulopoiesis, abundant megakaryocytes, and normoblastic erythropoiesis. Histiocytes contained much iron but erythroblast iron was reduced. Three stool samples gave negative reactions for occult blood. Urinalysis was normal except for mild pyuria. Roentgenograms of the chest showed no evidence of cardiac or active pulmonary disease. Prothrombin time was 12.4 seconds, serum albumin 1.2 g/dl, serum globulin 3.0 g/dl, serum alkaline phosphatase 75 units (normal range 30–80 units), SGOT 11 units, and SGPT 4 units.

At this stage of the diagnostic evaluation the mechanism of the patient's anemia was judged to be the anemia of chronic disorders. A radioisotopic scan of the liver and spleen, obtained because of the palpable left upper abdominal mass, showed both organs to be normal in size. Barium enema was normal. Upper gastrointestinal radiographs showed distorted gastric folds along the greater curvature and in the antrum of the stomach, probably due to a carcinoma. Roentgenograms of the small bowel were normal. At gastroscopy a large friable mass on the greater curvature was observed. Biopsies of the mass disclosed histologically a poorly differentiated adenocarcinoma. When informed of the diagnosis, the patient declined specific treatment. She developed marked ascites and edema and died about one month later.

Comment

In this unusual case carcinoma of the stomach appeared 45 years after the initial diagnosis of pernicious anemia. The gastric malignancy was responsible for an anemia of chronic disorders, leukocytosis, thrombocytosis, and severe hypoalbuminemia, presumably related to gastric loss of the protein.

The diverse causes of folic acid deficiency can be divided into four groups: (1) dietary deficiency, (2) impaired absorption, (3) increased metabolic demand for folic acid, and (4) therapy with folic acid antagonists (Table 8-5). Deficiency of folic acid is more frequently associated with malignancies than is deficiency of vitamin B$_{12}$. In persons with localized malignancies, values of the serum folate are usually normal. However, folate levels are commonly decreased in patients with disseminated neoplasms. Generally, the degree of folic acid deficiency is not sufficient to result in megaloblastic erythropoiesis. Treatment with folic acid rarely results in an improvement in the anemia of patients with a malignancy except when the marrow aspirate shows definite megaloblastic changes. Multiple

Table 8-5. Classification of Folic Acid Deficiency

Dietary deficiency
    Megaloblastic anemia of infancy
    Alcoholism
    Advanced neoplastic disease
Impaired small intestinal absorption
    Sprue, celiac disease
    Intestinal infiltrative diseases
    Crohn's disease
    Drug-related malabsorption
Increased metabolic requirements
    Infancy
    Pregnancy
    Chronically increased erythropoiesis
    Neoplastic disease
    Psoriasis
    Hemodialysis
Therapy with folic acid antagonists

myeloma and acute leukemia are the neoplasms most commonly associated with low values of the serum folate. Among patients with multiple myeloma, those with the highest amounts of production of paraprotein are the most likely to have decreased values of the serum folate (34).

There are three mechanisms for folic acid deficiency in patients with malignancies. The most common is dietary deficiency related to the anorexia common with advanced cancer. The minimum dietary requirement for folic acid is 50 μg per day. A second, albeit rare, mechanism is impaired absorption of folic acid in the small intestine due to a tumor such as a lymphoma. Third, folic acid deficiency may result from increased metabolic demands for the vitamin by the neoplasm. Such might be expected with highly proliferative processes such as leukemia and multiple myeloma (34).

Erythroleukemia is a leukemic process, usually acute but occasionally chronic, that can in its early stages be confused with megaloblastic anemias due to deficiency of either vitamin B_{12} or folic acid. Acute erythroleukemia is best classified as a variant of acute myeloblastic leukemia. Patients have a normocytic or macrocytic anemia, reticulocytopenia, thrombocytopenia, and, usually, granulocytopenia. The marrow aspirate discloses numerous erythroid precursors with megaloblastic features. In some cases very bizarre nuclear forms in erythroblasts and striking erythroid multinuclearity allow distinction from the classic megaloblastic picture of vitamin B_{12} or folic acid deficiency. Additionally, in erythroleukemia, usually there is an increased number of myeloblasts pointing toward the leukemic nature of the process. In contrast to vitamin B_{12} and folic acid deficiency, in which small numbers of nucleated red cells (less than 10 per 100 leukocytes) are found in the blood, in erythroleukemia there are sometimes large numbers of bizarre erythroblasts in the blood. The periodic acid-Schiff (PAS) reaction is positive in some cases of erythroleukemia, with large red cytoplasmic granules observed microscopically in the erythroblasts. On the other hand, the PAS reaction is negative in the marrow erythroid precursors of vitamin

B_{12} deficiency and folic acid deficiency. Results of ferrokinetic studies are consistent with ineffective erythropoiesis when performed in patients with erythroleukemia. Serum vitamin B_{12} levels are normal or elevated, while values for serum folate are normal or decreased. The natural course of erythroleukemia is characterized by diminishing numbers of erythroblasts in the blood and marrow with increasing numbers of myeloblasts in the marrow and sometimes in the blood. The clinical picture becomes that of acute myeloblastic leukemia. While most cases of erythroleukemia occur de novo, occasionally polycythemia vera, chronic myelogenous leukemia, or myelofibrosis undergo transformation to erythroleukemia during the preterminal phase of the illness.

Case 6

In a visit to her family physician a 39-year-old woman complained of fatigue, headaches, and palpitations of two weeks duration. Her hematocrit value was 13% and platelet count 28,000/mm^3. A bone marrow aspirate disclosed markedly megaloblastic erythropoiesis (Fig. 8-8). The serum vitamin B_{12} level was elevated, while the value of the serum folate was mildly decreased. Stage I Schilling test yielded normal results. She received transfusions of two units of packed red blood cells and treatment with folic acid orally and later parenterally. Her symptoms were relieved by the transfusions, but the anemia did not respond to folic acid therapy administered for 12 days. Because of the lack of response, her

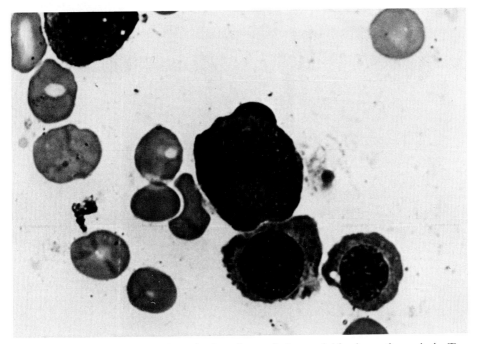

Figure 8-8. Bone marrow aspirate in Case 6 revealed megaloblastic erythropoiesis. Two polychromatophilic megaloblasts and one promegaloblast are pictured. (Magnification 1,250×.)

physician reviewed the marrow aspirate again and noted some immature leukocyte precursor cells (Fig. 8-9). The patient was then referred for hematologic consultation.

The only abnormal physical findings were marked pallor, small retinal hemorrhages, and ecchymoses of the lower extremities. The hemoglobin value was 6.4 g/dl, hematocrit 19%, platelet count 11,000/mm³, total leukocyte count 3,000/mm³, and differential count 19 segmented neutrophils, 1 band, 6 monocytes, and 74 lymphocytes. Examination of a peripheral blood film disclosed moderate anisocytosis with a moderate number of macrocytes and occasional teardrop red cells. Reticulocyte count was 0.1%. Bone marrow aspirate was hypercellular. Erythropoiesis was increased in amount and markedly megaloblastic. Monocytes were increased in number (20% of marrow cells) with many immature forms. Granulopoiesis was disorderly, with myeloblasts constituting 15% of the marrow cells. Few late granulocytic precursors were seen. Many of the erythroblasts had PAS-positive cytoplasmic granules. The diagnosis of erythroleukemia was made. The patient was treated with cytosine arabinoside and 6-thioguanine. During the first six weeks she sustained several hemorrhagic and infectious complications, but the leukemia then entered remission with attainment of normal peripheral blood counts. She received additional chemotherapy. After 5 years the leukemia remains in remission.

Comment

The patient had a severe megaloblastic anemia. Underlying leukemia was not suspected until vitamin B_{12} and folic acid deficiencies were excluded both by

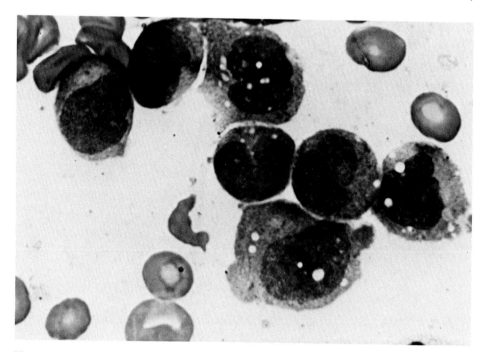

Figure 8-9. Immature monocytic precursors and blast cells in the bone marrow of a patient with erythroleukemia (Case 6). (Magnification 1,250×.)

diagnostic tests and failure of response to therapy. The case illustrates that erythroleukemia can prove difficult to differentiate from vitamin B_{12} or folic acid deficiency.

Drugs that inhibit DNA synthesis directly or indirectly may result in megaloblastic changes in the bone marrow. Folic acid antagonists cause deficiency of the folate coenzymes necessary for DNA synthesis. Pyrimethamine and trimethoprim are examples of folic acid antagonists that may induce a mild megaloblastic anemia. Antineoplastic folic acid antagonists such as methotrexate, an inhibitor of di-hydrofolate reductase, cause megaloblastic hematopoiesis. When the reaction is severe, the marrow is commonly not only megaloblastic but hypocellular as well. Other chemotherapeutic agents that may result in megaloblastic and hypoplastic marrow changes are the purine antagonists 6-mercaptopurine, 6-thioguanine, and azathioprine, and the inhibitors of deoxyribonucleotide synthesis cytosine arabinoside, hydroxyurea, and doxorubicin (Adriamycin).

SIDEROBLASTIC ANEMIA

The diagnostic hallmark of sideroblastic anemia is the recognition of ringed sideroblasts in marrow aspirates subjected to the Prussian blue reaction. Ringed sideroblasts are normoblasts in which the nucleus is encircled by Prussian blue-positive granules (Fig. 8-10). The unique appearance results from iron loading of the mitochondria surrounding the nucleus of the normoblast.

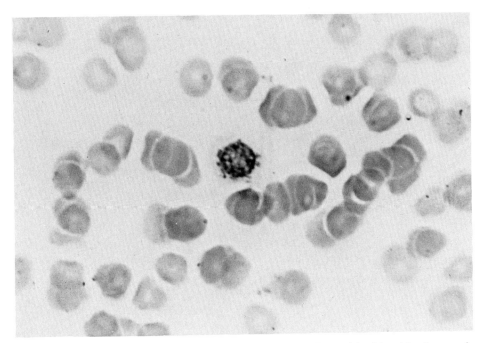

Figure 8-10. Prussian blue stain of the marrow of a patient with sideroblastic anemia reveals a "ringed" sideroblast. (Magnification $1,250\times$.)

Examination of the peripheral blood film commonly reveals a dimorphic red blood cell population with some erythrocytes distinctly hypochromic and microcytic while others are normocytic or macrocytic (Fig. 8-11). Usually the red cell indices are normochromic and normocytic, although they are occasionally macrocytic. The reticulocyte count is inappropriately low for the degree of anemia. Siderocytes, that is, hemosiderin-containing erythrocytes, may be observed with Prussian blue staining of blood films. Leukopenia and thrombocytopenia are variably noted.

Examination of a marrow aspirate discloses erythroid hyperplasia, sometimes a shift toward younger erythroid forms, and commonly megaloblastic nuclear features. Multinuclearity and nuclear pyknosis of erythroblasts are occasionally observed. Although infrequent, the discovery of a late normoblast with very poor hemoglobinization and coarse cytoplasmic basophilic stippling is very suggestive of sideroblastic anemia. In some patients there is a shift to earlier precursor cells in the granulocytic series. The Prussian blue reaction affords the diagnosis—ringed sideroblasts. Histiocytic iron is usually increased in amount.

The predominant mechanism of the anemia is ineffective erythropoiesis, exemplified by (1) erythroid hyperplasia much in excess of that expected by the reticulocyte count and (2) elevated plasma iron turnover with decreased incorporation of radioiron into new erythrocytes. When granulocytopenia and thrombocytopenia occur, they are usually due to ineffective hematopoiesis; the number of precursor cells in the marrow is generally ample. Values of leukocyte alkaline phosphatase are reduced in approximately one-half of patients.

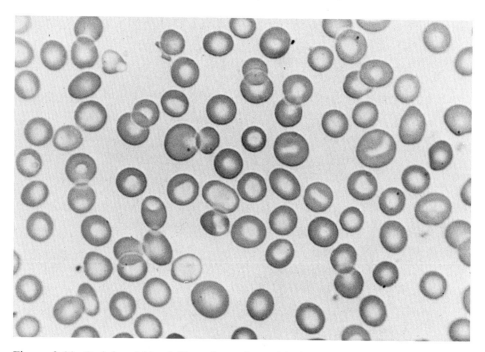

Figure 8-11. Peripheral blood film of a patient with sideroblastic anemia. Note that a majority of the erythrocytes are normochromic normocytic, some are hypochromic microcytic, and a few are macrocytic. (Magnification 800×.)

Table 8-6. Classification of Sideroblastic Anemia

Hereditary
Idiopathic acquired
Alcoholism
Drug-related
Lead poisoning
Hematologic disorders
  Myeloblastic leukemia
  Preleukemia
  Myelofibrosis
  Multiple myeloma
Carcinoma
Miscellaneous
  Rheumatoid arthritis
  Polyarteritis nodosa
  Myxedema

Frequently, an underlying cause cannot be identified in patients with sideroblastic anemia, and thus the illness is diagnosed as idiopathic acquired sideroblastic anemia. However, the physician should actively seek an etiology, because both prognosis and therapy are related to causation (Table 8-6). Hereditary cases are rare. The most common form of secondary sideroblastic anemia is that related to alcoholism. Such patients commonly have folic acid deficiency as well as sideroblastic anemia. Discontinuation of alcohol usually results in rapid improvement in the anemia. Additionally, the administration of pyridoxine and/or folic acid is often beneficial. Sideroblastic anemia may occur during the treatment of tuberculosis with isoniazid, pyrazinamide, or cycloserine and with the use of chloramphenicol (35). Ringed sideroblasts are sometimes found in the marrow aspirates of anemic patients with lead intoxication. Other disorders occasionally associated with sideroblastic anemia are rheumatoid arthritis, periarteritis nodosa, tuberculosis, hyperthyroidism, myxedema, uremia, and Hodgkin's disease (35). In these disorders a causal relationship of sideroblastic anemia to the nonhematologic disorder has not been clearly demonstrated. A small number of patients with coexistent sideroblastic anemia and carcinoma have been reported (36,37). In our clinic we have seen sideroblastic anemia in one patient with bronchogenic carcinoma and in one patient with metastatic squamous cell carcinoma of unknown primary site.

The association of sideroblastic anemia with certain hematologic disorders, particularly myeloblastic leukemia and myelofibrosis, is firmly established. At the time of diagnosis of acute myeloblastic leukemia or erythroleukemia, ringed sideroblasts are occasionally found in the bone marrow aspirate. More frequent and more important from a diagnostic standpoint are patients who are initially seen with a sideroblastic anemia, but months or a few years later develop unequivocal acute leukemia. The leukemia may be myeloblastic, monoblastic, or erythroleukemic in type. When the acquired Pelger-Hüet anomaly (Figs. 8-12 and 8-13) of the granulocytes accompanies sideroblastic anemia, almost invari-

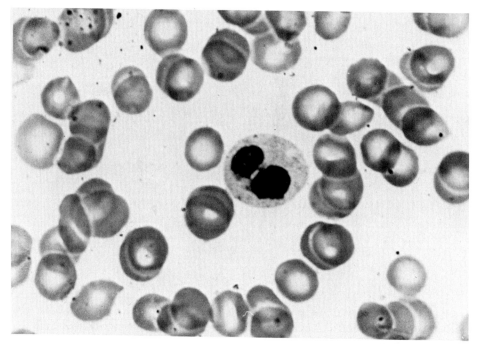

Figure 8-12. Bilobed neutrophilic granulocyte in the peripheral blood of a patient with sideroblastic anemia and the acquired Pelger-Hüet anomaly. (Magnification 1,250×.)

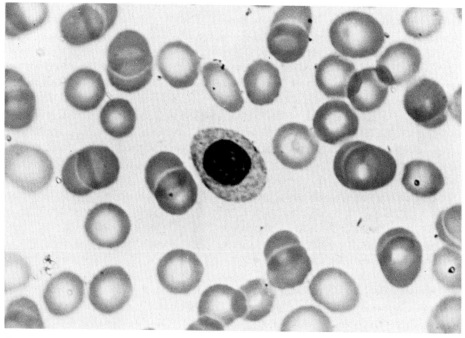

Figure 8-13. The acquired Pelger-Hüet anomaly. Failure of nuclear segmentation of a mature granulocyte is pictured. The granulocyte is called a Stodtmeister cell. (Magnification 1,250×.)

ably the illness terminates as acute leukemia. The leukemia is usually very poorly responsive to chemotherapy.

Case 7

An 82-year-old man was referred for evaluation of an anemia of three years duration. Previous bone marrow aspirates had been hypercellular, but no specific diagnosis had been made. Except for weakness due to the anemia, he had no symptoms. During the three years he had received 13 units of blood by transfusion. Except for pallor, there were no relevant physical findings. Neither the liver nor the spleen were enlarged.

His hemoglobin value was 8.6 g/dl, hematocrit 26%, reticulocyte count 0.9%, platelet count 210,000/mm^3, and total leukocyte count 4,900/mm^3, with a differential count of 34% mature granulocytes, 34% lymphocytes, and 32% monocytes. Approximately one-third of the granulocytes had nuclear characteristics of the acquired Pelger-Hüet anomaly. The erythrocytes were overal normochromic normocytic with some hypochromic microcytic forms. There was marked poikilocytosis with elliptocytes, teardrop erythrocytes, and schistocytes evident. Marrow aspirate was hypercellular. The myeloid to erythroid ratio was 4:1. Myelocytes predominated in the granulocytic series with a decreased number of more mature forms. Erythroid precursors showed poor hemoglobinization. The Prussian blue reaction disclosed numerous ringed sideroblasts.

The patient was treated with 200 mg daily pyridoxine and 40 mg daily fluoxymesterone. Later 1 mg daily folic acid was added. The anemia, however, did not improve and transfusions were required periodically. Six months after initial consultation his anemia was worse (hematocrit 20%) and thrombocytopenia (platelet count 44,000/mm^3) had appeared. Four months later the hematologic picture became frankly leukemic, with hematocrit 18%, platelet count 62,000/mm^3, and total leukocyte count 211,200/mm^3 with 92% monoblasts on differential count. He received treatment with cytosine arabinoside and 6-thioguanine, but his condition progressively deteriorated leading to death four weeks later.

Comment

In this patient sideroblastic anemia represented a preleukemic state to acute monoblastic leukemia. The presence of mature granulocytes with impaired nuclear segmentation (acquired Pelger-Hüet anomaly) was a valuable clue pointing to the ultimate leukemic outcome of the hematologic illness.

Sideroblastic anemia is seen in some patients with myelofibrosis. Among 148 patients with myelofibrosis seen by our group, 13 had sideroblastic erythropoiesis. A few patients have been reported in whom sideroblastic anemia appeared late in the course of polycythemia vera (38). These patients had pancytopenia and subsequently developed fulminant acute myeloid or myelomonocytic leukemia.

Sideroblastic anemia occasionally appears during the course of multiple myeloma (37,39). Some of these patients subsequently develop acute leukemia, usually myelomonocytic (40). Treatment of multiple myeloma, or lymphomas with alkylating agents such as melphalan or cyclophosphamide, is associated with a significantly increased incidence of acute leukemia (41). In patients treated chronically with alkylating drugs, sideroblastic anemia represents a preleukemic state (40,42).

AUTOIMMUNE HEMOLYTIC ANEMIA

Autoimmune hemolytic anemia (AHD) may be due to warm- or cold-reacting antibodies. Warm antibody hemolytic anemia is more common. This antibody shows maximum reactivity with erythrocytes at temperatures around 37°C. Specific antisera reveal that the erythrocytes are coated with an immunoglobulin, usually IgG and/or complement. The antibodies may be directed at a specific red cell antigen (such as an Rh group antigen) or no antigen specificity may be identified. Antibody-coated erythrocytes are removed by macrophages in the reticuloendothelial system, particularly the spleen, causing shortening of red cell life span.

Examination of the peripheral blood film commonly discloses many spherocytes and numerous polychromatophilic erythrocytes (Fig. 8-14). A brisk reticulocytosis is found. The direct Coombs' reaction is usually positive, indicating the presence of immunoglobulins and/or complement on the surface of erythrocytes. If free antibodies to erythrocytes are also present in the serum, the indirect Coombs' reaction will also be positive. Occasionally in patients with autoimmune hemolysis, the direct Coombs' reaction is negative because the number of molecules of antibody on the surface of erythrocytes is insufficient to be

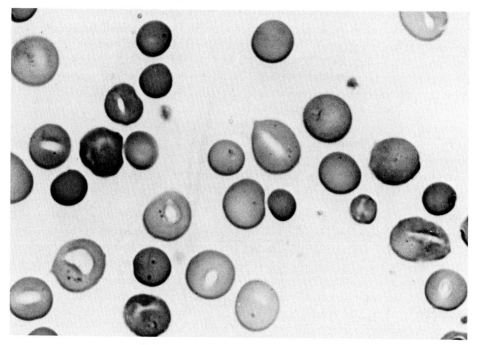

Figure 8-14. Spherocytes and polychromatophilic erythrocytes in the peripheral blood of a patient with autoimmune hemolytic anemia. (Magnification 1,250×.)

detected by the antiglobulin test. With a more sophisticated method, Gilliland and coworkers (43) demonstrated red cell antibodies in these patients.

Upon establishing warm antibody autoimmune hemolysis as the mechanism of an anemia, it is very important that the physician seek an underlying disorder responsible for AHD (Table 8-7). After careful diagnostic studies 25–50% of cases of AHD are classified as idiopathic. Among the most common causes of AHD are the collagen vascular disorders, particularly systemic lupus erythematosus. Evans' syndrome refers to the unusual association of idiopathic AHD and idiopathic thrombocytopenic purpura. The use of a number of drugs, such as alpha methyldopa, quinidine, and penicillin, can result in immune hemolysis.

In a review of 234 patients with AHD, Pirofsky (44) found an associated reticuloendothelial neoplasm in 114 or 48%. Chronic lymphocytic leukemia was the most frequent malignancy, accounting for 48 patients in Pirofsky's series. Ten to 20% of patients with chronic lymphocytic leukemia develop overt AHD at some point during the course of their illness. Thirty-seven percent are reported to have a positive direct Coombs' test (45). Other lymphomas, such as lymphocytic lymphoma, Hodgkin's disease, and histiocytic lymphoma, may be complicated by AHD (44,46–48). The incidence of AHD in Hodgkin's disease is approximately 3% (49). Usually the Hodgkin's disease is Stage III or IV at the time AHD appears. However, rarely AHD antedates the recognition of Hodgkin's disease (50). Less commonly, AHD is seen in patients with acute lymphoblastic leukemia, acute myeloblastic leukemia, chronic myelogenous leukemia, monocytic leukemia, multiple myeloma, and thymoma (44). The direct Coombs' test is positive in approximately one-third of patients with angioimmunoblastic lymphadenopathy. In one study, four of 25 patients with this disorder had overt autoimmune hemolytic anemia (51).

In patients with AHD associated with a reticuloendothelial malignancy, Pirofsky (44) reported the malignancy was discovered first in 61%, the AHD was diagnosed first in 7%, and the two conditions were found simultaneously in 32%. Therapy of the AHD should be initiated with corticosteroids (daily doses of 60–

Table 8-7. Classification of Autoimmune Hemolytic Anemia due to Warm Antibodies

Idiopathic acquired
Collagen vascular disorders
Evans' syndrome
Hematologic disorders
   Lymphoproliferative disorders
   Hodgkin's disease
   Immunoblastic lymphadenopathy
   Myeloproliferative disorders
Solid tumors
   Ovarian teratoma
   Carcinoma
Infection
Sarcoid
Drug-related

100 mg prednisone). Splenectomy can be beneficial when corticosteroid therapy fails. Control of the neoplastic process with chemotherapy or radiotherapy commonly ameliorates the hemolytic process (49).

An infrequent but therapeutically important association of AHD is that with ovarian teratoma. At least 16 such cases have been reported (52,53). While corticosteroid therapy is generally ineffective, surgical removal of the teratoma affords relief from the anemia and return of the positive Coombs' reaction to negative.

There have been 16 reported cases of Coombs' positive hemolytic anemia with carcinomas, four from our clinic (54). A wide variety of tumors have been associated with AHD. Because in more than 60% of affected patients the age was greater than 60 years, the possibility of occult carcinoma should be considered particularly in the evaluation of AHD in older patients. Symptoms of anemia rather than complaints related to a tumor mass commonly bring the patient to the doctor. Corticosteroid therapy is often ineffective in improving the anemia. When the neoplasm is localized to one site, removal of the tumor effects relief of the anemia and reversal of the direct Coombs' reaction to negative. In patients with extensive metastatic disease, chemotherapy and radiotherapy may cause lessening of hemolysis and improvement in the anemia.

In cold agglutinin hemolytic anemia, hemolysis results from the action of antibodies of IgM class, which cause agglutination of erythrocytes in the cold. These antibodies show maximum activity between 0 and 20°C. The antibodies are directed at the "I" or "i" antigens of red cells. The cold agglutinins may be polyclonal or monoclonal. In patients with cold agglutinins hemolysis is more likely to occur if the antibodies are present in high titer and have a wide range of thermal reactivity, with some activity for erythrocytes above 30°C. Affected patients may have Raynaud's phenomenon.

Gross agglutination of red cells may be recognized in some cases during preparation of a peripheral blood film. Reticulocytosis is present. The cold agglutinin test is positive. The direct Coombs' reaction may be positive or negative. Because hemolysis is, at least in part, intravascular, values of plasma hemoglobin, serum LDH, and serum glutamic oxaloacetic transaminase may be elevated, and hemoglobin and hemosiderin may be found in the urine.

Idiopathic cold agglutinin disease occurs predominantly in elderly patients, is associated with chronic hemolysis poorly responsive to corticosteroid therapy and splenectomy, and is frequently accompanied by a monoclonal peak on serum protein electrophoresis (Table 8-8). Polyclonal cold agglutinins are found in two-thirds of patients with mycoplasma pneumonia, but overt hemolytic anemia is uncommon. Hemolysis due to cold agglutinins is occasionally seen in patients with infectious mononucleosis or with systemic lupus erythematosus.

When associated with malignancies, the cold agglutinins are monoclonal. Malignancies associated with cold agglutinin-induced hemolysis are mainly the lymphoproliferative group. Cold agglutinins have been reported in patients with lymphocytic lymphoma, chronic lymphocytic leukemia, histiocytic lymphoma, Hodgkin's disease, multiple myeloma, Waldenström's macroglobulinemia, Kaposi's sarcoma, and chronic myelogenous leukemia (47,55,56). In the management of cold-agglutinin hemolysis, it is important to keep the patient warm. Although corticosteroids and splenectomy are commonly reported to be inef-

Table 8-8. Classification of Autoimmune Hemolytic Anemia due to Cold Antibodies

Cold agglutinins
    Idiopathic cold agglutinin disease
    Mycoplasma pneumonia
    Infectious mononucleosis
    Collagen vascular disorders
    Lymphoma
Paroxysmal cold hemoglobinuria
    Idiopathic
    Syphilis
    Postviral

fective, in some cases a good response is observed (56). Immunosuppressive drugs such as chlorambucil may be beneficial, but the response to therapy is slow.

MICROANGIOPATHIC HEMOLYTIC ANEMIA

Microangiopathic hemolytic anemia refers to the hemolytic anemia seen in patients with certain diseases of the microcirculation (57). A large variety of disorders may cause microangiopathic hemolytic anemia (Table 8-9). The hemolysis is predominantly intravascular. Thus, values of plasma hemoglobin, serum LDH, and serum glutamic oxaloacetic transaminase are usually elevated, and hemoglobin and hemosiderin may be found in the urine. Examination of the peripheral blood film provides the clue that leads to classification of an anemia in a

Table 8-9. Classification of Microangiopathic Hemolytic Anemia

Disseminated vascular disorders
    Thrombotic thrombocytopenic purpura
    Disseminated intravascular coagulation
    Purpura fulminans
    Disseminated carcinoma
Immune vascular disorders
    Systemic lupus erythematosus
    Polyarteritis nodosa
    Scleroderma
    Allergic vasculitis
Renal disorders
    Hemolytic uremic syndrome
    Renal cortical necrosis
    Malignant hypertension
    Acute glomerulonephritis
    Diabetic nephropathy
    Renal allograft rejection
Hemangiomas

particular patient as a microangiopathic hemolytic anemia. Fragmentation of erythrocytes is striking, with schistocytes, helmet cells, polychromasia, and microspherocytes evident (Fig. 8-15). In most affected patients, moderate to severe thrombocytopenia accompanies the anemia. The fragmentation of the red cells results from passage of the erythrocytes through diseased small blood vessels. Erythrocytic fragmentation with intravascular hemolysis also occurs in patients with certain cardiac problems, such as malfunctioning prosthetic valves, and after Teflon patch repairs of ostium primum defects. However, in these cardiac causes of erythrocyte fragmentation, platelet counts are usually normal.

Carcinoma is one of the more common causes of microangiopathic hemolytic anemia (57). Among 140 patients with metastatic carcinoma, Lohrmann and coworkers (58) found eight patients (5.7%) with features of microangiopathic hemolytic anemia. Disseminated intravascular coagulation with the formation of fibrin thrombi in the microvasculature is usually the cause of microangiopathic hemolytic anemia in persons with malignancy. However, in some patients, the underlying pathologic process is diffuse intravascular spread of neoplastic cells (Fig. 8-16) (58,59). Erythrocytes are damaged and fragmented as they pass through blood vessels partially occluded by fibrin thrombi or tumor. Neoplasms associated with microangiopathic hemolytic anemia are usually mucin-producing adenocarcinomas (60). Carcinoma of the stomach is the tumor most commonly associated with this type of hemolytic anemia. Among 12 cases reported by Brain

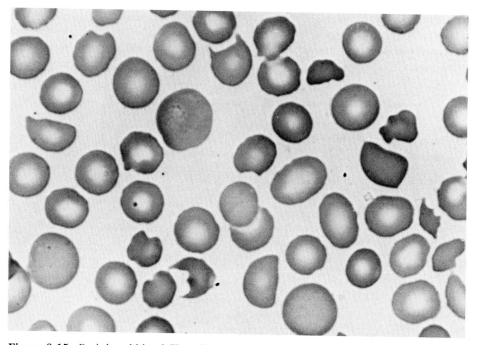

Figure 8-15. Peripheral blood film of a patient with microangiopathic hemolytic anemia associated with disseminated carcinoma of the stomach. Note the numerous fragmented erythrocytes. (Magnification 1,250×.)

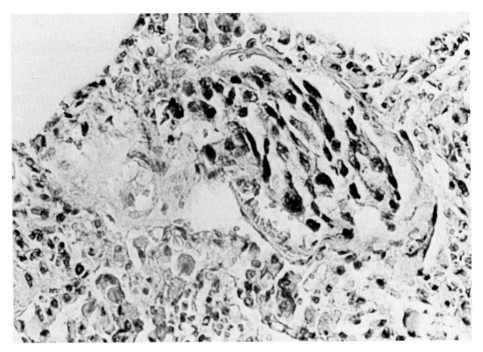

Figure 8-16. Metastatic carcinoma cells were found within pulmonary vessels at necropsy in this patient with microangiopathic hemolytic anemia due to carcinoma of the stomach. (Magnification 300×.)

and associates, in six the primary tumor was in the stomach (60). Cases have also been reported with carcinomas of the breast, pancreas, prostate, lung, colon, and gall bladder (57,58,60). When disseminated intravascular coagulation is the underlying cause of the hemolytic anemia, levels of coagulation factors I, II, V, and VIII are decreased causing prolongation of the prothrombin time and the partial thromboplastin time, and the level of fibrin degradation products in the serum is elevated. Administration of heparin can diminish formation of fibrin thrombi intravascularly and result in lessening of hemolysis.

Giant cavernous hemangiomas of infants and children, the Kasabach-Merritt syndrome, are commonly associated with thrombocytopenia (61). Platelets are sequestered and destroyed in the hemangioma. Fibrin thrombi form within the multiple vascular channels of the hemangioma resulting in the coagulation abnormalities characteristic of disseminated intravascular coagulation in some patients. Occasionally microangiopathic hemolytic anemia is also observed (62–64). In patients with hemangioendothelioma of the liver or the spleen, microangiopathic hemolytic anemia with thrombocytopenia can be a prominent feature (64). A woman with progressively increasing splenic size came to our clinic with moderate red cell fragmentation and mild thrombocytopenia. Radioisotopic splenic scan disclosed a cold defect. Splenectomy was performed with removal of a hemangioendothelioma. Anemia and thrombocytopenia disappeared after the splenectomy.

PAROXYSMAL NOCTURNAL HEMOGLOBINURIA

Classically in paroxysmal nocturnal hemoglobinuria (PNH), patients have episodes of intravascular hemolysis, particularly at night, resulting in hemoglobinuria. Most patients have irregular episodes of increased hemolysis lasting several days interspersed with periods of less intense hemolysis. However, in some patients the clinical picture is that of chronic continuous hemolysis without a history of hemoglobinuria. In these patients there is usually hemosiderinuria. Because of the substantial loss of iron in the urine by reason of hemoglobinuria and hemosiderinuria, patients with PNH may develop iron deficiency. Mild to moderate leukopenia and thrombocytopenia commonly accompany the anemia.

PNH is considered to be a clonal disorder of the bone marrow in which a population of red cells is produced with a membrane abnormality such that the erythrocytes are exceptionally sensitive to the lytic action of complement. Affected patients show laboratory evidence of intravascular hemolysis, such as elevated values of plasma hemoglobin and serum LDH, hemoglobinuria, and hemosiderinuria. The sucrose hemolysis test is positive. Normal erythrocytes do not hemolyze in an isotonic sucrose solution, but in the presence of a small amount of serum PNH red cells lyse when suspended in isotonic sucrose. Additionally, the acid hemolysis test (Ham's test) is positive in PNH because PNH erythrocytes are more susceptible than normal red cells to lysis at pH 6.5 in the presence of complement. Leukocyte alkaline phosphatase levels are commonly low in patients with PNH.

The cause of PNH in unknown. In some patients aplastic anemia appears during the course of PNH. In addition, the PNH defect of erythrocytes is occasionally identified in patients with either aplastic anemia or myelofibrosis. The chief relevance of PNH to malignancies is the occasional transformation of this hematologic disorder to acute leukemia, either acute myeloblastic leukemia or erythroleukemia (65–68). In three reported cases, acute myeloblastic leukemia was recognized two to seven years after the appearance of PNH (65–67). The reasons for the association of PNH with acute leukemia are unknown. Both PNH and acute myeloid leukemia may represent proliferation of abnormal clones of stem cells following marrow injury of undefined type.

HYPERSPLENISM

Hypersplenism refers to a clinical state in which there is excessive sequestering or destruction of blood cells in the spleen. Pancytopenia is usually present. In patients with hypersplenism, the degree of splenomegaly is generally substantial. With massive splenomegaly as much as one-quarter of the body's red cell mass can be sequestered in the spleen. Chromium-51 erythrocyte survival is reduced. External radioisotopic counting over the spleen discloses accumulation of radioactivity. The anemia is normochromic normocytic. There are no distinctive morphologic abnormalities of the erythrocytes disclosed by examination of the peripheral blood film. Marrow aspirates reveal hyperplasia of erythroid, granulocytic, and megakaryocytic elements. In patients in whom hypersplenism is the sole mechanism of anemia, leukopenia, and thrombocytopenia, the pancytopenia is corrected by splenectomy.

The causes of hypersplenism are numerous and diverse (Table 8-10). Most hematologic neoplastic disorders are associated with splenomegaly. However, hypersplenism is important as a mechanism of cytopenias in hematologic malignancies only when the extent of neoplastic infiltration in the spleen is extensive causing marked splenomegaly. Thus, hypersplenism is of little importance in acute leukemia because the spleen is usually not greatly enlarged. On the other hand, in advanced stages of chronic myelogenous leukemia, myelofibrosis, chronic lymphocytic leukemia, and lymphocytic lymphoma, both the degree of splenomegaly and the sequestration of blood cells in the spleen may be clinically important. The indications for splenectomy in these hematologic disorders include massive splenomegaly causing pressure symptoms, recurrent splenic infarctions, and severe cytopenias. While radiation therapy to the spleen decreases the size of this organ in patients with lymphocytic lymphoma, hypersplenism generally recurs (69). Splenectomy is the most definitive therapy.

Splenectomy is commonly accomplished during exploratory laparotomy performed for staging purposes in patients with Hodgkin's disease. Cytopenias due to hypersplenism occur in some patients with advanced Hodgkin's disease, mainly those with stage IV-B. Splenectomy usually results in relief from the cytopenias and improved tolerance to chemotherapy (70).

In patients with leukemic reticuloendotheliosis (LRE), or "hairy cell leukemia," substantial splenomegaly and pancytopenia commonly are found at the time the patient first sees the physician. Early splenectomy is warranted in this disorder and usually affords relief from cytopenias for a significant period of time. The diagnosis of LRE is suspected by a finding of "hairy cells" in the blood and confirmed by a marrow aspirate demonstrating infiltration of LRE cells. These cells are 10–18 μm in diameter and have oval or round nuclei and elongated

Table 8-10. Causes of Hypersplenism

Portal hypertension
   Hepatic disease, particularly cirrhosis
   Portal vein thrombosis
   Cavernous transformation of portal vein
Infiltrative diseases of the spleen
   Chronic lymphocytic leukemia
   Lymphocytic and histiocytic lymphomas
   Hodgkin's disease
   Leukemic reticuloendotheliosis
   Chronic myelogenous leukemia
   Myeloid metaplasia
   Gaucher's disease
Chronic infections
   Tuberculosis
   Histoplasmosis
   Brucellosis
Collagen disease
   Systemic lupus erythematosus
   Felty's syndrome

thin cytoplasmic protrusions, causing the "hairy" appearance. Histochemically, tartrate-resistant acid phosphatase activity is demonstrable in the LRE cells (71).

ERYTHROPHAGOCYTOSIS

In the rare neoplastic disorder, histiocytic medullary reticulosis (HMR), phago-cytosis of erythrocytes by histiocytes is the apparent mechanism of the anemia. The principal features of HMR are fever, generalized lymphadenopathy, hep-atomegaly, splenomegaly, anemia, leukopenia, and thrombocytopenia. Ap-proximately 80 patients with HMR have been reported. Usually the illness pro-gresses rapidly, with death occurring within a few weeks to a few months. The anemia is normochromic and normocytic. Radiochromium erythrocyte survival is shortened (72). Histologically, the lymph nodes show neoplastic proliferation of histiocytes with prominent erythrophagocytosis. Examination of a bone mar-row aspirate usually discloses intense phagocytosis of red blood cells by abnormal histiocytes (Fig. 8-17). Phagocytosis of erythrocytes, normoblasts, leukocytes, and platelets by neoplastic histiocytes in the bone marrow, spleen, liver, and lymph nodes probably accounts for the pancytopenia characteristically observed in HMR (73,74). Phagocytosis of erythrocytes, however, is not diagnostic of HMR because erythrophagocytosis by normal histiocytes is observed in a number of benign conditions, including autoimmune hemolytic anemia, tuberculosis, brucellosis,

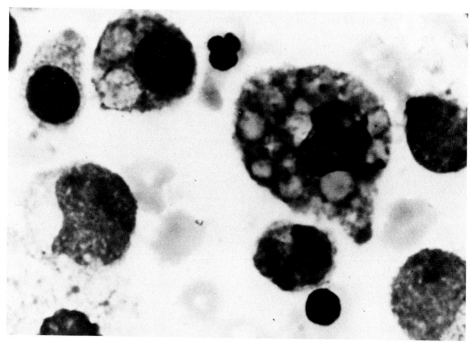

Figure 8-17. Bone marrow aspirate of a patient with histiocytic medullary reticulosis. Extensive phagocytosis of erythrocytes by abnormal histiocytes is observed. (Magnification 1,250×.)

typhoid, and other infections. Phagocytosis of leukocytes and platelets has been reported in a patient with miliary tuberculosis and in a patient with a presumed viral infection (75).

DILUTIONAL ANEMIA

Plasma volume is commonly increased in patients with Waldenström's macro-globulinemia and in those with multiple myeloma (76). The expanded plasma volume is due to increased plasma colloid oncotic pressure related to high cir-culating levels of abnormal immunoglobulin. Hematocrit values are often low in both macroglobulinemia and multiple myeloma, but in many of these patients the ^{51}Cr erythrocyte mass is normal, indicating that the low hematocrit values are simply due to expanded plasma volume. The term *dilutional anemia* is applied to this clinical state. True anemia may occur in both multiple myeloma and macroglobulinemia. Depressed erythropoiesis is the most common cause. He-molysis sometimes contributes to the anemia. In patients with macroglobuline-mia, iron deficiency may appear as a result of chronic bleeding provoked by the hyperviscosity due to high circulating levels of macroglobulins. Differentiation of true anemia from dilutional anemia in patients with macroglobulinemia or multiple myeloma requires measurement of the red blood cell mass of the body.

Dilutional anemia due to expanded plasma volume may also occur in patients with massive splenomegaly and can be a significant factor contributing to low venous hematocrit values along with splenic sequestration and destruction of erythrocytes. In patients affected with dilutional anemia associated with sple-nomegaly plasma volume gradually declines to normal after splenectomy. A proposed mechanism advanced by Hess et al. (77) to explain this dilutional anemia is a flow-induced portal hypertension with expansion of the portal vas-cular space. The resultant decreased effective intravascular volume stimulates the renin-angiotensin-aldosterone system and other renal hemodynamic changes, causing salt and water retention and expanded plasma volume.

ERYTHROCYTOSIS

Erythrocytosis, or polycythemia, is a disorder in which elevated values of the hemoglobin, hematocrit, and red blood cell count are found. Cases of erythro-cytosis may be classified into one of three groups: relative erythrocytosis, primary erythrocytosis (polycythemia vera), and secondary erythrocytosis.

Relative erythrocytosis is synonymous with spurious erythrocytosis, stress polycythemia, and pseudopolycythemia. In contrast to polycythemia vera and to the secondary erythrocytosis group, relative erythrocytosis is not a true erythrocytosis. Although values of the hematocrit and hemoglobin in venous blood are elevated, the red blood cell mass of the body as measured by the radiochromium technique is normal. Relative erythrocytosis occurs in patients with diminished plasma volume due to dehydration. In addition, relative erythro-cytosis is observed in some young to middle age adult men who are not dehy-drated. These patients are commonly tense, anxious, and at least mildly obese.

Hypertension, hypercholesterolemia, hyperuricemia, and cardiovascular thrombotic problems are common in these patients. The diagnosis is established by the constellation of findings of elevated hematocrit, normal ^{51}Cr erythrocyte mass, and normal or decreased radiolabeled albumin plasma volume.

Polycythemia vera is a disorder of the bone marrow in which there is increased erythropoiesis and, commonly, increased granulopoiesis and thrombopoiesis as well. The disease seems to be an autonomous overproduction of blood cells by the marrow rather than a marrow response to external stimuli. Urinary erythropoietin levels are low in polycythemia vera. Leukocytosis and thrombocytosis are present in more than 50% of patients and splenomegaly is detected in 75%. Other laboratory findings helpful in the diagnosis of polycythemia vera are hyperuricemia, increased leukocyte alkaline phosphatase, and elevated serum levels of vitamin B_{12}. A late complication of polycythemia vera, occurring in approximately 15% of patients, is acute leukemia. Usually the leukemia is acute myeloblastic in type, but sometimes myelomonocytic leukemia or erythroleukemia follow polycythemia vera. Radiophosphorus and alkylating agents, both commonly used in the treatment of polycythemia vera, appear to potentiate the development of acute leukemia, but occasional cases of leukemia are observed in patients not treated with either of these modalities.

There are numerous causes of secondary erythrocytosis (Table 8-11). In most instances excessive release of erythropoietin is responsible for the increased production of erythrocytes by the bone marrow. In contrast to polycythemia vera, the leukocyte and platelet counts are usually normal and splenomegaly is not expected.

For classification purposes secondary erythrocytosis is divided into two groups: (1) appropriately increased erythropoietin secretion due to a hypoxic stimulus, and (2) inappropriately increased erythropoietin secretion, that is, excessive secretion of the hormone not related to systemic hypoxia.

Hypoxia is the usual stimulus for increased erythropoietin secretion and thus is responsible for erythrocytosis in persons who live at high altitudes and in patients with cyanotic congenital heart disease, chronic pulmonary disease, hereditary methemoglobinemia, and carboxyhemoglobinemia due to excessive smoking. A rare cause is the inheritance of an abnormal hemoglobin that has an unusually high affinity for oxygen and therefore does not release oxygen easily in the tissues.

Erythropoietin secretion is elevated leading to erythrocytosis in a variety of nonneoplastic renal disorders. In patients affected with polycystic kidneys or solitary cysts, fluid from the cysts, as well as serum and urine, may demonstrate high erythropoietic stimulating activity. The reason for elevated erythropoietin production in certain patients with hydronephrosis is unclear but may be due to pressure on the remaining normal kidney causing tissue hypoxia. Similarly, renal hypoxia is a postulated mechanism for the erythrocytosis observed occasionally in patients with renal artery stenosis and in recipients of renal allografts undergoing transplant rejection.

Neoplasms are an important cause of erythrocytosis. In a comprehensive review of paraneoplastic erythrocytosis, Thorling (78) found hypernephroma to be the most common malignancy associated with erythrocytosis. At least 120 cases have been reported (79). The frequency of erythrocytosis in patients with

Table 8-11. Classification of Erythrocytosis

Relative erythrocytosis
Polycythemia vera
Secondary erythrocytosis
  Appropriate erythropoietin secretion
    Arterial hypoxia
      Cyanotic congenital heart disease
      Chronic pulmonary disease
      High altitude
    Tissue hypoxia without arterial hypoxia
      Methemoglobinemia
      Carboxyhemoglobinemia
      Abnormal hemoglobins with increased
        affinity for oxygen
  Inappropriate erythropoietin secretion
    Renal disorders
      Renal cysts
      Hydronephrosis
      Renal allograft rejection
    Tumors
      Hypernephroma
      Wilms' tumor
      Hepatoma
      Cerebellar hemangioblastoma
      Uterine myomas
      Hodgkin's disease
      Thymoma
      Oat cell carcinoma of lung
      Pheochromocytoma
      Aldosterone-secreting adenoma
      Cushing's syndrome
    Androgen therapy

hypernephroma is between 0.9 and 2.6% (78). Assays of serum and urine commonly reveal elevated erythropoietin levels in patients with erythrocytosis related to hypernephroma. It is generally accepted that hypernephroma cells produce erythropoietin. Extracts of tumor tissue showed a high level of erythropoietin in seven of nine cases of hypernephroma (79). When clinically the hypernephroma seems limited to the primary site, nephrectomy usually alleviates the erythrocytosis (78–80). However, erythrocytosis often reappears when the hypernephroma recurs (78). Occasionally, Wilms' tumors of the kidney (81) and renal adenomas, hemangiomas, and sarcomas have been associated with erythrocytosis (78). The mechanism of the erythrocytosis is probably a pressure effect of the tumor on normal renal tissue causing increased erythropoietin secretion.

The second most frequent organ serving as a primary site of a neoplasm associated with erythrocytosis is the liver. Thorling (78) found 64 cases. In most instances the tumor is a hepatoma (hepatocellular carcinoma). McFadzean and associates (82) observed that nearly 10% of patients in Hong Kong with hepatocellular carcinoma had hemoglobin values above 16.6 g/dl. Brownstein and Ballard (83) found that among 213 necropsy cases of hepatoma in New York City, 9.4% had hemoglobin levels above 16 g/dl and 2.8% had erythrocytosis, that is, hemoglobin values above 18 g/dl. Among patients with erythrocytosis related to a hepatoma, one-half have preexisting cirrhosis (83). The appearance of erythrocytosis in a patient with known cirrhosis is a clue to the diagnosis of a complicating hepatoma. Plasma or serum erythropoietin levels, when measured in patients with hepatoma and erythrocytosis, have been elevated in 50% (78,84). In a few cases erythropoietic active material has been extracted from tumor tissue (85,86). The mechanism of erythrocytosis due to hepatoma is probably inappropriate secretion of erythropoietin by the tumor (84). However, because erythropoietin has only infrequently been found in tumor extracts, alternative mechanisms have been proposed. For instance, it has been suggested that impaired liver function allows accumulation of erythropoietic substances produced in other organs.

The following case history is illustrative of the association of hepatoma with erythrocytosis.

Case 8

Hematologic consultation was requested on a 58-year-old mechanic who had an elevated value of the hemoglobin. The patient had entered the hospital because of dysphagia present for one year. Solid foods seemed to stick in the chest; this sensation was relieved by drinking liquids. The patient was otherwise asymptomatic. He specifically denied regurgitation of food, loss of weight, vomiting, and abdominal pain. There was no history of pulmonary, cardiac, hepatic, renal, or neurologic disorders. He had an extensive history of cigarette smoking and drank about six beers per week.

Three years previously the patient had been hospitalized for evaluation of hypertension. Review of those hospital records disclosed that at that time his hematocrit was 59% and hemoglobin 19.8 g/dl. Intravenous pyelogram and renal arteriogram were both normal.

Our physical examination revealed the blood pressure to be 170/108 mm Hg. Plethora of the skin and mucous membranes was observed. Grade two hypertensive changes were detected by funduscopic examination. Examination of the lungs and heart revealed that both were normal. The edge of the liver extended 12 cm below the right costal margin with total hepatic dullness to percussion 21 cm. The liver felt nodular in the right lateral area. No hepatic bruits or friction rubs were heard. The spleen was not palpable and no ascites was detected. Physical examination was otherwise unremarkable.

His hemoglobin value was 20.6 g/dl, hematocrit 63%, red blood cell count 6.73 million/mm^3, platelet count 275,000/mm^3, and total leukocyte count 7,300/mm^3, with a differential count of 62 segmented neutrophils, 1 eosinophil, 9 monocytes, and 28 lymphocytes. Urinalysis disclosed two to five red cells per high power field, but was otherwise normal. BUN was 17 mg/dl, prothrombin time 13.1 seconds, serum alkaline phosphatase 282 units (normal 30–80 units), total bilirubin 1.3 mg/dl, SGOT 83 units, and SGPT 31 units. Serum protein electrophoresis was normal. Serum iron was 73 μg/dl, with serum iron-binding capacity 327 μg/dl. Leukocyte alkaline phosphatase score was somewhat elevated at 168. Arterial oxygen saturation was 94%, with arterial PaO_2 81 mm Hg.

Radiographic studies of the upper gastrointestinal tract demonstrated a ring in the distal esophagus and a sliding hiatal hernia. The ring was visualized by esophagoscopy at 42 cm. A biopsy of this area showed chronic inflammatory changes. Roentgenograms of the chest and intravenous pyelogram were both normal, but films of bones demonstrated Paget's disease of the skull and one femur. Radioisotopic scans disclosed a normal spleen and a substantially enlarged right lobe of the liver containing a large cold area. By selective celiac angiography a massive malignant tumor, appearing to be a hepatoma, involving virtually the entire right lobe of the liver, was visualized (Fig. 8-18). Percutaneous liver biopsy yielded the histologic diagnosis of hepatocellular carcinoma. There were no cirrhotic changes. Urinary erythropoietin level was elevated. Urinary vanillyl mandelic acid level was normal.

A surgical consultant judged that the tumor was not resectable. The patient was treated with 5-fluorouracil, but died four months later.

Comment

This patient had asymptomatic erythrocytosis for more than three years before a hepatoma was discovered. It is very likely that the hepatoma was responsible for the erythrocytosis. No other reasonable alternative cause was found during the diagnostic evaluation of the patient. The case illustrates that erythrocytosis can be an early important sign of hepatocellular carcinoma.

Erythrocytosis has been reported in at least 50 patients with cerebellar hemangioblastoma (78). Affected patients generally see their physicians with symptoms due to direct effects of the tumor mass rather than for complaints related to erythrocytosis. When measured, serum erythropoietin levels have been elevated in less than one-half of cases. However, in each of five patients in whom cyst fluid was tested, strong erythropoietic activity was found (78,87). The erythropoietin obtained from cyst fluid seems to be identical to normal human erythropoietin in respect to molecular weight and electrophoretic mobility, and it is neutralized by an antibody raised in rabbits to human erythropoietin (88). Among 26 patients who survived an operation with complete removal of the hemangioblastoma, erythrocytosis disappeared in all of them (78). With recurrence of tumor, erythrocytosis commonly reappears.

Erythrocytosis is occasionally associated with uterine myomas. Approximately 30 such cases have been reported. The tumors are very large in size. Removal of the tumor relieved the erythrocytosis in 18 of 20 cases (78). In a few but not all patients, erythropoietin production by the tumor has been demonstrated (89,90). An alternative explanation for increased serum and urinary levels of erythropoietin is secretion of the hormone by the kidneys due to compression of the renal blood supply by the tumor or hydronephrosis resulting from ureteral obstruction by the tumor.

Several other tumors are on rare occasions associated with erythrocytosis. Examples are oat cell carcinoma of the lung, Hodgkin's disease, thymoma (91), pheochromocytoma, and adrenal adenoma. Resection of an undifferentiated carcinoma of the lung relieved the erythrocytosis in one patient, but later, with

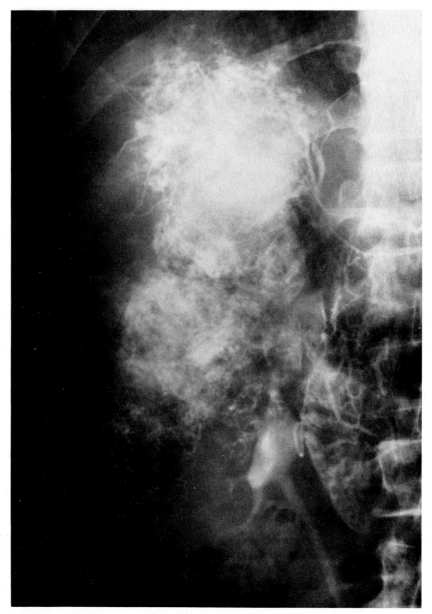

Figure 8-18. Extensive involvement of the right lobe of the liver demonstrated by celiac angiography in Case 8.

recurrence of the tumor, elevated values of the hematocrit returned (92). One patient with Hodgkin's disease has been reported in whom erythrocytosis was severe (hematocrit value 71%) in the early phase of the illness (93). True erythrocytosis has been reported in patients with pheochromocytoma. In one patient with four pheochromocytomas, erythropoietic-stimulating activity was demonstrated in tumor extracts and the erythrocytosis disappeared after removal of the pheochromocytomas (94,95). In addition, low plasma volume in patients with pheochromocytoma can cause a relative erythrocytosis. Surgical removal of an aldosterone-secreting adrenal adenoma resulted in return of elevated serum erythropoietin levels to normal and resolution of erythrocytosis in one patient (96). In patients with Cushing's syndrome, steroidal hormones, particularly androgens, are probably responsible for erythrocytosis. Leukocytosis is commonly found in these patients, presumably due to the stimulatory effect of corticosteroids on granulopoiesis.

REFERENCES

1. Ellman L: Bone marrow biopsy in the evaluation of lymphoma, carcinoma and granulomatous disorders. *Am J Med* 60:1, 1976.
2. Brunning RD, Bloomfield CD, McKenna RW, et al: Bilateral trephine bone marrow biopsies in lymphoma and other neoplastic diseases. *Ann Intern Med* 82:365, 1975.
3. Myers CE, Chabner BA, DeVita VT, et al: Bone marrow involvement in Hodgkin's disease: Pathology and response to MOPP chemotherapy. *Blood* 44:197, 1974.
4. Hansen HH, Muggia FM: Early detection of bone-marrow invasion in oat-cell carcinoma of the lung. *N Engl J Med* 284:962, 1971.
5. Veenema RJ: Bone marrow acid phosphatase determination for prostate cancer metastasis. *JAMA* 235:1615, 1976.
6. Katayama I, Finkel HE: Leukemic reticuloendotheliosis: A clinicopathologic study with review of the literature. *Am J Med* 57:115, 1974.
7. Coughlin C, Greenwald ES, Schraft WC, et al: Myelofibrosis associated with multiple myeloma. *Arch Intern Med* 138:590, 1978.
8. Case Records of the Massachusetts General Hospital. Case 21-1963. *N Engl J Med* 268:672, 1963.
9. Wasser JS, Yolken R, Miller DR, et al: Congenital hypoplastic anemia (Diamond-Blackfan syndrome) terminating in acute myelogenous leukemia. *Blood* 51:991, 1978.
10. Steinherz PG, Canale VC, Miller DR: Hepatocellular carcinoma, transfusion-induced hemochromatosis and congenital hypoplastic anemia (Blackfan-Diamond syndrome). *Am J Med* 60:1032, 1976.
11. Krantz SB: Pure red-cell aplasia. *N Engl J Med* 291:345, 1974.
12. Jepson JH, Lowenstein L: Panyhypoplasia of the bone marrow I: Demonstration of a plasma factor with anti-erythropoietin-like activity. *Can Med Assoc J* 99:99, 1968.
13. Rogers BHG, Manaligod JR, Blazek WV: Thymoma associated with pancytopenia and hypogammaglobulinemia: Report of a case and review of the literature. *Am J Med* 44:154, 1968.
14. Al-Mondhiry H, Zanjani ED, Spivack M, et al: Pure red cell aplasia and thymoma: Loss of serum inhibitor of erythropoiesis following thymectomy. *Blood* 38:576, 1971.
15. Pierre RV: Preleukemic states. *Semin Hematol* 13:73, 1974.
16. Abeloff MD, Waterbury L: Pure red blood cell aplasia and chronic lymphocytic leukemia. *Arch Intern Med* 134:721, 1974.
17. Kitahara M: Pure RBC aplasia associated with chronic granulocytic leukemia. *JAMA* 240:376, 1978.
18. Gilbert EF, Harley JB, Anido V, et al: Thymoma, plasma cell myeloma, red cell aplasia and malabsorption syndrome. *Am J Med* 44:820, 1968.
19. Field EO, Caughi MN, Blackett NM, et al: Marrow-suppressing factors in the blood in pure red-cell aplasia, thymoma and Hodgkin's disease. *Br J Haematol* 15:101, 1968.
20. Mitchell ABS, Pinn G, Pegrum GD: Pure red cell aplasia and carcinoma. *Blood* 37:594, 1971.

21. Dosik H, Hsu LY, Todara GJ, et al: Leukemia in Fanconi's anemia: Cytogenetic and tumor virus susceptibility studies. *Blood* 36:341, 1970.

22. Swift M, Zimmerman D, McDounough ER: Squamous cell carcinomas in Fanconi's anemia. *JAMA* 216:325, 1971.

23. Bernstein MS, Hunter RL, Yachnin S: Hepatoma and peliosis hepatis developing in a patient with Fanconi's anemia. *N Engl J Med* 284:1135, 1971.

24. Brauer MJ, Dameshek W: Hypoplastic anemia and myeloblastic leukemia following chloramphenicol therapy. *N Engl J Med* 277:1003, 1967.

25. Cohen T, Creger WP: Acute myeloid leukemia following seven years of aplastic anemia induced by chloramphenicol. *Am J Med* 43:762, 1967.

26. Dougan L, Woodliff HJ: Acute leukemia associated with phenylbutazone treatment: A review of the literature and report of a further case. *Med J Aust* 1:217, 1965.

27. Vigliani EC, Saita G: Benzene and leukemia. *N Engl J Med* 271:872, 1964.

28. Rosner F, Grünwald H: Hodgkin's disease and acute leukemia: Report of eight cases and review of the literature. *Am J Med* 58:339, 1975.

29. Coleman CN, Williams CJ, Flint A, et al: Hematologic neoplasia in patients treated for Hodgkin's disease. *N Engl J Med* 297:1249, 1977.

30. Zamcheck N, Grable E, Ley A, et al: Occurrence of gastric cancer among patients with pernicious anemia at the Boston City Hospital. *N Engl J Med* 252:1103, 1955.

31. Chanarin I: *The Megaloblastic Anaemias.* Oxford, Blackwell Scientific Publications, 1969.

32. Hoskins LC, Loux HA, Britten A, et al: Distribution of ABO blood groups in patients with pernicious anemia, gastric carcinoma and gastric carcinoma associated with pernicious anemia. *N Engl J Med* 273:633, 1965.

33. Harris AI, Greenberg H: Pernicious anemia and the development of carcinoid tumors of the stomach. *JAMA* 239:1160, 1978.

34. Hoffbrand AV, Hobbs JR, Kremenchuzky S, et al: Incidence and pathogenesis of megaloblastic erythropoiesis in multiple myeloma. *J Clin Pathol* 20:699, 1967.

35. Hines, JD, Grasso JA: The sideroblastic anemias. *Semin Hematol* 7:86, 1970.

36. Lee GR, Cartwright GE, Wintrobe MM: The response of free erythrocyte protoprophyrin to pyridoxine therapy in a patient with sideroachrestic (sideroblastic) anemia. *Blood* 27:557, 1966.

37. MacGibbon BH, Mollin DL: Sideroblastic anaemia in man: Observations on seventy cases. *Br J Haematol* 11:59, 1965.

38. Meytes D, Katz D, Ramot B: Preleukemia and leukemia in polycythemia vera. *Blood* 47:237, 1976.

39. Catovsky D, Shaw MT, Hoffbrand AV, et al: Sideroblastic anaemia and its association with leukaemia and myelomatosis: Report of five cases. *Br J Haematol* 20:385, 1971.

40. Khaleeli M, Keane WM, Lee GR: Sideroblastic anemia in multiple myeloma: A preleukemic change. *Blood* 41:17, 1973.

41. Rosner F, Grunwald H: Multiple myeloma terminating in acute leukemia: Report of 12 cases and review of the literature. *Am J Med* 57:927, 1974.

42. Kyle RA, Pierre RV, Bayrd ED: Multiple myeloma and acute leukemia associated with alkylating agents. *Arch Intern Med* 135:185, 1975.

43. Gilliland BC, Baxter E, Evans RS: Red-cell antibodies in acquired hemolytic anemia with negative antiglobulin serum tests. *N Engl J Med* 285:252, 1971.

44. Pirofsky B: Autoimmune hemolytic anemia and neoplasia of the reticuloendothelium; with a hypothesis concerning etiologic relationships. *Ann Intern Med* 68:109, 1968.

45. Zacharski LR, Linman JW: Chronic lymphocytic leukemia versus chronic lymphosarcoma cell leukemia. *Am J Med* 47:75, 1969.

46. Dausset J, Colombani J: The serology and prognosis of 128 cases of autoimmune hemolytic anemia. *Blood* 14:1280, 1959.

47. Dacie JV: *The Haemolytic Anaemias: Congenital and Acquired. Part II: The Auto-Immune Haemolytic Anaemias.* London, Churchill, 1962.

48. Pirofsky B: Clinical aspects of autoimmune hemolytic anemia. *Semin Hematol* 13:251, 1976.

49. Eisner E, Ley AB, Mayer K: Coombs'-positive hemolytic anemia in Hodgkin's disease. *Ann Intern Med* 66:258, 1967.

50. Bowdler AJ, Glick IW: Autoimmune hemolytic anemia as the herald state of Hodgkin's disease. *Ann Intern Med* 65:761, 1966.

51. Pangalis GA, Moran EM, Rappaport H: Blood and bone marrow findings in angioimmunoblastic lymphadenopathy. *Blood* 51:71, 1978.

52. Barry KG, Crosby WH: Auto-immune hemolytic anemia arrested by removal of an ovarian teratoma: Review of the literature and report of a case. *Ann Intern Med* 47:1002, 1957.

53. Dawson MA, Talbert W, Yarbro JW: Hemolytic anemia associated with an ovarian tumor. *Am J Med* 50:552, 1971.

54. Spira MA, Lynch EC: Autoimmune hemolytic anemia and carcinoma: An unusual association. *Am J Med* 67:753, 1979.

55. Pruzanski W, Shumak KH: Biologic activity of cold-reacting autoantibodies. *N Engl J Med* 297:583, 1977.

56. Isbister JP, Cooper DA, Blake HM, et al: Lymphoproliferative disease with IgM lambda monoclonal protein and autoimmune hemolytic anemia: A report of four cases and review of the literature. *Am J Med* 64:434, 1978.

57. Brain MC, Dacie JV, O'Hourihane D O'B: Microangiopathic haemolytic anaemia: The possible role of vascular lesions in pathogenesis. *Br J Haematol* 8:358, 1962.

58. Lohrmann HP, Adam W, Heymer B, et al: Microangiopathic hemolytic anemia in metastatic carcinoma: Report of eight cases. *Ann Intern Med* 79:368, 1973.

59. Lynch EC, Bakken CL, Casey TH, et al: Microangiopathic hemolytic anemia in carcinoma of the stomach. *Gastroenterology* 52:88, 1967.

60. Brain MC, Azzopardi JG, Baker LRI, et al: Microangiopathic haemolytic anaemia and mucin-forming adenocarcinoma. *Br J Haematol* 18:183, 1970.

61. Kasabach HH, Merritt KK: Capillary hemangioma with extensive purpura: Report of a case. *Am J Dis Child* 59:1063, 1940.

62. Propp RP, Scharfman WB: Hemangioma-thrombocytopenia syndrome associated with microangiopathic hemolytic anemia. *Blood* 28:623, 1966.

63. Inceman S, Tangun Y: Chronic defibrination syndrome due to a giant hemangioma associated with microangiopathic hemolytic anemia. *Am J Med* 46:997, 1969.

64. Alpert LI, Benisch B: Hemangioendothelioma of the liver associated with microangiopathic hemolytic anemia: Report of four cases. *Am J Med* 48:624, 1970.

65. Jenkins DE Jr, Hartmann RC: Paroxysmal nocturnal hemoglobinuria terminating in acute myeloblastic leukemia. *Blood* 33:274, 1969.

66. Holden D, Lichtman H: Paroxysmal nocturnal hemoglobinuria and acute leukemia. *Blood* 33:283, 1969.

67. Kaufmann RW, Schechter GP, McFarland W: Paroxysmal nocturnal hemoglobinuria terminating in acute granulocytic leukemia. *Blood* 33:287, 1969.

68. Carmel R, Coltman CA Jr, Yatteau RF, et al: Association of paroxysmal nocturnal hemoglobinuria with erythroleukemia. *N Engl J Med* 283:1329, 1970.

69. Shukla SK, Evans JT, Mittelman A: Splenectomy or radiation and splenectomy for hypersplenism in lymphosarcoma. *J Surg Oncol* 8:99, 1976.

70. Lowenbraun S, Ramsey HE, Serpick AA: Splenectomy in Hodgkin's disease for splenomegaly, cytopenias and intolerance to myelosuppressive chemotherapy. *Am J Med* 50:49, 1971.

71. Yam LT, Li CY, Finkel HE: Leukemic reticuloendotheliosis: The role of tartrate-resistant acid phosphatase in diagnosis and splenectomy in treatment. *Arch Intern Med* 130:248, 1972.

72. Lynch EC, Alfrey CP: Histiocytic medullary reticulosis: Hemolytic anemia due to erythrophagocytosis by histiocytes. *Ann Intern Med* 63:666, 1965.

73. Natelson EA, Lynch EC, Hettig RA, et al: Histiocytic medullary reticulosis: The role of phagocytosis in pancytopenia. *Arch Intern Med* 122:223, 1968.

74. Seligman BR, Rosner F, Lee SL, et al: Histiocytic medullary reticulosis. *Arch Intern Med* 129:109, 1972.

75. Chandra P, Chaudhery SA, Rosner F, et al: Transient histiocytosis with striking phagocytosis of platelets, leukocytes and erythrocytes. *Arch Intern Med* 135:989, 1975.

76. Kopp WL, MacKinney AA Jr, Wasson G: Blood volume and hematocrit value in macroglobulinemia and myeloma. *Arch Intern Med* 123:394, 1969.

77. Hess CE, Ayers CR, Sandusky WR, et al: Mechanism of dilutional anemia in massive splenomegaly. *Blood* 47:629, 1976.

78. Thorling EB: Paraneoplastic erythrocytosis and inappropriate erythropoietin production. *Scand J Haematol* [Suppl] 17:1, 1972.

79. Hammond D, Winnick S: Paraneoplastic erythrocytosis and ectopic erythropoietins. *Ann NY Acad Sci* 230:219, 1974.

80. Damon A, Holub DA, Melicow MM, et al: Polycythemia and renal carcinoma: Report of ten new cases, two with long hematologic remission following nephrectomy. *Am J Med* 25:182, 1958.

81. Thurman WG, Grabstald H, Lieberman PH: Elevation of erythropoietin levels in association with Wilms' tumor. *Arch Intern Med* 117:280, 1966.

82. McFadzean AJS, Todd D, Tsang KC: Polycythemia in primary carcinoma of the liver. *Blood* 13:427, 1958.

83. Brownstein MH, Ballard HS: Hepatoma associated with erythrocytosis: Report of eleven new cases. *Am J Med* 40:204, 1966.

84. Davidson CS: Hepatocellular carcinoma and erythrocytosis. *Semin Hematol* 13:115, 1976.

85. Santer MA, Waldmann TA, Fallon HJ: Erythrocytosis and hyperlipemia as manifestations of hepatic carcinoma. *Arch Intern Med* 120:735, 1967.

86. Nakao K, Kimura K, Miura Y, et al: Erythrocytosis associated with carcinoma of the liver (with erythropoietin assay of tumor extract). *Am J Med Sci* 251:161, 1966.

87. Waldmann TA, Levin EH, Baldwin M: The association of polycythemia with a cerebellar hemangioblastoma: The production of an erythropoiesis stimulating factor by the tumor. *Am J Med* 31:318, 1961.

88. Waldmann TA, Rosse WF, Swarm RL: The erythropoiesis-stimulating factors produced by tumors. *Ann NY Acad Sci* 149:509, 1968.

89. Wrigley PFM, Malpas JS, Turnbull AL, et al: Secondary polycythaemia due to a uterine fibromyoma producing erythropoietin. *Br J Haematol* 21:551, 1971.

90. Ossias AL, Zanjani ED, Zalusky R, et al: Case report: Studies on the mechanism of erythrocytosis associated with a uterine fibromyoma. *Br J Haematol* 25:179, 1973.

91. Sundström C: A case of thymoma in association with erythrocytosis. *Acta Pathol Microbiol Scand* [Section A] 80:235, 1972.

92. Donati RM, McCarthy JM, Lange RD, et al: Erythrocythemia and neoplastic tumors. *Ann Intern Med* 58:47, 1963.

93. Brownstein MH, Scherl BA: Hodgkin's disease with erythrocytosis: Report of a case. *Arch Intern Med* 117:689, 1966.

94. Bradley JE, Young JD Jr, Lentz G: Polycythemia secondary to pheochromocytoma. *J Urol* 86:1, 1961.

95. Waldmann TA, Bradley JE: Polycythemia secondary to pheochromocytoma with production of an erythropoiesis stimulating factor by the tumor. *Proc Soc Exp Biol Med* 108:425, 1961.

96. Mann DL, Gallagher NI, Donati RM: Erythrocytosis and primary aldosteronism. *Ann Intern Med* 66:335, 1967.

9
Abnormalities of White Blood Cells, Platelets, and Hemostasis

Clarence P. Alfrey, Jr., Martin R. White, and Paul W. Zelnick

Nonhematopoietic cancers may have marked effects on leukocytes, platelets, and blood coagulation. We have reviewed reports of observed changes in each of these elements and have attempted to determine the significance of the change relative to the extent of the disease or prognosis.

LEUKEMOID REACTIONS

A leukemoid reaction is present when a patient's blood findings resemble leukemia but are due to a nonleukemic disease state. Firm limits of leukocyte abnormalities are difficult to define for a leukemoid reaction because the blood findings in leukemia are quite variable. Marked leukocytosis caused by carcinoma is uncommon. In general, leukemoid reactions caused by carcinomas are myeloid (1–3), although lymphocytic leukemoid reactions have been reported with metastatic melanoma and breast adenocarcinoma. Myeloid leukemoid reactions with cancers may consist of either a marked leukocytosis with a shift to the left or a picture of variable degrees of leukocytosis accompanied by significant myeloid immaturity in the peripheral blood.

Chen and Walz (2) studied 24 patients with cancer who had leukocytosis. Primary carcinoma of the lung, pancreas, stomach, bladder, and rectum predominated. Evaluations of the marrow differentials showed a modest left shift of maturity in the myeloid series. Only 33% of these patients had evidence of bone marrow metastases. Fahey (4) found three cases of marked granulocytosis (white blood cell count—WBC—greater than 50,000/mm³) with mild left shift in 160 cases of lung carcinoma (1.8%). Two of these cases had metastatic disease outside the thorax, but none had marrow metastases demonstrated. Two additional patients with cancer of the lung had significant suppurative infections, an alternative explanation for the marked leukocytosis seen. Banerjie and Narang (5) found leukocytosis in 23% of patients with malignancies. Postobstructive bronchopneumonia and/or atelectasis were present in the patients with lung cancer, leading to the suggestion that infection may be the principal cause of leukocytosis in patients with tumors of the lung. Robinson (6) studied 12 patients with cancer who had a WBC greater than 20,000: eight cases had a small number of myelocytes present in the peripheral blood; all had myeloid predominance in the differential blood counts. He was able to demonstrate significantly elevated colony-stimulating factor (CSF) in the serum and urine in these patients. The two tumor masses tested were devoid of CSF activity. Polymorphonuclear leukocytosis is not a common feature of carcinomatosis; when present it suggests an infection or other complication and is not indicative of marrow metastasis.

Leukoerythroblastosis refers to the presence of immature white cells of the myeloid series (usually myelocytes) and nucleated red cells in the circulating blood, with or without anemia (7). Initially this finding was thought to be most frequently seen with space-consuming lesions of the bone marrow, especially metastatic carcinomas (3,8), but in more recent series, hemolysis, hemorrhage, severe infections, and hematologic malignancies have accounted for most cases, with only 6–15% being caused by marrow involvement by carcinoma (7,9,10). However, the presence of leukoerythroblastosis in patients with cancer almost always indicates that the bone marrow is involved by the tumor (11–16), and when patients with carcinoma metastatic to the bone marrow have been carefully studied, 19–53% had leukoerythroblastosis (11,12,14–19). Carcinomas of the prostate, breast, lung, and gastrointestinal tract were the most frequently associated tumors, but virtually any tumor that metastasizes to the bone marrow could be involved (7,9,10,12,14).

Clinically most patients with leukoerythroblastosis secondary to carcinoma have a normocytic, normochromic anemia, frequently with hemoglobins less than 9 g percent (7,9,12,13,15,18). Many also have moderate to marked anisocytosis and poikilocytosis, with many of the poikilocytes being teardrop cells (20,21). A mild reticulocytosis is often noted (7,20,22). Most will have normal white blood cell counts, but mild leukopenia to moderate leukocytosis may be seen (3,9,13,20,22,23) and thrombocytopenia is not uncommon (3,20–22,24).

Several mechanisms have been proposed to explain the presence of immature erythroid and myeloid cells in the peripheral circulation of these patients. Bone marrow biopsies usually reveal extensive fibrosis and new bone formation and occasionally necrosis associated with the metastatic foci of tumor (17); some investigators have proposed that the extensive marrow replacement by this sclerosing and infiltrating process causes an altered anatomic arrangement of the marrow leading to the release of immature cells (21). However, others have noted no relationship between either the site or degree of marrow involvement by tumor and the presence of leukoerythroblastosis (3,8,22,24). In recent studies in which autopsies were performed, the patients were all noted to have extensive marrow involvement by metastatic carcinoma with marked displacement of normal marrow elements, frequently with extensive fibrosis, and all also had extramedullary hematopoiesis involving the spleen and occasionally the liver, kidney, and lymph nodes (14,22). This suggests that the presence of the tumor cells in the marrow depresses hematopoiesis resulting in anemia that stimulates extramedullary foci of hematopoiesis, with release of immature cells from the sites of extramedullary hematopoiesis or occasionally from the altered bone marrow (23).

The treatment of leukoerythroblastic anemia is that of the primary tumor, and the anemia may remit if the tumor is responsive to therapy (22–24).

BONE MARROW METASTASES

Bone marrow metastasis occurs in an appreciable number of patients with carcinoma. The most common tumors found in marrow biopsy and aspirate studies are breast, prostate, and lung. Virtually every cancer, however, can metastasize to the marrow. The diagnostic utility of the marrow biopsy is superior to the aspirate, with the biopsy being positive in 90% of cases while the marrow aspirate is positive in only 49% (17). Pathologic features commonly occurring in marrow biopsies are bone marrow necrosis, fibrosis adjacent to malignant cells, and proliferation of new trabecular bone (25). The fibrosis may be very extensive, and extramedullary splenic hematopoiesis may occur (3,20,26).

Leukopenia is commonly defined as a white blood cell count (WBC) less than 4,500 per mm^3. Granulocytopenia is present where there are less than 3,000 polymorphonuclear leukocytes per mm^3. Lymphopenia is present when there are less than 1,500 lymphocytes per mm^3. Even with extensive marrow infiltration with carcinoma, leukopenia is uncommon. Only 8% of patients with documented marrow invasion by carcinoma had leukocyte counts less than 4,000/mm^3 (17). Banerjie found an incidence of 12% of patients with carcinoma having WBC between 2,500 and 4,500/mm^3 (5). Only two of eight patients with extensive myelofibrosis and marrow metastases had leukopenia (20). Riesco (27) studied leukocyte counts and survival in patients with carcinoma presumed cured by surgery, chiefly cervical and breast carcinoma, without evidence of metastatic disease. Granulocytopenia was present in 22% of the patients. However, neither granulocytosis or granulocytopenia was predicative of five-year survival.

Lymphocytopenia, however, is relatively common with extensive carcinoma and further does not appear to predict a poor overall prognosis. Shillitoe (28) reviewed 687 random blood counts, identifying 87 with lymphocytopenia. Nine of these patients had carcinoma. Zacharski and Linman (29), however, found that 42.7% of those patients with absolute lymphocytopenia had cancer. Twenty-two percent of patients with unresectable gastrointestinal carcinomas had lymphocyte counts less than 1,000/mm^3. Riesco (27) found that the lymphocyte count was the hematologic variable that best predicted five-year cure rate; lymphocytopenia was a relatively poor prognostic sign. Lee et al. (30) found similar results. Using lymphocyte counts and nitrochlorobenzene sensitization as measures of immunocompetence, they found that disease progression for carcinomas was much more common in those patients unable to become sensitized to DNCB and who had less than 1,000 lymphocytes per mm^3. Termini (31) found that patients with lung cancer had fewer peripheral lymphocytes than normal subjects (1799 vs. 2071 lymphocytes per mm^3). Eighteen percent of those with cancer had absolute lymphocytopenia, while only 4% of normal subjects were lymphocytopenic. Lee (32) reviewed the relationship of subpopulations of T and B cells and carcinoma. Extensive cancer was more commonly associated with lymphocytopenia than limited disease. Some reduction of the precentage of T cells had been reported, especially following radiotherapy.

EOSINOPHILIA

An absolute eosinophil count of more than 300 per mm^3 is the customary definition of eosinophilia. As a rule, eosinophilia associated with cancers usually accompanies granulocytosis. Eosinophilia is also most commonly seen with extensive disease and particularly with tumor necrosis (33). A specific eosinophilic infiltration around tumor or necrotic tumor masses is not demonstrable. The cause may be an immunologic stimulus of host toward cancerous tissue. Robinson (6) found that seven of 12 cases with cancer and granuloctyosis also had some degree of eosinophilia. Four of these cases had greater than 10% and over 1,000 eosinophils per mm^3. Assays for CSF failed to reveal any specific stimulus for evolution of eosinophilic colonies. All of these seven cases had extensive metastatic disease; five had liver involvement. Viola et al. (34) reported a case of striking eosinophilia-associated cancer. Their review of the literature revealed instances of eosinophilia associated with carcinomas from multiple organs and usually with widely metastatic disease. Colonic, lung, and gastric carcinomas were the most commonly found tumors associated with eosinophilia. Several instances have been reported in which normal eosinophil counts were present until metastatic disease occurred (35).

MONOCYTOSIS

Monocytosis is defined as more than 800 monocytes per mm^3 of blood. Barrett (36) compared the monocyte counts of 100 normal controls against patients with a variety of types of carcinoma. There was a twofold increase in the average monocyte count in patients with cancer. Maldonado and Hanlon (37) found that 13 of 82 patients with absolute monocytosis had carcinoma. Riesco (27) found that 21% of 589 cases with unselected carcinomas of limited extent had monocytosis. The presence of monocytosis does not appear to affect the prognosis, nor does it appear more frequently with extensive disease (27,36).

LEUKEMIA

Leukemogenesis appears to be one of the effects of cancer therapy. Over the past 20 years, the development of leukemia has been noted in populations receiving alkylating agents and irradiation. For example, large retrospective (38) studies have shown an apparent increase in the leukemia risk factors for those receiving alkylating agents for ovarian cancer. Studies of groups of patients receiving both chemotherapy and irradiation for lymphoma appear to show an increase in risk of leukemia (39). There is uncertainty whether therapy causes leukemia or whether a leukemic potential of the primary malignancy is uncovered by the relative longevity of those receiving therapy.

Insight into the question of whether patients with leukemia have a predeliction to development of carcinoma may be gained from two studies of patients with leukemias. These patients appeared to have significant risk of developing skin cancers, but were no more prone to other carcinomas. Gunz and Angus (40) found a 12-fold increased risk of skin cancer in their population with chronic lymphocytic leukemia, but no increased risk in acute and chronic leukemias for other cancers. Berg (41) found similar results with an overall increased risk of sevenfold for skin cancer for both myeloid and lymphoid leukemia. He, however, found a small but significant increase in the risk of prostatic cancer.

Of particular interest to the question of leukemogenesis is the observation of leukemia in patients receiving immunosuppressive or cytotoxic medicines for nonmalignant diseases, for example, lupus erythematosus, nephritis, and rheumatoid arthritis (42,43). In addition to the expected pancytopenia routinely observed with use of alkylating agents, immunosuppressives, and radiotherapy, these agents are capable of inducing major chromosomal aberrations (42–46).

Mitelman et al. (47) found a significant relation of chromosomal aberrations with marrow toxin exposure in adults with acute nonlymphocytic leukemia. The exposure consisted of petroleum products, solvents, and radiation. The group of patients without significant exposure by history had little chromosomal abnormality. This may argue that agents that can cause major chromosomal aberrations may cause leukemia. The leukemogenic potential of irradiation is well accepted. Perhaps the most poignant demonstration of this is the increase in chronic and acute myelogenous leukemia within six years in survivors within 1,500 meters of the atomic blasts in Hiroshima and Nagasaki (48).

Several recent studies of large numbers of patients receiving alkylating agents with or without radiotherapy highlight the risk of inducing leukemia. Reimer et al. (38) compared patient populations with ovarian carcinoma; 13,309 women treated before the use of intensive chemotherapy regimens showed no increase in leukemia. Neither was there an increase in those patients treated with radiotherapy alone. Analysis of a more recent group of 5,455 women, of which 80% were treated with alkylating agents, showed 13 cases of acute nonlymphocytic leukemia. The expected number of cases for this group was 0.62—a 21-fold increase. Agents used for chemotherapy were melphalan (5), chlorambucil (3), cyclophosphamide (3), thiotepa, and uracil mustard (1 each). The duration of administration was from 10 to 90 months. The interim from the start of therapy to the onset of leukemia was 26 to 90 months. Nine of the 13 patients developed pancytopenia lasting 1 to 12 months prior to the diagnosis of acute leukemia.

The occurrence of leukemia with lymphoproliferative and myelomatous disease has also been noted. Rosner and Grunwald (49) reported on leukemia in patients treated for myeloma. They found 12 cases of acute nonlymphocytic leukemia occurring 5 to 120 months after therapy with melphalan was begun. They found 46 additional cases reported in the literature. Eleven of these cases had the diagnosis of leukemia made at the time of presentation for the myeloma. Three instances were found in which leukemia occurred without treatment with alkylating agents or irradiation.

Coleman et al. (39) reported the occurrence of leukemia following intensive therapy for Hodgkin's disease. No instances of acute nonlymphocytic leukemia

(AN-LL) occurred in the groups treated with chemotherapy or radiation alone. In the group treated with a combination of chemotherapy and radiation, however, there was a 2.9% chance of developing AN-LL at five years and 3.9% chance at seven years after treatment. This corroborated the earlier report by Arseneau et al. (50), who reported a higher relative risk of developing AN-LL in the group receiving a combination of "intensive" chemotherapy and radiotherapy.

THROMBOCYTOSIS

Thrombocytosis commonly accompanies carcinoma. The thrombocytosis seen with cancers appears to be a reactive phenomenon and of itself does not appear to contribute to thrombosis or bleeding diathesis, as is the case with myeloproliferative disorders. While the finding of thrombocytosis may mean the patient has carcinoma, it does not imply extensive disease.

A recent report (51) showed that 31 of 80 patients found to have an elevated platelet count also had carcinoma. The original 80 patients were identified from a review of the peripheral smears of 14,400 patients. The remainder had miscellaneous inflammatory disorders. Similar results were found (52) in a study of 100 consecutive patients with greater than 500,000 platelets per mm^3. Thirty-six patients were shown to have carcinoma. Interestingly, 25 patients had "expected thrombocytosis" by virtue of splenectomy or myeloproliferative diseases. Thus, of the 75 remaining patients with unexplained thrombocytosis, 51% had carcinoma. Only one of the 36 patients with carcinoma had thrombotic disease with pulmonary emboli. Silvis et al. (53) found thrombocytosis in 60% of patients with lung cancer. There was no difference in platelet counts between the 8.9% of patients with thrombophlebitis and those without. Hagedorn et al. (54) found that 30% of patients with inoperable lung cancer had thrombocytosis. There were no cases of thrombocytosis in the seven cases with bone marrow metastases. Contreras et al. (17) found only 10% of patients with proven bone marrow metastases had thrombocytosis. Sun et al. (55) found a 12% incidence to thrombocytosis in patients specifically referred for clinical bleeding, prolonged clotting times, or screening postoperatively; 50% of these patients had widely metastatic disease.

THROMBOCYTOPENIA

Thrombocytopenia is less common than thrombocytosis; however, its presence usually connotes extensive disease. Two mechanisms for reduction of platelets in widely metastatic carcinoma are (1) marrow replacement with tumor and (2) platelet consumption associated with chronic intravascular coagulation.

Banerjie and Narang (5) found 12% of patients with a variety of carcinomas to have thrombocytopenia. No information is given about the extent of disease or data about coagulation abnormalities. Contreras et al. (17) found that 39% of patients with bone marrow metastases were thrombocytopenic. Six of the seven patients with extensive myelofibrosis associated with metastatic carcinoma reported by Kiely and Silverstein (20) were thrombocytopenic. Hagedorn et al. (54) found a 4% incidence of thrombocytopenia in patients with inoperable carcinoma of the lung, but an 8% incidence in those with metastatic disease, principally metastases in the lymph nodes. Likewise, Silvis et al. (53) found only 2.56% of patients with lung cancer had thrombocytopenia in a group with relatively limited disease.

Thrombocytopenia is particularly common in patients with ongoing consumptive coagulopathy. Slichter and Harker (56) have shown that platelet life spans were reduced in patients with carcinoma. Those dying of cancer within two weeks of the study had platelet half-survival of approximately 24 hours (normal 80–100 hours). Brain et al. (57) reported 12 patients with mucin-forming adenocarcinoma with multiple coagulation abnormalities. Ten of the 12 patients were moderately to severely thrombocytopenic.

ALTERATIONS OF COAGULATION

Alterations of coagulation in patients with cancer may occur in any histologic type of carcinoma, but are particularly common in patients with adenocarcinoma. This may be due to thromboplastin-like material elaborated by the malignant tissue. Carcinomas of the prostate gland, stomach, pancreas, breast, and lung are the more common offenders. In general, the more extensive the spread of malignancy, the more severe the coagulation abnormalities.

Miller et al. (58) studied 50 consecutive patients with carcinoma and lymphoma, 39 and 11 patients respectively. The carcinomas arose chiefly from breast, colon, stomach, and lung, though histologic types were unspecified. The majority had at least one major abnormality in coagulation studies. Whole blood clotting times and recalcification clotting times were reduced for the group when compared to normals. However, prothrombin times were longer than normal in patients with metastatic cancers. Factor assays for fibrinogen, prothrombin, and factors V, VIII, IX, and XI were elevated in most patients. The fibrinogen and factor VIII levels were both about two-times greater for the group than levels for normal controls. Twelve patients had evidence of systemic fibrinolysis. Only one patient had clinical bleeding, and only one patient with prostatic carcinoma had thrombosis with emboli. Hagedorn et al. (54) found multiple abnormalities of coagulation in patients with inoperable lung cancer. One-third of the patients had increased fibrinogen–fibrin split products, and all patients had elevated fibrinogen levels. The patients with the highest fibrinogen levels had the most extensive metastatic disease, including those with liver metastases.

Slichter and Harker (56) found that fibrinogen and platelet half-lives in the circulation were concomitantly reduced in patients with carcinoma. The absolute plasma level of fibrinogen was unpredictable with respect to extent of disease, but the plasma half-life was much shorter in those with the most extensive metastatic disease. Even in those patients with marked thrombocytopenia and markedly increased fibrinogen turnover, the fibrinogen levels were normal. The host is capable of maintaining adequate levels of fibrinogen even with high rates of consumption. These authors were able to localize the site of fibrinogen utilization to the tumor mass in two instances using radioactive fibrinogen tracer.

They also demonstrated that heparin administration could reduce the consumption of fibrinogen in patients with cancers.

Patients with widely metastatic disease may have an ongoing intravascular coagulation syndrome with depletion of clotting factors and clinical bleeding. Lohrmann et al. (59) reported on eight cases with adenocarcinoma from prostate, colon, and undetermined origin. All had severe thrombocytopenia with evidence of ongoing microangiopathic hemolysis. Only two of the eight had mildly reduced fibrinogen levels. Intravascular platelet fibrin thrombi and tumor emboli were found at autopsy in six of seven patients. A study of coagulation alterations in 61 patients with cancer (55) showed that 82% had elevated fibrinogen split products, 11% were hypofibrinogenemic, and 57% had a prolongation of the partial thromboplastin time. Paracoagulation tests for circulating clottable fibrinogen degradation products were positive in 55% of the cases. This population was highly skewed in that one-third had prostatic carcinoma. Mertens et al. (25) found that those patients with prostatic carcinoma who had elevated fibrinogen split products or positive paracoagulation tests had more postoperative bleeding from prostatic surgery.

Brain et al. (57) studied 12 patients with microangiopathic hemolysis. Eleven of these patients had mucin-positive adenocarcinomas: six from stomach, two from breast, one from lung, and three from unidentified sources. Ten of the 12 were thrombocytopenic. The fibrinogen catabolic rate was markedly increased in four patients studied. The fibrinogen levels were normal or increased. Increased fibrinogen split products were present in five of six tested. Pineo et al., in a later publication (60), demonstrated that mucin extracted as a crude homogenate from adenocarcinomas from a variety of primary sites acted as a powerful thromboplastin-like material. It was high in carbohydrate and sialic acid and low in lipid content, as opposed to tissue thromboplastin, which activates factor VII. This mucin extract corrected clotting in systems deficient in factors XI, IX, VII, and VIII. It was inert against fibrinogen and prothrombin preparations and lacked identifiable enzymatic activity of its own. It appeared to activate factor X. Interestingly, reduction of sialic acid content lessened the coagulant activity. Further, injection of this material into rabbits caused a precipitous defibrination syndrome, with microthrombi in small blood vessels. This finding was corroborated by Sakuragawa et al. (61).

The major clinical expression of a coagulation abnormality may be bleeding as noted above, but thrombosis may also herald ongoing procoagulant consumption. Ambrus et al. (62) studied thrombophlebitis in patients with cancer. They observed 209 thrombophlebitic events in 1,126 patients, which was a significant increase over the expected 95 events. Patients with pancreatic, gastrointestinal, and lung cancers had a 50-, 18-, and five-fold increased incidence, respectively, of thrombophlebitis over the average incidence for the whole group. While pancreatic tumors were associated with the highest risk of phlebitis, gastrointestinal adenocarcinomas and lung cancers accounted for many more individual cases. Circulating tumor cells were found in a small number of patients but occurred equally often in those with and those without phlebitis. In this series, thrombophlebitis was the sign that led to the diagnosis of malignancy in only 9 of 1,126 patients.

Sack et al. (63) reported 10 cases with disordered coagulation associated with malignancy. Four were patients with widely metastatic carcinoma who had venous thrombosis, arterial embolic phenomenon, and evidence of disseminated intravascular coagulation (DIC). Two of these patients had nonbacterial thrombotic endocarditis (NBTE) found at autopsy. The remaining six patients had migratory thrombophlebitis with evidence of DIC. Thrombophlebitis preceded the diagnosis of cancer by as much as six months in these cases. Two of 10 suffered significant bleeding.

The finding of arterial emboli in patients with cancer is another manifestation of a disordered coagulation state. Kim et al. (64) found 36 cases of NBTE in a review of 4,783 autopsies. The pathologic appearance of the cardiac valve lesions is a bland fibrin-platelet verrucous deposit. Culture of these lesions was negative. The diagnosis was not suspected before death in the majority of cases. Of the 36 cases, 13 had carcinoma. Histologic evidence of premortem intravascular coagulation was found in 11 of the 18 patients with NBTE and cancer. Rosen and Armstrong (65) found a 1% incidence of NBTE in patients dying of cancer. Seventy-five patients out of 7,840 autopsies were found to have culture negative, platelet-fibrin depositions on heart valves. They pointed out that approximately one-third of these patients had preexisting heart disease, atherosclerosis with cardiomegaly, cardiomegaly alone, or evidence of rheumatic valvular damage. In both of the above studies, emboli were widely disbursed through the vital organs. Sufficiently large emboli were present in one-third of the cases to have contributed to the immediate cause of death.

REFERENCES

1. Aisenberg AC, Castleman B: Case records of the Massachusetts General Hospital. *N Engl J Med* 270:1302, 1964.

2. Chen HP, Walz DV: Leukemoid reaction in the bone marrow associated with malignant neoplasm. *Am J Clin Pathol* 29:345, 1958.

3. Pisciotta AV: Clinical and pathologic effects of space-occupying lesions of the bone marrow. *Am J Clin Pathol* 22:915, 1950.

4. Fahey RJ: Unusual leukocyte responses in primary carcinoma of the lung. *Cancer* 4:930, 1951.

5. Banerjie RN, Narang RM: Hematological changes in malignancy. *Br J Haematol* 13:829, 1967.

6. Robinson WA: Granulocytosis in neoplasia. *Ann NY Acad Sci* 230:212, 1974.

7. Burkett LL, Cox ML, Fields ML: Leukoerythroblastosis in the adult. *Am J Clin Pathol* 44:494, 1965.

8. Vaughn JM: Leuco-erythroblastic anaemia. *J Pathol Bacteriol* 42:541, 1936.

9. Retief FP: Leuco-erythroblastosis in the adult. *Lancet* 1:639, 1964.

10. Weick JK, Hagedorn AB, Linman JW: Leukoerythroblastosis: Diagnostic and prognostic significance. *Mayo Clin Proc* 49:110, 1974.

11. Broghamer WL Jr, Keeling MM: The bone marrow biopsy, osteoscan and peripheral blood in non-hematopoietic cancer. *Cancer* 40:836, 1977.

12. Chernow B, Wallner SF: Variables predictive of bone marrow metastasis. *Cancer* 42:2373, 1978.

13. Clifton JA, Philipp RJ, Ludovic E, et al: Bone marrow and carcinoma of the prostate. *Am J Med Sci* 224:121, 1952.

14. Delsol G, Guiu-Godfrin B, Guiu M, et al: Leukoerythroblastosis and cancer frequency, prognosis, and physiopathologic significance. *Cancer* 44:1009, 1979.

15. Jonsson V, Rundles RW: Tumor metastases in bone marrow. *Blood* 6:16, 1951.

16. Sundberg RD: Differential diagnosis of anemias which present peripheral leukoerythroblastotic reactions. *Am J Med Tech* 22:34, 1956.

17. Contreras E, Ellis LD, Lee RE: Value of the bone marrow biopsy in the diagnosis of metastatic carcinoma. *Cancer* 29:778, 1972.

18. Pittman G, Tung KSK, Hoffman GC: Metastatic cells in bone marrow: Study of 83 cases. *Cleveland Clin Q* 38:55, 1971.

19. Stonier PF, Evans PV: Carcinoma cells in bone marrow aspirates. *Am J Clin Pathol* 45:722, 1966.

20. Kiely JM, Silverstein MJ: Metastatic carcinoma simulating agnogenic myeloid metaplasia and myelofibrosis. *Cancer* 24:1041, 1969.

21. Mettier SR: Hematologic aspects of space consuming lesions of the bone marrow (myelophthisic anemia). *Ann Intern Med* 14:436, 1940.

22. West CD, Ley AB, Pearson DH: Myelophthisic anemia in cancer of the breast. *Am J Med* 18:923, 1955.

23. Clifford GO: The clinical significance of leukoerythroblastic anemia. *Med Clin North Am* 50:779, 1966.

24. Eriksson S, Killander J, Wadman B: Leuco-erythroblastic anaemia in prostatic cancer. *Scand J Haematol* 9:648, 1972.

25. Mertens BF, Greene LF, Bowie EJW, et al: Fibrinolytic split products (FSP) and ethanol gelation test in preoperative evaluation of patients with prostatic disease. *Mayo Clin Proc* 49:642, 1974.

26. Erf LA, Herbut PA: Primary and secondary myelofibrosis. *Ann Intern Med* 21:863, 1944.

27. Riesco A: Five year cancer cure: Relation to total amount of peripheral lymphocytes and neutrophils. *Cancer* 25:135, 1970.

28. Shillitoe AJ: The common causes of lymphocytopenia. *J Clin Pathol* 3:321, 1959.

29. Zacharski LR, Linman JW: Lymphocytopenia: Its causes and significance. *Mayo Clin Proc* 46:168, 1971.

30. Lee YN, Sparks FC, Eilber FR, et al: Delayed cutaneous hypersensitivity and peripheral lymphocyte counts in patients with advanced cancer. *Cancer* 35:748, 1975.

31. Termini BA: Lymphocytopenia in malignant disease. *Md State Med J* 21:71, 1972.

32. Lee YN: Peripheral lymphocyte count and subpopulations of T & B lymphocytes in benign and malignant diseases. *Surg Gynecol Obstet* 144:435, 1977.

33. Miller WM, Adcook KJ, Moniot AL, et al: Hypereosinophilia with lung nodules due to thyroid carcinoma. *Chest* 71:789, 1977.

34. Viola MV, Chung EDB, Mukhopadhyay MG: Eosinophilia and metastatic Carcinoma. *Med Ann DC* 41:1, 1972.

35. Isaacson NH, Rapoport P: Eosinophilia in malignant tumors: Its significance. *Ann Intern Med* 25:893, 1946.

36. Barrett O: Monocytosis in malignancy. *Ann Intern Med* 73:991, 1970.

37. Maldonado JE, Hanlon DG: Monocytosis: A current appraisal. *Mayo Clin Proc* 40:248, 1966.

38. Reimer RR, Hoover R, Fraumeni JF, et al: Acute leukemia after alkylating agent therapy for ovarian cancer. *N Engl J Med* 297:177, 1977.

39. Coleman CN, Williams CJ, Flint A, et al: Hematologic malignancy in patients treated for Hodgkin's disease. *N Engl J Med* 297:1249, 1977.

40. Gunz FW, Angus HB: Leukemia and cancer in the same patient. *Cancer* 18:145, 1965.

41. Berg JW: The incidence of multiple primary cancers. *JNCI* 38:741, 1967.

42. Mooy JMV, Hagenouvw-Taal JC, Lameijer LDF, et al: Chronic granulocytic leukemia in a renal transplant recipient. *Cancer* 41:7, 1978.

43. Tolchin SF, Winkelstein A, Rodnan GP, et al: Chromosome abnormalities from cyclophosphamide therapy in rheumatoid arthritis and progressive systemic sclerosis (scleroderma). *Arthritis Rheum* 17:375, 1974.

44. Bridge MF, Melamed MR: Leukocyte chromosome abnormalities in advanced non-hematopoietic disease. *Cancer Res* 32:2212, 1972.

45. Karchmer RK, Amare M, Larsen WE, et al: Alkylating agents as leukemogens in multiple myeloma. *Cancer* 33:1103, 1974.

46. Hutchinson GB: Late neoplastic changes following medical irradiation. *Cancer* 37:1102, 1976.

47. Mitelman F, Brandt L, Nilsson PG: Relation among occupational exposure to potential mutagenic/carcinogenic agents. *Blood* 52:1229, 1978.

48. Bizzozero OJ, Johnson KG, Ciscco A: Radiation-related leukemia in Hiroshima and Nagasaki, 1946–1964. *N Engl J Med* 274:1095, 1966.

49. Rosner F, Grunwald H: Multiple myeloma terminating in acute leukemia. *Am J Med* 57:927, 1974.

50. Arseneau JC, Sponzo RW, Levin DL, et al: Nonlymphomatous malignant tumors complicating Hodgkin's disease possible association with intensive chemotherapy. *N Engl J Med* 287:1119, 1972.

51. Levin J, Conley CL: Thrombocytosis associated with malignant disease. *Arch Intern Med* 114:497, 1964.

52. Davis WM, Ross AOM: Thrombocytosis and thrombocythemia. *Am J Clin Pathol* 59:244, 1973.

53. Silvis SE, Turkbas N, Doscherholmen A: Thrombocytosis in patients with lung cancer. *JAMA* 211:1852, 1970.

54. Hagedorn AB, Bowie EJW, Elveback LR, et al: Coagulation abnormalities in patients with inoperable lung cancer. *Mayo Clin Proc* 49:467, 1974.

55. Sun NCJ, Bowie EJW, Kazmier FS, et al: Blood coagulation studies in patients with cancer. *Mayo Clin Proc* 49:467, 1974.

56. Slichter SJ, Harker LA: Hemostasis in malignancy. *Ann NY Acad Sci* 230:252, 1974.

57. Brain MC, Azzopardi JG, Baker LR, et al: Microangiopathic haemolytic anemia and mucin-forming adenocarcinoma. *Br J Haematol* 18:183, 1970.

58. Miller SP, Sanchez-Avalos J, Stefanski T, et al: Coagulation disorders in cancer. *Cancer* 20:1452, 1967.

59. Lohrmann H, Adam W, Heymer B, et al: Microangiopathic hemolytic anemia in metastatic carcinoma: 8 cases. *Ann Intern Med* 79:368, 1973.

60. Pineo GF, Regeoczi E, Hatton MWC, et al: The activation of coagulation by extracts of mucus: A possible pathway of intravascular coagulation accompanying adenocarcinomas. *J Lab Clin Med* 82:255, 1973.

61. Sakuragawa N, Takahashi K, Hoshiyama M, et al: The extract from the tissue of gastric cancer as procoagulant in disseminated intravascular coagulation syndrome. *Thromb Res* 10:457, 1977.

62. Ambrus JL, Ambrus CM, Pickern J, et al: Hematologic changes and thromboembolic complications of neoplastic diseases and their relationship to metastasis. *J Med* 6:433, 1975.

63. Sack GH, Levin J, Bell WR: Trousseau's syndrome and other manifestations of chronic disseminated coagulopathy in patients with neoplasma. *Medicine* 1:1, 1977.

64. Kim H, Suzuki M, Lie JT, et al: NBTE and DIC: Autopsy study of 36 cases. *Arch Pathol Lab Med* 101:65, 1977.

65. Rosen P, Armstrong D: Nonbacterial thrombotic endocarditis in patients with malignant neoplastic diseases. *Am J Med* 54:23, 1973.

10
Disorders
of Serum Proteins

Edward C. Lynch

MONOCLONAL IMMUNOGLOBULINS

In healthy persons the serum immunoglobulins are constituted by a large number of different proteins (polyclonal immunoglobulins) directed at a wide variety of antigens. Based upon physiochemical and immunochemical studies, five classes of immunoglobulins are recognized—immunoglobulins G, A, M, D, and E. In certain clinical states, large amounts of a single immunoglobulin are elaborated. Structurally and electrophoretically this protein is homogenous. It is termed a monoclonal immunoglobulin or an "M-protein." The presence of an M-protein in the serum is generally recognized by serum protein electrophoresis. Usually a narrow monoclonal spike is found in the gamma or beta region. The M-protein can be classified by class of immunoglobulin (Ig) (G, A, M, D, or E) by immunoelectrophoresis and quantitated by radial immunodiffusion studies. Occasionally, the amount of the M-protein is insufficient to recognize by serum protein electophoresis; it is found with immunoelectrophoresis.

Serum protein electrophoresis is a very commonly applied laboratory test in clinical medicine. An M-protein is identified in the serum of 0.9% of the adult population above the age of 25 years and of 3% above the age of 70 years (1). Careful evaluation of a patient with an M-protein in the serum or urine is indicated since malignancies, particularly of the lymphoid-plasmacytic line, are a frequent cause of M-proteins (Table 10-1).

Subunits or fragments of immunoglobulins may appear in large amounts in the serum or urine in certain disease states. The most important of these are the Bence Jones proteins. These proteins are monoclonal light chains (either kappa or lambda type) with molecular weights of 22,500 in the monomeric form. They can exist as dimers or mixtures of monomers and dimers. Because of their low molecular weights, Bence Jones proteins are filtered by the glomeruli and are found principally in the urine rather than the serum. Renal clearance of Bence Jones proteins is inversely related to molecular size and varies between 9 and 50% of the creatinine clearance (2). The proteins have the unusual property of precipitation between 50 to 60°C in acid media (pH 5.0). The proteins resolubilize on heating to 90–100°C. A few other urinary proteins have heat solubility characteristics similar to light chains. An example is transferrin, which

219

Table 10-1. Classification of Causes of Monoclonal Immunoglobulins

---

Multiple myeloma
Primary amyloidosis
Macroglobulinemia
Heavy-chain diseases
Lymphocytic lymphoma
Chronic lymphocytic leukemia
Other leukemias
Carcinoma
Benign monoclonal gammopathy
Cold agglutinin disease
Pyoderma gangrenosum
Lichen myxedematosus
Hyperparathyroidism
Chronic inflammatory disorders

---

precipitates at 59°C and redissolves at 95°C. Light chains are specifically identified in the urine through the discovery of a monoclonal "fast gamma" protein by electrophoresis of the urinary proteins followed by a reaction of this monoclonal protein to specific antisera directed at light chains.

Multiple Myeloma

Multiple myeloma is a progressive neoplastic proliferation of plasma cells, principally in the bone marrow. Patients are commonly anemic. Loss of calcium from bones is usually evident radiographically, either in the form of discrete osteolytic lesions or diffuse demineralization. Complications include severe bone pain, hypercalcemia, and renal failure. Abnormalities of immunoglobulins are found in nearly all patients with multiple myeloma. M-protein is discovered by serum electrophoresis in approximately 75–80% of patients (2–5). Between 65 and 70% of the M-proteins are of the IgG class with most of the remainder IgA (2–5). Rarely the characteristic clinical picture of multiple myeloma is associated with a monoclonal serum protein of IgM, IgD, or IgE class or even with two M-proteins in the serum. Among patients with multiple myeloma, approximately 20% (11–26%) do not have a serum M-protein but do have monoclonal light chains in the urine (2,3,5–7). This variant is called *light-chain myeloma*. The amount of light chains in the blood is usually too small to detect by serum protein electrophoresis, except when renal insufficiency is present.

By the heat precipitation method, 40–55% of patients with multiple myeloma have Bence Jones proteinuria (4). Using urinary protein electrophoresis and immunoelectrophoresis, light chains are found in the urine in 70–75% of patients. Using highly specific antisera the percentage of patients with monoclonal light chains in the urine is increased to 80–85%. The light chains are kappa type in 60–70% of cases (2,3); the remainder are lambda type.

One to two percent of patients with multiple myeloma have neither a serum M-protein nor light chains in the urine (nonsecretory multiple myeloma), but are deficient in circulating immunoglobulins. Rarely cases of multiple myeloma have been described with no detectable abnormalities of the immunoglobulins.

When patients with multiple myeloma are classified according to the type of immunoglobulin abnormality, certain differences are noted among groups. The prognosis is best for the group of patients with IgG myeloma who have no Bence Jones proteinuria. Their disease tends to be more chronic than that observed in other types of multiple myeloma. They often show marked reduction in the level of polyclonal immunoglobulins and have serious infections. The mean survival time is shorter in IgA myeloma than in IgG myeloma (5). In patients with a serum M-component, mean survival is less in patients with Bence Jones proteinuria than for those without light chains in the urine (5). Patients with light-chain myeloma, that is, light chains in the urine but no serum M-protein component, have a higher incidence of renal disease and of amyloidosis and more difficulty with bone disease and hypercalcemia than do patients with IgG or IgA multiple myeloma (5,6,8). Severe azotemia is at least twice as frequent in light-chain disease as in IgG or IgA myeloma. Among patients with light-chain myeloma or IgG myeloma, but not those with IgA myeloma, survival time is shorter for the group with lambda light chain proteinuria than for the group with kappa light chains in the urine (5).

Less than 200 cases of IgD multiple myeloma have been reported (9). As a group these patients are younger than those with IgG or IgA myeloma and have a more severe form of multiple myeloma. They show a higher incidence of lymphadenopathy, hepatosplenomegaly, extramedullary tumors, and amyloidosis. Bence Jones proteinuria occurs in almost all patients and azotemia (67% of patients) is very common (9). The amount of the serum M-protein is generally less than in IgG or IgA myeloma. Lambda light chains are found in 90% of patients with IgD myeloma (9).

Approximately 30 patients have been reported in whom two monoclonal proteins were identified in the serum (10). Usually one protein is IgM, while the other is IgG or IgA. The clinical picture is quite heterogenous, with patients variously showing manifestations of multiple myeloma, plasmacytoma, macroglobulinemia, or a lymphoma-type illness.

Quantitation of the M-protein in serum and urine is important. Response to chemotherapy can be accurately gauged by changes in the concentration of the M-protein because in a specific patient the amount of the M-protein correlates well with the extent of the tumor cell mass.

When a serum M-protein is present in substantial amounts, rouleaux formation of the erythrocytes is evident by examination of a peripheral blood film (Fig. 10-1). Large amounts of M-protein in the serum may result in the hyperviscosity syndrome. Clinical manifestations include cutaneous hemorrhages, mucous membrane bleeding, retinal hemorrhages, impaired vision, neurologic deficits, cardiac failure, and renal insufficiency. Plasma volume is expanded. Serum viscosity can be measured with an Ostwald viscosimeter tube, in which the viscosity of serum is compared with that of water. The value of viscosity for water is 1.0 and for normal serum 1.6. Patients vary considerably in their threshold for experiencing clinical symptoms due to hyperviscosity. However, signs of the hyperviscosity syndrome usually do not appear unless the relative serum viscosity is increased to a value of 4 or above. While the hyperviscosity syndrome is very

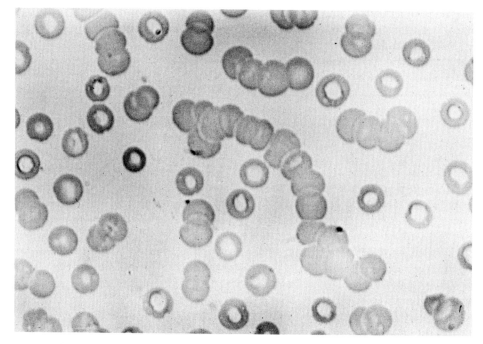

Figure 10-1. Rouleaux formation of the erythrocytes in the peripheral blood of a patient with multiple myeloma. (Magnification 800X.)

common in patients with macroglobulinemia, it only occurs in 2–4% of patients with multiple myeloma (11). In multiple myeloma an increase in viscosity sufficient to cause the hyperviscosity syndrome is usually due to very high blood levels of IgG, aggregates of IgG in the blood, or polymerization of IgA M-proteins (12). Plasmapheresis is an effective form of treatment for relief of symptoms due to hyperviscosity. Because the systemic distribution of IgM is such that 80% is intravascular, plasmapheresis can easily reduce the blood viscosity and alleviate symptoms in patients with macroglobulinemia. More intensive plasmapheresis is required when an IgG paraprotein is responsible for symptoms due to hyperviscosity because only 40% of the body's IgG is intravascular (13). The easiest means of accomplishing plasmapheresis is through the use of a blood cell separator, although it can be accomplished by withdrawal of the patient's blood into donor packs with return of the red cells to the patient following centrifugation of the blood.

"Myeloma kidney" is a unique form of renal insufficiency characterized by atrophy of renal tubular cells, dilatation of distal and collecting tubules, and intratubular deposits of eosinophilic or polychromatophilic-staining, protein-containing casts (7). Light chains in the glomerular filtrate seem to be one important factor in altering renal function and producing the histologic lesions of myeloma kidney (14,15).

The renal Fanconi syndrome has been reported in 18 adults with Bence Jones proteinuria accompanying multiple myeloma or primary amyloidosis (16). Usually the diagnosis of the Fanconi syndrome preceded the recognition of the plasmacytic disorder. None of the patients had an M-protein in the serum. The Fanconi syndrome is characterized by proximal tubular dysfunction resulting in glycosuria, aminoaciduria, phosphaturia, acidosis, and osteomalacia.

Case 1

A 49-year-old man was seen on March 18, 1969 complaining of severe pain of four months duration in the area of the lumbar spine. Roentgenograms disclosed osteolytic lesions in the fourth and fifth lumbar vertebrae. Peripheral blood counts were normal. Serum protein electrophoresis revealed a monoclonal peak in the gamma region amounting to 3.9 g/dl. This monoclonal protein was identified as IgG kappa by immunoelectrophoresis. Electrophoresis of the urinary proteins demonstrated no light chains. Examination of a bone marrow aspirate showed that 16% of the nucleated cells of the marrow were plasma cells. The diagnosis of multiple myeloma was made. Following radiotherapy amounting to 2,000 rads to the lower lumbar spine, the patient noted almost complete disappearance of pain.

During the subsequent 11 years changes in the amount of the M-protein quantitated by serum protein electrophoresis were closely related to changes in his symptoms and alterations in his chemotherapeutic program (Fig. 10-2). Chemotherapy was initiated in April 1969 with a regimen of 0.2 mg/kg/day melphalan and 2.0 mg/kg/day prednisone for 4 days each month (Fig. 2A). A marked decline in the serum M-protein was detected. After six months the doses of melphalan and prednisone were reduced by 50%. The patient was essentially asymptomatic until October 1972, when he noted easy fatigability, excessive bruising, and mild bone pain. At this time an increase in the serum M-protein was found (Fig. 2B). During the following year he continued four-day courses of chemotherapy each month with melphalan at an increased dosage of 0.15

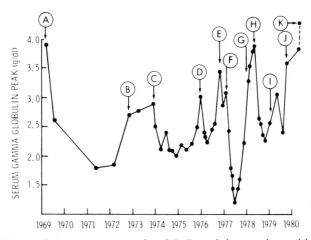

Figure 10-2. Values of the serum monoclonal IgG peak in a patient with multiple myeloma observed during a period of 11 years. Points A through K are explained in the report of Case 1.

mg/kg/day and prednisone 1.0 mg/kg/day. His symptoms did not change but were mild in degree. The serum M-protein spike slowly increased in amount.

In November 1973 the chemotherapeutic program was changed to four-day courses every six weeks consisting of cyclophosphamide, 500 mg/M^2 intravenously on day 1, and 6 mg/M^2 melphalan and 60 mg/M^2 prednisone orally on days 1–4 (Fig. 2C). A marked fall in the serum M-protein occurred and the patient was asymptomatic until December 1975, when sharp lumbar pains appeared requiring radiotherapy (Fig. 2D), which relieved the pain.

The patient continued on the same chemotherapeutic program and had few symptoms until November 1976, when intense pain in the iliac crests was experienced (Fig. 2E). With radiotherapy the pain lessened. Chemotherapy with VBAP was initiated in January 1977 (Fig. 2F). In this regimen 1.0 mg vincristine was given intravenously on day 1, 30 mg/M^2 Adriamycin and 30 mg/M^2 BCNU (carmustine) were given intravenously on day 2, and prednisone was taken orally in the dosage of 60 mg/M^2 daily on days 2–5. He received nine courses of VBAP at three-week intervals between January and July 1977. A marked decline in the level of the serum M-protein was observed, and the patient had only mild symptomatology related to the multiple myeloma. During the following six months (July–December 1977) he received no chemotherapy and felt well until late December, when pain in the lower right ribs appeared (Fig. 2G). Radiotherapy was administered to the ribs. Within the next four months severe pain in the sternum and cervical spine led to additional radiotherapy. In June 1978 four-day courses of VMCP chemotherapy, administered at three-week intervals, were initiated (Fig. 2H). 1.0 mg vincristine was administered on day 1. On days 2–5, the patient took orally 125 mg/M^2 cyclosphosphamide, 6 mg/M^2 melphalan and 60 mg/M^2 prednisone. A substantial fall in the amount of the serum M-protein was demonstrated, and the patient experienced thereafter only mild pains in his bones.

Bone pain increased in March 1979, and, although VMCP chemotherapy was continued, moderate bone pain persisted and the level of the serum M-protein increased (Fig. 2I). In July 1979 vincristine was discontinued because of peripheral neuropathy. By October 1979 severe pain in the hips was present, and the value of the serum M-protein had increased further. Additional radiotherapy to painful areas was used. Chemotherapy with Adriamycin, BCNU, cyclophosphamide, and prednisone was initiated in December 1979 (Fig. 2J). No benefit was received. He experienced intense bone pain in multiple sites during the first three months of 1980. The level of the serum M-protein rose to 5.4 g/dl in late March 1980 (Fig. 2K). He contracted disseminated herpes zoster of the skin and died of pneumonia due to *Klebsiella* species on April 4, 1980.

Comment

The clinical course of this patient's illness illustrates the close correlation of accentuated clinical symptomatology with increases in the level of the serum M-protein and the decline in both symptoms and the level of the M-protein during and after effective chemotherapy. The protracted course of the multiple myeloma in this patient over a period of 11 years reflects the more favorable prognosis with IgG myeloma and the unusual sensitivity of his malignant disease to chemotherapy.

Case 2

A 68-year-old man was hospitalized for neurologic evaluation. During the two months before admission increasingly frequent episodes of confusion were observed by family members. He became weak, lethargic, slept excessively, and had frequent falls. He had no history of headache, visual difficulties, or localizing neurologic symptoms. He denied pain, bleeding from all organ systems, fever, and weight loss.

Physical examination disclosed normal vital signs. He was very disoriented, somnolent, and had a poor memory. His gait was mildly ataxic and there was mild weakness of both lower extremities. Funduscopic examination disclosed marked dilatation of retinal veins but no retinal hemorrhages or papilledema. No enlargement of lymph nodes, liver, or spleen was detected. No tenderness of bones was elicited. Physical examination was otherwise unremarkable.

The hemoglobin level was 9.8 g/dl, hematocrit 30%, platelet count 141,000/ mm^3, and total leukocyte count 7,100/mm^3 with a normal differential count. Routine urinalysis gave normal results. BUN was 20 mg/dl, serum creatinine 1.9 mg/dl, serum sodium 131 mEq/liter, serum potassium 3.4 mEq/liter, serum chloride 98 mEq/liter, serum CO_2 34 mEq/liter, serum calcium 10.9 mg/dl, serum phosphorus 2.7 mg/dl, and serum uric acid 12.5 mg/dl.

A neurologic consultant considered the patient to have a diffuse encephalopathy. An electroencephalogram showed very slow wave activity consistent with bilateral diffuse encephalopathy. Roentgenograms of the chest and skull and computerized axial tomography of the brain were normal. When an intravenous pyelogram disclosed osteolytic lesions of the pelvis and a serum protein electrophoresis revealed a monoclonal spike in the gamma region, attention was turned toward the diagnosis of multiple myeloma. Total serum protein was 14.4 g/dl, with albumin 4.3 g/dl and a gamma spike of 7.2 g/dl. Immunoelectrophoresis and immunodiffusion studies showed the monoclonal protein to be IgG. The excretion of protein in the urine was 264 mg/24 hours. Monoclonal light chains were demonstrated by immunoelectrophoresis of the urinary proteins. The diagnosis of multiple myeloma was confirmed by examination of a bone marrow aspirate showing 57% of the marrow cells to be plasma cells.

Serum viscosity was measured at 4.0 using an Ostwald viscosimeter tube. Following plasmapheresis by means of a cell separator with the removal of 1,000 ml of plasma, the patient's neurologic symptoms substantially improved. A second plasmapheresis with removal of 750 ml led to return of the patient to his usual mental status. At the conclusion of this plasmapheresis total serum protein was 9.9 g/dl with a serum albumin value of 2.9 g/dl. Relative serum viscosity was 2.3 and serum creatinine 1.2 mg/dl. Treatment of the multiple myeloma with melphalan and prednisone was initiated.

Comment

In this patient the symptoms indicated a diffuse encephalopathic process. Identification of hyperviscosity, due to multiple myeloma, as the cause of the neurologic deficits enabled the return of the patient to good mental function after reduction of blood viscosity by plasmapheresis. The narrow anion gap of 2 is commonly seen in patients with very high concentrations of monoclonal immunoglobulins in the serum.

Primary Amyloidosis

Systemic amyloidosis has historically been classified as primary, secondary, and familial. Primary amyloidosis is generally considered to be a plasma cell dyscrasia. The amyloid of primary amyloidosis is made up of two major proteins, one of which consists of light chain fragments of immunoglobulins. The amyloid found in the organs of some patients with multiple myeloma is similar structurally to that of primary amyloidosis. In contrast, the principal protein of secondary amyloidosis is not an immunoglobulin. It is a protein known as amyloid A protein. Secondary amyloidosis is associated with chronic disorders such as rheumatoid arthritis, Hodgkin's disease, chronic ulcerative colitis, leprosy, osteomyelitis, and tuberculosis. Amyloidosis is seen as a familial form in familial Mediterranean fever (FMF) and in patients with the Portuguese type of limb neuropathy. Amyloidosis of FMF resembles secondary amyloidosis clinically and histologically, while the Portuguese type is characterized by amyloid deposits in peripheral nerves. Localized amyloidosis refers to infiltration of a single organ by amyloid.

Kyle and Bayrd (17) reported 236 patients with amyloidosis seen during a 13-year period at the Mayo Clinic. Fifty-six per cent were classified as primary amyloidosis, 26% were associated with multiple myeloma, 8% were secondary amyloidosis, 9% were localized amyloidosis, and 1% were familial.

Monoclonal immunoglobulins are commonly found in the serum and monoclonal light chains are frequently detected in the urine in primary amyloidosis, but M-proteins are not usually present in the secondary or familial forms of amyloidosis (18). Plasma cells, sometimes with atypical features, are generally discovered in increased numbers in aspirates of marrow. Histologically, amyloid is deposited in many organs, including skin, tongue, gums, heart, joints, skeletal muscle, gastrointestinal tract, nerves, kidneys, liver, spleen, and bone marrow. Clinical problems include purpura due to skin involvement, macroglossia, cardiomyopathy with cardiac failure and conduction defects, arthritis, carpal tunnel syndrome, gastrointestinal hemorrhage, malabsorption, protein-losing enteropathy, peripheral neuropathy, autonomic neuropathy, nephrotic syndrome, hepatomegaly, and splenomegaly. The diagnosis of amyloidosis depends on the histologic demonstration of infiltration of organs with amyloid. Sites most likely to yield a diagnosis by biopsy are the rectum and the gums.

Case 3

A 66-year-old banker was hospitalized with the symptom of edema. Eight months earlier he had noted the insidious appearance of malaise, weakness, and bilateral pedal edema. Because the extent of the edema increased, two months later he saw a physician who found hypertension (never noted previously), proteinuria, and an elevated value of the blood urea nitrogen. The patient gave no history of nephritis, hematuria, prior renal or cardiac disease, or the use of medications.

The only abnormalities noted on physical examination were the blood pressure of 210/110 mm Hg and four plus dependent edema extending up to the knees.

Hematocrit value was 35%, total leukocyte count 9,900/mm^3 with a normal differential count, and platelet count 249,000/mm^3. Urinalysis disclosed specific gravity 1.014, protein four plus, and sugar negative. Examination of the urinary sediment revealed 1–2 red cells and 2–4 leukocytes per high power field with many oval fat bodies. Blood urea nitrogen was 27 mg/dl and serum creatinine was 2.6 mg/dl. Values of the fasting blood sugar, serum alkaline phosphatase, total serum bilirubin, SGOT, and SGPT were normal. Roentgenograms of the chest and an electrocardiogram revealed no abnormalities. A drip intravenous pyelogram with nephrotomograms showed the kidneys to be normal in size.

The value of the serum albumin was 1.8 g/dl. A monoclonal peak was discovered by serum protein electrophoresis. This peak was IgG. Quantitation of the serum immunoglobulins revealed IgG 2,300 mg/dl, IgA 85 mg/dl, and IgM 150 mg/dl. The urinary loss of protein varied between 8.9 and 12.3 g per day. Although 60% of the urinary protein was albumin, 24% of the protein was present as a gamma monoclonal spike, shown subsequently to be light chains. No osteolytic lesions were detected radiographically. Examination of a bone marrow aspirate showed 10% of the marrow cells to be plasma cells. Histologic examination of a rectal biopsy demonstrated Congo red positive material in the walls of blood vessels in the submucosa. With polarized light the "apple-green" birefringence characteristic of amyloid was seen.

Comment

The patient had the clinical picture of the nephrotic syndrome of uncertain causation. The discovery of monoclonal immunoglobulins in the serum and urine suggested that amyloidosis was a strong diagnostic possibility. The presence of amyloid was confirmed by rectal biopsy.

Macroglobulinemia

In 1944 Waldenström (19) first described macroglobulinemia, a disorder in which he found an abnormal amount of a 19 S globulin with a molecular weight above 1,000,000 in the serum. Subsequently the globulin was discovered to be monoclonal immunoglobulin M (IgM). The disorder is a neoplastic proliferative process of B lymphocytes. Morphologically the cells have the appearance of lymphocytes or immature plasma cells or of an intermediate form commonly called *plasmacytoid lymphocytes*. These cells infiltrate particularly the bone marrow, lymph nodes, liver, and spleen and are responsible for the production of the monoclonal IgM found in the serum.

The diagnosis of Waldenström's macroglobulinemia is established by the findings of a monoclonal immunoglobulin spike of at least 1 g/dl by serum protein electrophoresis, the identification of this protein as monoclonal IgM by immunoelectrophoresis, and the presence of clinical abnormalities characteristic of the disorder. The IgM peaks are frequently in the "fast" gamma region on serum protein electrophoresis, but sometimes are in the beta or slow gamma regions. In some patients with monoclonal IgM proteins in the serum, the disorder is asymptomatic and nonprogressive; thus, these patients have a benign monoclonal gammopathy of IgM type. Approximately 25% of patients with Waldenström's macroglobulinemia have monoclonal light chains in the urine. The light chains are kappa type in 80% of cases. In one-third of patients, cryoprecipitable IgM (cryoglobulin) is present in the serum; these patients sometimes have Raynaud's phenomenom.

Histologically the liver, spleen, lymph nodes, and, sometimes, the kidneys are extensively infiltrated by lymphocytes, lymphocytoid cells, and plasma cells (20). The bone marrow aspirate, although usually nondiagnostic, shows a similar infiltration. Ten to 90% of the marrow cells are lymphoid or plasmacytic. It is often difficult to distinguish the abnormalities of the marrow in macroglobulinemia from those of lymphocytic lymphoma. Tissue mast cells are frequently increased in number in the marrow in macroglobulinemia.

Hepatomegaly is present clinically in 55–77% of patients with macroglobulinemia, splenomegaly in 45–71%, and lymphadenopathy in 45–49% (20,21). In contrast to multiple myeloma, only 7% have osteolytic lesions (20).

The major symptoms experienced by patients with Waldenström's macroglobulinemia are fatigue and weakness (44%), weight loss (23%), bleeding (44%), neurologic abnormalities (11%), and visual disturbances (8%) (21). These symptoms are related to the IgM monoclonal protein and more particularly to the hyperviscosity of the blood due to the protein. MacKenzie and Fudenberg (20) found the level of the total serum proteins to be 10.0 g/dl or higher in 17 of 40 patients with macroglobulinemia. Relative serum viscosity values were above 4.0 in 14 of 34 patients. Plasma volume is usually substantially increased. Low values of the hemoglobin are common (89% of cases) and can be due to the expanded plasma volume, blood loss, or myelophthisis. Rouleaux formation of the erythrocytes is often very prominent, particularly when the value of the serum IgM is quite high. Visual complaints include loss of vision and conjunctival hemorrhages. The earliest ophthalmoscopic finding is dilated retinal veins. Later, sausage-like segmentation of the veins appears, often accompanied by retinal hemorrhages. Cerebral symptoms are usually related to hyperviscosity and include headache, lethargy, vertigo, confusion, disorientation, and even coma. Polyneuropathy is occasionally seen in macroglobulinemia. Increased blood viscosity may contribute to the appearance of either cardiac or renal failure in patients with macroglobulinemia. Both expanded plasma volume and anemia can also be important in the development of congestive heart failure.

Bleeding from mucous membranes is particularly prominent in patients with macroglobulinemia. Thus, epistaxis, oral bleeding, and conjunctival hemorrhages are commonly seen. Some patients bleed chronically from the gastrointestinal tract and develop an iron deficiency anemia. Purpura and easy bruisability are frequent. Disordered hemostasis is particularly noticeable in patients who have overt symptoms of the hyperviscosity syndrome. Two mechanisms account for the impaired hemostatis. Platelet function is defective due to coating of platelets by the IgM protein. In addition, the IgM protein inhibits fibrin monomer aggregation, thus blocking the conversion of fibrinogen to fibrin.

Plasmapheresis offers a very effective immediate form of therapy for Waldenström's macroglobulinemia (12,13). Symptoms due to hyperviscosity generally improve rapidly and bleeding ceases.

MacKenzie and Fudenberg (20) pointed out that Waldenström's macroglobulinemia is frequently associated with other malignancies. While the majority were lymphomas, eight of their 40 patients developed carcinomas. Usually the lymphoma or carcinoma appeared months to years after the recognition of macroglobulinemia.

Case 4

A 78-year-old man was hospitalized because of anemia, first discovered seven months earlier. During the month before hospitalization he experienced frequent epistaxis and melena and received transfusions. Physical examination upon admission to the hospital disclosed scattered ecchymoses, very dilated retinal veins, numerous retinal hemorrhages, and the spleen palpable 2 cm beneath the left costal margin. The liver was not enlarged and no enlarged lymph nodes were found. There were no petechiae.

Hemoglobin level was 6.4 g/dl, hematocrit 19%, reticulocyte count 3.4%, platelet count 29,000/mm^3, and total leukocyte count 6,500/mm^3, with 50 segmented neutrophils, 5 bands, 1 metamyelocyte, 36 lymphocytes, and 8 monocytes on differential count. Examination of a peripheral blood film revealed a highly "proteinaceous" background on the slide, marked rouleaux of the erythrocytes, and three normoblasts per 100 leukocytes. Many of the lymphocytes were plasmacytoid in appearance. Both the bone marrow aspirate and the needle biopsy were very hypercellular. Forty-five percent of the nucleated cells of the marrow were lymphoid cells, many of which showed plasmacytoid features.

Total serum protein level was 10.7 g/dl. Serum protein electrophoresis disclosed a monoclonal peak in the gamma region, with the gamma globulins amounting to 6.1 g/dl. By immunoelectrophoresis the monoclonal protein was identified as IgM kappa class. Quantitation of the serum immunoglobulins revealed an IgM level of 6,400 mg/dl. No cryoglobulins were demonstrable in the serum. Relative serum viscosity was 4.1. Light chains were not found in the urine. Plasma volume was 56.7 mg/kg, a moderately increased value.

The patient was given transfusions of packed red blood cells and platelets. Three liters of plasma were removed by plasmapheresis. The value of serum viscosity decreased to 2.1. Gastrointestinal and nasal bleeding ceased. Retinal hemorrhages disappeared. Chemotherapy was initiated with a program using cyclophosphamide, vincristine, and prednisone. During the next four months values of the serum monoclonal peak varied between 1.9 and 2.8 g/dl and the relative serum viscosity ranged between 1.8 and 2.4. The treatment program was then changed to chlorambucil orally with good control of IgM production and improvement in the anemia and thrombocytopenia. Subsequent complications included an autoimmune hemolytic anemia (responsive to treatment with prednisone) seven months after the original hospitalization and pneumonia two months later. The patient eventually died of left ventricular failure and cardiac arrhythmias 18 months after the initial diagnosis of macroglobulinemia.

Comment

Hemorrhagic manifestations and anemia were the dominant abnormalities in this patient with Waldenström's macroglobulinemia. Erythropoiesis and thrombopoiesis were both substantially reduced because of heavy infiltration of the marrow by lymphoid cells. Plasmapheresis and platelet transfusions resulted in cessation of bleeding. Chemotherapy effected control of the paraproteinemia.

Heavy-Chain Diseases

The heavy-chain diseases are uncommon proliferative disorders of plasmacytic or lymphoid origin in which the infiltrating cells synthesize and secrete a portion of the heavy chains of immunoglobulins, rather than a complete immunoglobulin. Three heavy-chain diseases have been recognized: gamma-heavy-chain disease, in which the monoclonal protein is of IgG class; alpha-heavy-chain disease, with a monoclonal IgA protein; and mu-heavy-chain disease, in which the heavy chain is of the IgM class. No heavy-chain diseases of IgD or IgE class have been identified yet. Most patients with gamma- or mu-heavy-chain disease are more than 40 years old, but alpha-heavy-chain disease has a peak incidence in the second and third decades of life. About 60–65% of patients with heavy-chain disease are men.

The clinical picture of *gamma-heavy-chain disease* is that of a malignant lymphoma (22). Generalized lymphadenopathy is usually present. Splenomegaly and hepatomegaly are found in at least 70% of affected patients. A majority of patients have an unusual physical finding—a swollen, erythematous palate due to involvement of the lymphatic tissue of Waldeyer's ring. No abnormalities of bones are found radiographically. Fever is a very common symptom (75% of cases). Anemia is found in virtually all patients, leukopenia in 60%, and thrombocytopenia in about one-half. In many patients plasma cells or atypical lymphocytes are seen in the peripheral blood. Rarely plasma cell leukemia appears in the terminal phase of the illness. Examinations of bone marrow aspirates commonly reveal increased plasma cells and sometimes increased lymphocytes or eosinophils. The histologic appearance of lymph nodes and other organs in patients with gamma-heavy-chain disease is not diagnostic. Usually infiltration with plasma cells and lymphocytes is found, often associated with eosinophils and histiocytes. Respiratory infection is the most frequent cause of death (23).

The monoclonal protein, that is, gamma-heavy-chain protein, migrates on serum protein electrophoresis in the gamma-beta region (22). On immunoelectrophoresis the protein reacts with antisera to IgG but not to antisera for light chains. Quantitatively the serum monoclonal protein exceeds 1 g/dl in about one-half of patients. Usually there is an associated substantial diminution in the levels of normal serum immunoglobulins. Although gamma-heavy chains can be detected in the urine by immunoelectrophoresis in most cases, the excretion of the protein exceeds 1 g/24 hours in only about 20% of patients. The diagnosis of gamma-heavy-chain disease can be established only by demonstrating a protein in the serum and/or the urine that reacts on immunoelectrophoresis with antisera directed at IgG but not with antisera for light chains.

Alpha-heavy-chain disease is the most frequent of the three heavy-chain diseases. In its characteristic clinical presentation, the illness appears as an abdominal lymphoma with primarily enteric involvement. The disorder has been termed "Mediterranean lymphoma" because most cases have been from that area; however, patients with similar disorders have been observed in other parts of the world (24). Histologically, there is massive infiltration of lymphocytes, plasma cells, and histiocytes in the lamina propria of the intestines and mesenteric lymph nodes. Villous atrophy occurs. The patient has chronic diarrhea, abdominal pain, excessive fecal loss of water and electrolytes, and the clinical manifestations of a malabsorption syndrome such as loss of weight, steatorrhea, and hypocalcemia (25). Large abdominal masses are sometimes felt and intestinal obstruction may occur. Clubbing of the fingers is occasionally observed. Osteolytic bone lesions are not seen. The bone marrow, peripheral lymph nodes, liver, and spleen are usually not involved by the process, but abnormal plasma cells are occasionally recognized in the peripheral blood and bone marrow. In a rare form of alpha-heavy-chain disease the infiltration of plasma cells and lymphocytes occurs in the respiratory tract rather than the gastrointestinal tract. Alpha-heavy-chain disease is usually progressive to death but complete clinical remissions occasionally occur. In the later stages of the illness overt histologic features of reticulum cell sarcoma or of an immunoblastic lymphoma may be recognized (25,26).

Serum protein electrophoresis usually demonstrates hypoalbuminemia and hypogammaglobulinemia. In about one-half of affected patients a broad band is detected in the alpha-2-beta region (25). Recognition of the alpha-heavy chains depends on immunoelectrophoresis of the serum proteins. The abnormal serum protein reacts with antisera to IgA but not with light-chain antisera. Because some complete IgA myeloma paraproteins also fail to precipitate with light-chain antisera, confirmation of the diagnosis of alpha-heavy-chain disease in some patients is dependent upon purification of the abnormal serum protein (25). Serum levels of normal IgA, IgG, and IgM are usually decreased. In most patients the alpha-heavy chain is excreted in the urine but usually in small amounts. Concentrated samples of urine must be analyzed to detect the abnormal protein. Large amounts of the alpha-heavy-chain protein are present in jejunal fluid (25).

Mu-heavy-chain disease is very rare. Clinically the disorder closely resembles chronic lymphocytic leukemia (CLL) (27,28). Affected patients have less peripheral lymphadenopathy than usually found in CLL, but show considerable involvement of the liver, spleen, and intra-abdominal lymph nodes. Pathologic fractures and amyloidosis may complicate the illness (27). In addition to numerous small lymphocytes, vacuolated plasma cells are found in the bone marrow (28).

Generally serum protein electrophoresis shows only hypogammaglobulinemia. However, an anomalous protein is present in some cases. The diagnosis rests upon detecting by immunoelectrophoresis of the serum proteins a rapidly moving component that reacts with antisera to mu-chains but not with antisera to light chains. Because intact macroglobulins unreactive to antisera to light chains are sometimes encountered, the definitive diagnosis of mu-chain disease requires further characterization of the protein by ultracentrifugation or gel filtration. Rarely the abnormal protein has been identified in the urine. In most patients with mu-heavy-chain disease large amounts of Bence Jones proteinuria occur (28).

Lymphomas and Chronic Lymphocytic Leukemia

Diffuse lymphocytic lymphoma (DLL) and chronic lymphocytic leukemia (CLL) are among the more common causes of serum IgM paraproteins (29–31). In fact, the frequency of serum IgM peaks in these two disorders is approximately 100 times greater than that found in the general population. A mild, but significant increase in serum IgG M-proteins also occurs in DLL and CLL. Alex-anian (29) found the frequency of serum IgM peaks to be 9.7% in DLL, 4.1% in CLL, and 2.1% in reticulum cell sarcoma (RCS), while the incidence of serum IgG peaks was 3.0% in DLL, 1.0% in CLL, and 0.8% in RCS. One among 266 patients with CLL had an IgA serum paraprotein. When chemotherapy of DLL or CLL resulted in a 50% or greater reduction in the monoclonal IgM com-ponent, all overt clinical manifestations of the disease disappeared. Alexanian (29) observed no increase in frequency in monoclonal immunoglobulin peaks in 218 patients with Hodgkin's disease or 292 patients with nodular lymphomas compared to the normal population.

In patients with DLL and CLL who have serum IgM peaks, quantitatively the serum monoclonal IgM is considerably less than usually found in patients with Waldenström's macroglobulinemia. These patients with DLL or CLL do not have clinical findings related to hyperviscosity. Rather they have the usual clinical picture of DLL or CLL. The IgM paraprotein is occasionally cold-precipitable (cryoglobulin), or is a cold agglutinin resulting in a hemolytic anemia (31,32).

In approximately 95% of patients with CLL, immunofluorescent studies have demonstrated immunoglobulins on the surface of the lymphocytes (33). Mono-clonal IgM is bound to the cell surface in 80% of cases. IgG is the surface immunoglobulin of the lymphocytes in approximately 10% of patients with CLL. Rarely the lymphocytes of CLL have surface-bound IgA. These findings indicate that in most cases of CLL, immunoglobulins are produced by the neoplastic cells. Thus, the occurrence of monoclonal immunoglobulins in the serum of patients with CLL is not surprising. That it occurs in only a few, rather than most, patients with CLL appears to be mainly a matter of the quantity of the monoclonal immunoglobulin produced by the neoplastic clone. In most patients this quantity is insufficient to be detected by serum protein electrophoresis.

Occasionally Bence Jones protein is found in the urine of patients with DLL or CLL. Burke and associates (34) reported two patients with lymphosarcoma, light chains in the urine, and the clinical picture of "myeloma kidney."

Other Leukemias

Isolated instances of patients with other forms of leukemia accompanied by a serum monoclonal protein have been reported. In one patient a monoclonal IgM was associated with hairy cell leukemia (35). In this case the hairy cells had surface IgM and the properties of B lymphocytes. Rarely IgG paraproteins have been found in the sera of patients with acute lymphoblastic leukemia (36,37), monocytic leukemia (38), and chronic myelogenous leukemia (39). The causal relationship of the leukemia to the paraprotein is uncertain.

Carcinoma

At the present time the data is insufficient to ascertain to what extent carcinomas may be responsible for, or associated with, serum M-proteins. In an extensive study published in 1968, Migliore and Alexanian (40) found the incidence of serum monoclonal peaks in patients with cancer (of nonlymphoid origin) did not differ from that expected in the normal population. Among 5,066 patients referred for evaluation of a suspected neoplasm, monoclonal gammopathy in the absence of overt evidence of multiple myeloma was found in only 0.65%. Control of the tumor with surgery or radiotherapy did not alter the concentration of the M-protein. More recently Solomon (41) summarized several studies that point to some degree of relationship of epithelial cell tumors to serum monoclonal immunoglobulins. Among 806 patients with serum M-components studied by Isobe and Osserman (42), 128 had nonreticular neoplasms. The frequency of adenocarcinomas of the rectosigmoid, lung, prostate, and gall bladder was twice as great in patients with serum M-proteins as in patients with no monoclonal proteins. When an M-component is found in a patient with a carcinoma, it is usually of IgG class. The origin of the serum M-proteins may be the plasma cells and lymphocytes that surround masses of neoplastic cells (41). In studies of tumors of five patients in whom a serum M-component accompanied a carcinoma, Williams and colleagues (43) stained tumor tissue with immunofluorescent techniques and showed plasma cells containing monoclonal immunoglobulin clustered about or interspersed among nonstaining tumor cells.

An example of a globulin spike observed on serum protein electrophoresis that is not immunoglobulin in nature is the alpha-2-globulin spike of hyperhaptoglobinemia, which may be seen with cancers such as renal cell carcinoma (44).

Benign Monoclonal Gammopathy

The most frequent explanation for a monoclonal immunoglobulin peak discovered by serum protein electrophoresis is the clinical state, benign monoclonal gammopathy (idiopathic or essential paraproteinemia). Affected patients have no findings supportive of the diagnosis of any of the other disorders that cause monoclonal proteins, such as multiple myeloma, macroglobulinemia, or primary amyloidosis. In contrast to these plasma cell dyscrasias, clinical abnormalities related to the paraprotein do not develop in patients with benign monoclonal gammopathy, and no significant changes in the amount of the serum M-protein occur as the years pass. However, approximately 10% of patients whose illness is initially classified as benign monoclonal gammopathy subsequently develop overt clinical manifestations of multiple myeloma, macroglobulinemia, primary amyloidosis, or a lymphoproliferative disorder. Because the physician cannot predict which patients with an asymptomatic monoclonal gammopathy will eventually develop a symptomatic and progressive plasma cell dyscrasia, some authors prefer the term "monoclonal gammopathy of undetermined significance" to the more frequently used term "benign monoclonal gammopathy" (45). One-half to two-thirds of all monoclonal serum proteins initially fall into the group, monoclonal gammopathy of undetermined significance.

Patients with benign monoclonal gammopathies may have an M-protein of IgG, IgA, or IgM class. Approximately 75% of M-protein peaks are IgG, 10% IgA, and 15% IgM (45). Almost always the monoclonal peak, estimated by serum protein electrophoresis, is less than 3 g/dl (46). However, many patients with multiple myeloma or macroglobulinemia have serum M-protein levels of less than 3 g/dl. Benign monoclonal gammopathy cannot be clearly separated from multiple myeloma or macroglobulinemia by the quantitation of the serum M-component. Bachmann (47) found that 78% of patients with more than 2 g/dl of IgG M-protein and 82% with more than 1 g/dl of IgA M-protein had multiple myeloma. Macroglobulinemia was diagnosed in 67% of patients with an IgM monoclonal protein greater than 2 g/dl. Monoclonal serum proteins rarely disappear. Kyle (45) observed this occurrence in only two patients of 243 with monoclonal peaks. Usually patients with benign monoclonal gammopathy have little or no detectable monoclonal light chains in the urine. Among 42 patients with benign monoclonal gammopathy studied by Dammacco and Waldenström (48), 23.8% had light chains in the urine, but in none was the amount greater than 60 mg/liter. However, rarely substantial quantities of Bence Jones protein have been found in the urine of patients with serum monoclonal peaks in whom all other available data indicate a benign monoclonal gammopathy. In two such patients followed for a period of seven years, Kyle et al. (49) measured daily excretion of Bence Jones protein in excess of 1 g. Other features of benign monoclonal gammopathy, which contrast with the clinical picture of multiple myeloma, are normal values of the hemoglobin and the lack of hypercalcemia and osteolytic lesions of bone. Patients with benign monoclonal gammopathies usually have less than 10% plasma cells in the bone marrow, whereas the marrow aspirate commonly shows more than 20% plasma cells in patients with multiple myeloma. Nevertheless, quantitation of plasma cells in the marrow is not a completely reliable diagnostic indicator because the neoplastic process in multiple myeloma is spotty, and samples procured from some areas may show low numbers of plasma cells.

Constancy over an extended period of time of the serum M-component is the most important indicator that the process is benign monoclonal gammopathy and not a progressive plasma cell dyscrasia (50). It is essential that asymptomatic patients with serum M-proteins be followed for many years to assess accurately the significance of their monoclonal peaks. In this regard the extensive study by Kyle (45) of 243 patients with monoclonal gammopathy of undetermined significance followed for at least five years is particularly relevant. Fifty-seven percent showed no significant change in the serum monoclonal component, 11% developed a progressive plasma cell dyscrasia or a lymphoproliferative disorder, 9% demonstrated a more than 50% increase in the monoclonal protein or the appearance of a monoclonal urine protein but did not have clinical findings of a progressive plasma cell disorder, and 23% died during the five-year interval without evidence of multiple myeloma, macroglobulinemia, or amyloidosis. Among the 27 patients in whom a proliferative disorder was recognized, multiple myeloma appeared in 18, macroglobulinemia in four, primary amyloidosis in four, and chronic lymphocytic leukemia in one. The mean interval from recognition of the monoclonal gammopathy to appearance of the plasma cell dyscrasia was 64 months for patients with multiple myeloma, 103 months for those with macroglobulinemia, and 92 months for those with amyloidosis. The frequency of the development of a plasma cell dyscrasia, or a more than 50% increase in the serum M-protein, was 18% for patients who had IgG M-proteins, 28% for those with IgA M-proteins, and 25% for those with IgM M-proteins. The mean amount of the initial M-peak for the 27 patients who subsequently developed a progressive plasma cell dyscrasia was 1.8 g/dl, the same value observed for the 137 patients who showed no change in their M-protein over the five-year period.

Kyle (45) found that such factors as the hemoglobin level, the presence of small amounts of light chains in the urine, the serum levels of uninvolved immunoglobulins, and the number of plasma cells in the bone marrow were not useful in the initial evaluation of an asymptomatic patient to predict whether a progressive plasma cell dyscrasia would subsequently appear. The mean number of plasma cells seen in the bone marrow was 3.0% for those with a nonprogressive disorder and 3.6% for those in whom a progressive disorder later appeared. In both groups the range in the number of plasma cells in the marrow was 1–10%.

Miscellaneous Disorders

Chronic idiopathic cold agglutinin disease is a disorder affecting the elderly. Chronic hemolysis due to monoclonal IgM antibodies is observed. The antibodies react with the I antigen of erythrocytes. Occasionally the IgM antibodies are present in sufficient concentration in the serum to be identified as an M-peak on serum protein electrophoresis. Monoclonal IgM cold agglutinins may also be seen in patients with lymphoproliferative disorders (32).

Pyoderma gangrenosum is a rare dermatologic disorder in which tender, red, nodular or pustular lesions appear, usually on the lower extremities, followed by necrosis of the lesions and formation of painful ulcers. The ulcers have undermined edges and distinctive red-purple borders (51). They can become quite large. Forty per cent of patients with pyoderma gangrenosum have ulcerative colitis. The disorder may also be associated with regional enteritis and with an arthritis that resembles rheumatoid arthritis, but usually with negative results on tests for rheumatoid factor. Rarely pyoderma gangrenosum accompanies acute leukemia, myelofibrosis, or Hodgkin's disease. Corticosteroid therapy is effective in promoting healing of the ulcers. In some patients with pyoderma gangrenosum monoclonal serum proteins of IgA, IgG, or IgM class have been detected by electrophoresis (52). We cared for one patient with severe pyoderma gangrenosum and a long history of rheumatoid-like arthritis in whom an IgM monoclonal cryoglobulin was identified in the serum. The disorder does not exhibit features of the common plasma cell dyscrasias, such as multiple myeloma, macroglobulinemia, or primary amyloidosis.

A second dermatologic condition associated with a monoclonal immunoglobulin in the serum is lichen myxedematosus, also called papular mucinosis. Papular or plaque lesions appear on the face, trunk, and extremities of affected patients. The skin has a cobblestone appearance. The dermis is infiltrated with mucopolysaccharides with accompanying fibroblastic proliferation. Serum protein electrophoresis commonly reveals a monoclonal peak usually located to the cathodal side of the normal gammaglobulin region (53). The protein, regularly IgG lambda class, is quite basic (54). Plasmacytosis of the marrow occurs rarely. Light chains in the urine and osteolytic lesions of bone have not been observed. The course of the illness is chronic and free of the classic manifestations of multiple myeloma.

At least seven patients have been reported in whom primary hyperparathyroidism and a benign monoclonal gammopathy of either IgG or IgA class coexisted (55). No causal relationship has been conclusively demonstrated to date. The protein abnormality disappeared in only one of five patients after parathyroidectomy. The clinical importance of the coexistence of the two disorders relates to diagnostic confusion with multiple myeloma, a disease commonly causing an M-protein in the serum and hypercalcemia.

When sera from large numbers of patients have been subjected to protein electrophoresis, a substantial number are found to have M-proteins without evidence of plasma cell dyscrasias, neoplasms, or any other clear explanation for the protein abnormality. Conventionally the abnormality is assigned tentatively to the group, benign monoclonal gammopathy. Reviewing clinical records of 239 such patients, Isobe and Osserman (42) concluded that this group has an increased incidence of chronic inflammatory disorders. Examples are chronic biliary tract disease (cholecystitis and cholelithiasis), chronic urinary tract infections, tuberculosis, and syphilis (42,56). However, it remains unproved as to whether chronic inflammation can be responsible for a monoclonal gammopathy in humans.

CRYOGLOBULINEMIA

Cryoglobulins are immunoglobulins that precipitate in the cold (4°C) and redissolve with warming. Based upon clinical studies of 86 patients with cryoglobulinemia accompanied by immunochemical studies of the cryoproteins, Brouet and coworkers (57) classified cryoglobulins as three groups. Type I cryoglobulins are those consisting of isolated monoclonal immunoglobulins, usually either IgM or IgG. Type II cryoglobulins are mixed cryoglobulins characterized by a monoclonal component (usually IgM) possessing antibody activity directed at polyclonal IgG. Similar to type II, most type III cryoglobulins are also immunoglobulin-anti-immunoglobulin immune complexes. These type III cryoproteins consist of mixed polyclonal cryoglobulins of one or more immunoglobulin classes, sometimes complexed with nonimmunoglobulin proteins, such as components of the complement system or lipoproteins.

The main disorders associated with cryoglobulinemia are the collagen vascular disorders, hepatitis B antigenemia, immunohematologic conditions such as autoimmune hemolytic anemia and idiopathic thrombocytopenic purpura, and proliferative diseases of the B-lymphocyte system, such as multiple myeloma, Waldenström's macroglobulinemia, chronic lymphocytic leukemia, lymphocytic lymphoma, and immunoblastic lymphadenopathy (58). Cryoglobulins are occasionally found in patients with infections such as infectious mononucleosis, cytomegalovirus infection, leprosy, subacute bacterial endocarditis, and syphilis (59). In approximately 30% of patients with cryoglobulinemia, no associated disease is found. These patients are classified as having essential cryoglobulinemia. Patients with essential cryoglobulinemia usually have type III cryoglobulins. Patients with multiple myeloma or Waldenström's macroglobulinemia may have type I or II cryoglobulins, while those with chronic lymphocytic leukemia or lymphocytic lymphoma have type II or III cryoglobulins. The incidence of cryoglobulinemia in multiple myeloma is approximately 5%. Patients with an essential monoclonal cryoglobulinemia of IgG type occasionally later develop classic multiple myeloma (60).

The most common symptoms attributable to cryoglobulinemia are Raynaud's phenomenon and vascular purpura, each occurring in about 50% of patients with cryoglobulinemia (57). The purpuric lesions usually appear first on the lower extremities. Skin biopsies reveal the changes of acute vasculitis. Cold-precipitated urticaria and livedo reticularis are occasionally experienced by patients with cryoglobulinemia. Skin necrosis of distal areas, such as the toes, fingers, ears, or tip of the nose, occurred in 14% of Brouet's 86 cases (57). Peripheral neuropathy and diffuse glomerulonephritis are sometimes associated with cryoglobulinemia and may pose serious problems to affected patients. Renal failure may occur. Histologically, the kidneys show membraneous or membrano-proliferative glomerulonephritis. The pathogenesis of the glomerulonephritis is related to deposition of immune complexes in the glomerular basement membrane.

PYROGLOBULINS

Pyroglobulins are immunoglobulins that precipitate when serum is heated to 56°C. They do not dissolve with further heating or subsequent cooling of the serum. Pyroglobulinemia is quite uncommon. When found, the pyroglobulins are generally of IgG class but occasionally IgM or IgA (4). They are usually associated with either multiple myeloma, macroglobulinemia, or a lymphocytic lymphoma (4,61,62). Pyroglobulins do not ordinarily result in any clinical abnormalities, although rare instances of the hyperviscosity syndrome and interference with the conversion of fibrinogen to fibrin have been seen with pyroglobulinemia (63,64).

IMMUNOGLOBULIN DEFICIENCY

The immunoglobulin deficient states are classified as congenital or acquired (Table 10-2). Many of these disorders are associated with an increased incidence of malignancy. *Severe combined immunodeficiency* (Swiss-type agammaglobulinemia) is a congenital disorder in which infants lack both T and B lymphocytes. Death

Table 10-2. Classification of Immunoglobulin Deficiency

Congenital
   Severe combined immunodeficiency
   Congenital agammaglobulinemia
   Selective deficiencies of immunoglobulins A and G
   Wiskott-Aldrich syndrome
   Ataxia telangiectasia
Acquired
   Common variable immunodeficiency
   Secondary immunoglobulin deficiency
      Nephrotic syndrome
      Gastrointestinal disorders
      Chronic lymphocytic leukemia
      Lymphocytic lymphoma
      Multiple myeloma
      Thymoma

usually occurs within the first two years of life. In a few patients lymphoma or leukemia has appeared (65). In patients with *congenital agammaglobulinemia* (Bruton-type agammaglobulinemia) B cells are lacking but T-cell function is normal. Plasma cells are absent in lymph nodes, spleen, and bone marrow. Patients are deficient in all five classes of immunoglobulins. The disorder is inherited as an X-linked recessive trait. Sinus and pulmonary infections are common. Administration of gammaglobulin is effective in preventing infections. Although four cases of leukemia and one case of lymphoma have been reported in patients with congenital agammaglobulinemia, it is not yet clear whether this actually represents an increased propensity for development of neoplasms in the disorder. Other congenital immunoglobulin deficient conditions are the *selective deficiencies of immunoglobulins A and G* (IgA and IgG). Four patients with selective IgA deficiency subsequently developed a malignancy (one lymphoma, one leukemia, one carcinoma of the stomach, and one carcinoma of the lung) (65). The causal relationship of IgA deficiency to the appearance of the neoplasms is not established.

The *Wiskott-Aldrich syndrome* is characterized by thrombocytopenia, eczema, recurrent infections, and a diminished concentration of serum IgM with normal serum levels of IgG and IgA. The inheritance is X-linked. Approximately 10% of patients with Wiskott-Aldrich syndrome develop a reticuloendothelial malignancy, either lymphoma or leukemia (65).

Patients with *ataxia telangiectasia* have cerebellar ataxia during infancy, followed later by the appearance of telangiectasias of the face, ears, eyelids, and conjunctivae. The disease is inherited as an autosomal recessive trait. Cellular immunity is defective, and most patients are deficient in both serum and secretory IgA (66). Severe respiratory infections occur frequently. In a 1972 review of the literature of reported cases of ataxia telangiectasia, 42 patients were found to have developed malignancies (65). This number represents about 10% of all patients with ataxia telangiectasia. The majority of the malignancies were classified in the lymphoma group, principally lymphocytic lymphoma, reticulum cell sarcoma, and Hodgkin's disease (65,66). Eight cases of leukemia have been reported (65).

Common variable immunodeficiency is a condition also referred to as primary acquired agammaglobulinemia or idiopathic late-onset immunoglobulin deficiency. The age of onset varies from the second to the sixth decade. Mean age of onset in one study of 50 patients was 30.7 years (67). In contrast to congenital agammaglobulinemia, sex distribution of cases is even. In most instances no hereditary pattern of the disorder is evident but occasionally multiple cases occur within a family. Serum concentrations of IgG are invariably decreased, but frequently IgG levels are not as low as are found in patients with congenital agammaglobulinemia. In most patients values of serum IgA and IgM are also decreased.

Patients with common variable immunodeficiency are prone to contract sinus, middle ear, and pulmonary infections. In some bronchiectasis develops. Other frequently associated abnormalities include chronic diarrhea, malabsorption, lymphoid hyperplasia of the small bowel, intestinal giardiasis, and achlorhydria. Less frequently patients with common variable immunodeficiency develop pernicious anemia, Sjögren's syndrome, arthritis, eczema, vitiligo, hyperthyroidism, or spontaneous hypothyroidism.

The incidence of neoplasms is distinctly increased in patients with common variable immunodeficiency, and death is frequently related to malignant disease. In a review of the literature, 24 cases of malignancy were found in patients with common variable immunodeficiency (65). Seventeen were lymphomas. Later Hermans et al (67), reviewing their 50 patients with idiopathic late-onset immunodeficiency, reported that 12 developed neoplasms. Four had adenocarcinoma of the stomach, four thymoma (one with complicating lymphocytic lymphoma), one lymphoblastic lymphoma of the rectum and cecum, one adenocarcinoma of the sigmoid colon, one squamous cell carcinoma of the lung, and one agnogenic myeloid metaplasia. Malignant neoplasms were responsible for death in seven of the nine patients followed by Hermans and coworkers. The risk for the development of neoplasia in common variable immunodeficiency is among the highest of the immunodeficiency states in humans.

Waldmann and coworkers (68) have presented studies indicating that in some patients with common variable immunodeficiency a population of suppressor T lymphocytes interferes with immunoglobulin secretion by B lymphocytes. The function of T lymphocytes is deranged in some patients as judged by skin tests for delayed hypersensitivity and phytohemagglutinin stimulation of lymphocytes in vitro. Altered function of T lymphocytes may be responsible for the increased propensity for neoplasia in individuals with common variable immunodeficiency.

Secondary Acquired Immunoglobulin Deficiency

Hypogammaglobulinemia occurs in patients with the nephrotic syndrome, by reason of loss of immunoglobulins in the urine, and with certain disorders of the stomach and small intestines because of loss of immunoglobulins into the lumen of the gastrointestinal tract (protein-losing enteropathy). Malignancies of the B-lymphocyte system (particularly multiple myeloma, chronic lymphocytic leukemia, and lymphocytic lymphoma) and thymomas are the other disorders commonly associated with acquired immunoglobulin deficiency. In these disorders the immunoglobulin deficiency is due to a failure of synthesis of immunoglobulins.

Patients with multiple myeloma almost invariably have depressed levels of polyclonal immunoglobulins in the serum. Antibody formation in response to antigenic stimulation is impaired (69). Patients are particularly susceptible to respiratory and urinary tract infections. Pneumococci (70) and gram-negative bacteria (71) are prone to cause infections. The principal reason for the low levels of circulating polyclonal immunoglobulins is decreased synthesis. Broder et al (72) found that when lymphocytes of patients with multiple myeloma are stimulated in vitro with pokeweed mitogen, immunoglobulin synthesis is much less than that of normal lymphocytes. In some patients with multiple myeloma they demonstrated circulating mononuclear cells that suppressed immunoglobulin synthesis by normal lymphocytes in culture. Thus, one mechanism of the depressed polyclonal immunoglobulin synthesis in multiple myeloma appears to be inhibition of B-lymphocyte function by suppressor cells.

Deficiency of gammaglobulin is detected by serum protein electrophoresis in approximately one-third to 50% of patients with chronic lymphocytic leukemia (CLL) or lymphocytic lymphoma (73,74). When levels of the specific immunoglobulins (IgG, IgM, and IgA) are quantitated, an even greater incidence of decreased values is found. Immunoglobulin deficiency is correlated with the duration and extent of the lymphoproliferative disease. In chronic lymphocytic leukemia low immunoglobulin levels are more likely to be found in patients with high numbers of lymphocytes in the blood and those with lymphadenopathy and hepatosplenomegaly (75). The incidence of infection is greater in patients with CLL who have low immunoglobulin levels (75).

Approximately 6% of patients with a thymoma have hypogammaglobulinemia (76). Such patients may exhibit, in addition, certain findings known to be associated with thymomas, such as myasthenia gravis, pure erythroid aplasia, pancytopenia, immunohemolytic anemia, and chronic diarrhea (77–79). Discovery of hypogammaglobulinemia may precede or follow the recognition of a thymoma.

HYPOALBUMINEMIA

There are four mechanisms by which hypoalbuminemia may develop in patients with malignancies: (1) protein malnutrition, (2) reduced synthesis of albumin in the liver related to hepatic involvement by the neoplasm, (3) protein-losing enteropathy, and (4) urinary loss of albumin due to the nephrotic syndrome. Hypoalbuminemia resulting from deficient dietary intake of protein is usually seen only in markedly anorexic patients during the late stages of malignancies. In patients with hepatic metastatic disease, synthesis of albumin is generally reasonably well preserved until there is extensive replacement of the liver by the malignancy. Loss of albumin and gammaglobulin through the gastrointestinal tract, causing hypoalbuminemia and hypogammaglobulinemia, has been reported in patients with adenocarcinoma of the stomach and with lymphomas of the stomach or small intestine (80,81). The nephrotic syndrome causing hypoalbuminemia has been described in Hodgkin's disease, other lymphomas, multiple myeloma, and a variety of carcinomas. Lipoid nephrosis occurs in some patients with Hodgkin's disease. Renal amyloidosis is seen in some patients with multiple myeloma and occasionally in patients with Hodgkin's disease. The nephrotic syndrome occurring in association with carcinoma usually has the histologic features of membraneous or membranoproliferative glomerulonephritis.

REFERENCES

1. Axelsson U, Bachmann R, Hällén J: Frequency of pathological proteins (M-components) in 6995 sera from an adult population. *Acta Med Scand* 179:235, 1966.
2. Pruzanski W, Ogryzlo MA: Abnormal proteinuria in malignant disease. *Adv Clin Chem* 13:335, 1970.
3. Zawadski ZA, Edwards GA: M-components in immunoproliferative disorders: Electrophoretic and immunologic analysis of 200 cases. *Am J Clin Pathol* 48:418, 1967.
4. Kyle RA, Greipp PR: The laboratory investigation of monoclonal gammopathies. *Mayo Clin Proc* 53:719, 1978.
5. Cooperative Study by Acute Leukemia Group B: Correlation of abnormal immunoglobulin with clinical features of myeloma. *Arch Intern Med* 135:46, 1975.

6. Stone MJ, Frenkel EP: The clinical spectrum of light chain myeloma: A study of 35 patients with special reference to the occurrence of amyloidosis. *Am J Med* 58:601, 1975.

7. Zlotnick A, Rosenmann E: Renal pathologic findings associated with monoclonal gammopathies. *Arch Intern Med* 135:40, 1975.

8. Shustik C, Bergsagel DE, Pruzanski W: K and λ light chain disease: Survival rates and clinical manifestations. *Blood* 48:41, 1976.

9. Jancelewicz Z, Takatsuki K, Sugai S, et al: IgD multiple myeloma: Review of 133 cases. *Arch Intern Med* 135:87, 1975.

10. Pruzanski W, Underdown B, Silver EH, et al: Macroglobulinemia-myeloma double gammopathy: A study of four cases and a review of the literature. *Am J Med* 57:259, 1974.

11. Somer T: Hyperviscosity syndrome in plasma cell dyscrasias. *Adv Microcirc* 6:1, 1975.

12. Block KJ, Maki DG: Hyperviscosity syndromes associated with immunoglobulin abnormalities. *Semin Hematol* 10:113, 1973.

13. Perry MC, Hoagland HC: The hyperviscosity syndrome. *JAMA* 236:392, 1976.

14. Solomon A, Fahey JL: Bence Jones proteinemia. *Am J Med* 37:206, 1964.

15. Solomon A: Bence-Jones proteins and light chains of immunoglobulins. *N Engl J Med* 294:91, 1976.

16. Maldonado JE, Velosa JA, Kyle RA, et al: Fanconi syndrome in adults: A manifestation of a latent form of myeloma. Am J Med 58:354, 1975.

17. Kyle RA, Bayrd ED: Amyloidosis: Review of 236 cases. *Medicine* (Baltimore) 54:271, 1975.

18. Cathcart ES, Ritchie RF, Cohen AS, et al: Immunoglobulins and amyloidosis: An immunologic study of sixty-two patients with biopsy-proved disease. *Am J Med* 52: 93, 1972.

19. Waldenström J: Incipient myelomatosis or "essential" hyperglobulinemia with fibrinogenopenia: A new syndrome? *Acta Med Scand* 117:216, 1944.

20. MacKenzie MR, Fudenberg HH: Macroglobulinemia: An analysis for forty patients. *Blood* 39:874, 1972.

21. McCallister BD, Bayrd ED, Harrison EG Jr, et al: Primary macroglobulinemia: Review with a report of thirty-one cases and notes on the value of continuous chlorambucil therapy. *Am J Med* 43:394, 1967.

22. Frangione B, Franklin EC: Heavy chain diseases: Clinical features and molecular significance of the disordered immunoglobulin structure. *Semin Hematol* 10:53, 1973.

23. Block KJ, Lee L, Mills JA, et al: Gamma heavy chain disease: An expanding clinical and laboratory spectrum. *Am J Med* 55:61, 1973.

24. Pittman FE, Tripathy K, Isobe T, et al: IgA heavy chain disease: A case detected in the western hemisphere. *Am J Med* 58:424, 1975.

25. Seligmann M: Immunochemical, clinical, and pathological features of α-chain disease. *Arch Intern Med* 135:78, 1975.

26. Guardia, J, Rubies-Prat J, Gallart MT, et al: The evolution of alpha heavy chain disease. *Am J Med* 60:596, 1976.

27. Forte FA, Prelli F, Yount WJ, et al: Heavy chain disease of the μ (γ M) type: Report of the first case. *Blood* 36:137, 1970.

28. Franklin EC: μ-chain disease. *Arch Intern Med* 135:71, 1975.

29. Alexanian R: Monoclonal gammopathy in lymphoma. *Arch Intern Med* 135:62, 1975.

30. Moore DF, Migliore PJ, Shullenberger CC, et al: Monoclonal macroglobulinemia in malignant lymphoma. *Ann Intern Med* 72:43, 1970.

31. Krauss S, Sokal JE: Paraproteinemia in the lymphomas. *Am J Med* 40:400, 1966.

32. Isbister JP, Cooper DA, Blake HM, et al: Lymphoproliferative disease with IgM lambda monoclonal protein and autoimmune hemolytic anemia. *Am J Med* 64:434, 1978.

33. Aisenberg AC, Bloch KJ, Long JC: Cell-surface immunoglobulins in chronic lymphocytic leukemia and allied disorders. *Am J Med* 55: 184, 1973.

34. Burke JF, Flis R, Lasker N, et al: Malignant lymphoma with "myeloma kidney" acute renal failure. *Am J Med* 60:1055, 1976.

35. Golde DW, Saxon A, Stevens RH: Macroglobulinemia and hairy-cell leukemia. *N Engl J Med* 296:92, 1977.

36. Stoop JW, Zegers BJM, van der Heiden C, et al: Monoclonal gammopathy in a child with leukemia. *Blood* 32:774, 1968.

37. Lindquist KJ, Ragab AH, Osterland CK: Paraproteinemia in a child with leukemia. *Blood* 35:213, 1970.

38. Poulik MD, Berman L, Prasad AS: "Myeloma protein" in a patient with monocytic leukemia. *Blood* 33:746, 1969.

39. Ritzmann SE, Stoufflet EJ, Houston EW, et al: Coexistent chronic myelocytic leukemia, monoclonal gammopathy and multiple chromosomal abnormalities. *Am J Med* 41:981, 1966.

40. Migliore P, Alexanian R: Monoclonal gammopathy in human neoplasia. *Cancer* 21:1127, 1968.

41. Solomon A: Homogeneous (monoclonal) immunoglobulins in cancer. *Am J Med* 63:169, 1977.

42. Isobe T, Osserman EF: Pathologic conditions with plasma cell dyscrasias: A study of 806 cases. *Ann NY Acad Sci* 190:507, 1971.

43. Williams RC Jr, Bailly RC, Howe RB: Studies of "benign" serum M-components. *Am J Med Sci* 257:275, 1969.

44. McPhedran P, Finch SC, Nemerson YR, et al: Alpha-2 globulin "spike" in renal carcinoma. *Ann Intern Med* 76:439, 1972.

45. Kyle RA: Monoclonal gammopathy of undetermined significance: Natural history in 241 cases. *Am J Med* 64:814, 1978.

46. Ritzmann SE, Loukas D, Sakai H, et al: Idiopathic (asymptomatic) monoclonal gammopathies. *Arch Intern Med* 135:95, 1975.

47. Bachmann R: The diagnostic significance of the serum concentration of pathological proteins (M-components). *Acta Med Scand* 178:801, 1965.

48. Dammacco F, Waldenström J: Bence-Jones proteinuria in benign monoclonal gammapathies: Incidence and characteristics. *Acta Med Scand* 184:403, 1968.

49. Kyle RA, Maldonado JE, Bayrd ED: Idiopathic Bence Jones proteinuria: A distinct entity. *Am J Med* 55:222, 1973.

50. Waldenström JG: Benign monoclonal gammapathies, in *Multiple Myeloma and Related Disorders, vol I*. New York, Harper & Row, 1973.

51. Lazarus GS, Goldsmith LA, Rocklin RE, et al: Pyoderma gangrenosum, altered delayed hypersensitivity, and polyarthritis. *Arch Dermatol* 105:46, 1972.

52. Cream JJ: Pyoderma gangrenosum with a monoclonal IgM red cell agglutinating factor. *Br J Dermatol* 84:223, 1971.

53. Shapiro, CM, Fretzin D, Norris S: Papular mucinosis. *JAMA* 214:2052, 1970.

54. James K, Fudenberg H, Epstein WL, et al: Studies on a unique diagnostic serum globulin in papular mucinosis (lichen myxedematosus). *Clin Exp Immunol* 2:153, 1967.

55. Schnur MJ, Appel GB, Bilezikian JP: Primary hyperparathyroidism and benign monoclonal gammopathy. *Arch Intern Med* 137:1201, 1977.

56. Michaux JL, Heremens JF: Thirty cases of monoclonal immunoglobulin disorders other than myeloma or macroglobulinemia: A classification of diseases associated with the production of monoclonal-type immunoglobulins. *Am J Med* 46:562, 1969.

57. Brouet JC, Clauvel JP, Danon F, et al: Biologic and clinical significance of cryoglobulins: A report of 86 cases. *Am J Med* 57:775, 1974.

58. Schultz DR, Yunis AA: Immunoblastic lymphadenopathy with mixed cryoglobulinemia: A detailed case study. *N Engl J Med* 292:8, 1975.

59. Barnett EV, Bluestone R, Cracchiolo A, et al: Cryoglobulinemia and disease. *Ann Intern Med* 73:95, 1970.

60. Grey HM, Kohler PF: Cryoimmunoglobulins. *Semin Hematol* 10:87, 1973.

61. Stefanini M, McConnell EE, Andracki EG, et al: Macropyroglobulinemia. *Am J Clin Pathol* 54:94, 1970.

62. Patterson R, Roberts M, Rambach W, et al: An IgM pyroglobulin associated with lymphosarcoma. *Am J Med* 48:503, 1970.

63. Sugai S: IgA pyroglobulin, hyperviscosity syndrome and coagulation abnormality in a patient with multiple myeloma. *Blood* 39:224, 1972.

64. McCann SR, Zinneman HH, Oken MM, et al: IgM pyroglobulinemia with erythrocytosis presenting as hyperviscosity syndrome, I: Clinical features and viscometric studies. *Am J Med* 61:316, 1976.

65. Waldmann TA, Strober W, Blaese RM: Immunodeficiency disease and malignancy: Various immunologic deficiencies of man and the role of immune processes in the control of malignant disease. *Ann Intern Med* 77:605, 1972.

66. Peterson RDA, Cooper MD, Good RA: Lymphoid tissue abnormalities associated with ataxia-telangiectasia. *Am J Med* 41:342, 1966.

67. Hermans PE, Diaz-Buxo JA, Stobo JD: Idiopathic late-onset immunoglobulin deficiency: Clinical observations in 50 patients. *Am J Med* 61:221, 1976.

68. Waldmann TA, Durm M, Broder S, et al: Role of suppressor T cells in pathogenesis of common variable hypogammaglobulinemia. *Lancet* 2:609, 1974.

69. Fahey JL, Scoggins R, Utz JP, et al: Infection, antibody response and gamma globulin components in multiple myeloma and macroglobulinemia. *Am J Med* 35:698, 1963.

70. Glenchur H, Zinneman HH, Hall WH: A review of fifty-one cases of multiple myeloma: Emphasis on pneumonia and other infections as complications. *Arch Intern Med* 103:173, 1959.

71. Meyers BR, Hirschman SZ, Axelrod JA: Current patterns of infection in multiple myeloma. *Am J Med* 52:87, 1972.

72. Broder S, Humphrey R, Durm M, et al: Impaired synthesis of polyclonal (non-paraprotein) immunoglobulins by circulating lymphocytes from patients with multiple myeloma: Role of suppressor cells. *N Engl J Med* 293:887, 1975.

73. Ultmann JE, Fish W, Osserman E, et al: The clinical implications of hypogammaglobulinemia with chronic lymphocytic leukemia and lymphocytic lymphosarcoma. *Ann Intern Med* 51:501, 1959.

74. Zacharski LR, Linman JW: Chronic lymphocytic leukemia versus chronic lymphosarcoma cell leukemia: Analysis of 496 cases. *Am J Med* 47:75, 1969.

75. Fiddes P, Penny R, Wells JV, et al: Clinical correlations with immunoglobulin levels in chronic lymphatic leukaemia. *Aust NZ J Med* 2:346, 1972.

76. Souadjian JV, Enriquez P, Silverstein MN: The spectrum of diseases associated with thymoma: Coincidence or syndrome? *Arch Intern Med* 134:374, 1974.

77. Conn HO, Quintiliani R: Severe diarrhea controlled by gamma globulin in a patient with agammaglobulinemia, amyloidosis, and thymoma. *Ann Intern Med* 65:528, 1966.

78. Mongan ES, Kern WA Jr, Terry R: Hypogammaglobulinemia with thymoma, hemolytic anemia, and disseminated infection with cytomegalovirus. *Ann Intern Med* 65:548, 1966.

79. Rogers BHG, Manaligod JR, Blazek WV: Thymoma associated with pancytopenia and hypogammaglobulinemia: Report of a case and review of the literature. *Am J Med* 44:154, 1968.

80. Jeffries GH, Holman HR, Sleisenger MH: Plasma proteins and the gastrointestinal tract. *N Engl J Med* 266:652, 1962.

81. Werdegar D, Adler H, Watlington C: Enteric protein loss with hypoproteinemia in diffuse lymphosarcoma of the bowel. *Ann Intern Med* 59:207, 1963.

11
Metabolic Abnormalities in Cancer Patients

Montague Lane

The metabolic abnormalities that are observed in cancer patients may be due to a broad range of etiologic factors operating singly or in combination. Some of the factors may have been preexisting conditions, for example, diabetes, renal insufficiency, liver disease, cardiac disorders, endocrine problems, and gastrointestinal and pancreatic diseases, which often are complicated by the development of cancer. The drugs used in the treatment of these preexisting disorders superimpose other potential sources of metabolic changes. Metabolic disturbances related to cancer may be a consequence of (*1*) local growth and extension of the primary tumor and compromise of its organ of origin or of structures and organs that it impinges upon or invades, (*2*) similar effects caused by its metastases, (*3*) hormonal effects if tumors are of endocrine origin, and (*4*) remote effects due to humoral factors released by the tumor that normally are not produced by its cells of origin (paraneoplastic syndromes). Additional metabolic abnormalities may develop as a consequence of treatment with surgery, radiotherapy, and chemotherapy. Thus, an understanding of an individual patient's clinical problems is dependent upon a careful analysis of the patient's prior and present history, the physical examination, and the results of laboratory investigations. It also requires knowledge of internal medicine, of the natural history of malignant tumors, and of cancer therapy.

The organizational approach of this book is to focus on the clinical presentation of cancer as it involves various organ systems. In this chapter the same approach is used, when possible, by focusing on the effects of disordered metabolism as they are seen in practice, for example, malnutrition, hypokalemia, hypernatremia, and acidosis, and to delineate the distinguishing features of the possible causes of these disorders. This approach differs from standard expositions in which subjects such as the paraneoplastic syndromes are individually catalogued and described. Some of these syndromes that result in metabolic disorders are discussed in this chapter. Other chapters deal with the paraneoplastic syndromes that relate primarily to specific organ systems. No effort is made here to be comprehensive, and only sufficient detail is offered for a functional approach to the recognition and analysis of metabolic disturbances. The reader is referred to other texts for specifics relating to the structures, biochemistry, receptor assay, and radioimmunoassay of hormonal products of tumors.

MALNUTRITION

Malnutrition is a general term that encompasses a spectrum of disorders ranging from asymptomatic biochemical abnormalities to cachexia. Its symptomatology may be nonspecific or may reflect aspects of the pathophysiologic events leading to its development.

Malnutrition may be the consequence of obvious anatomic and physiologic disruptions resulting from the progressive growth of a primary tumor or its metastases. Impaired dietary intake may be caused by anorexia from ulcerated and infected nonobstructing tumors of the upper aerodigestive tract, by dysphagia from obstructing tumors, by odynophagia from painful lesions in these locations, or by tumors that produce trismus or painful mastication. Intrinsic tumors of the stomach and intestines, extrinsic tumors that impinge upon these structures (such as in the liver, mesenteric nodes, omentum, pancreas, kidney), and ascites reduce the capacity for food, delay or even obstruct its passage, and cause anorexia, nausea, easy satiety, and vomiting. Maldigestion and malabsorption may result from tumors invading the gastrointestinal tract, the pancreas, and the biliary tract or from the production of fistulas. Abnormal external fluid, electrolyte, and protein losses may be secondary to obstructing lesions that cause vomiting, internal and external fistulas, ulceration, or inflammation of the bowel, and enteropathies due to bowel and lymphatic invasion or congestion of lymphatic vessels. Internal losses may occur into "third spaces" as pleural and peritoneal transudates and exudates. Tumors require nutrients for their growth. If food intake is inadequate to provide sufficient nutrition for tumor and host, malnutrition will develop; tumors continue to grow in the malnourished host. If the liver is replaced by tumor, there is inadequate production of essential proteins, decreased glycogen storage, hypoglycemia (occasionally), and reduced steroid hormone catabolism, all of which contribute to the development of cachexia.

Malnutrition may also be due to humoral effects of neoplasms. The so-called anorexia-cachexia syndrome is believed to be due to humoral products of tumors, since it bears no relationship to tumor mass, histology, location, or anatomical effects, and can be relieved by removal of the tumor. Presumably, tumor products are responsible for the multiple derangements that inexorably produce malnutrition and cachexia through effects on taste, appetite, and multiple metabolic events. These substances adversely affect appetite either by impairing stimulatory influences or by increasing inhibitory influences on the appetite centers in the central nervous system (1,2,3). Taste thresholds for test substances that correlate with the desire for specific foods, such as meats and sweets, are altered adversely (4). Factors influencing appetite include the blood glucose concentration, the concentration and balance of blood amino acids, the state of body lipids, the concentration of various metabolites in the serum, and the balance of body hormones. In cancer patients many of these factors are altered to adversely affect appetite. Glucose tolerance is frequently impaired; insulin resistance has been observed (5). Postprandial glucose is abnormally increased and the rate of glucose utilization is decreased. These chemical abnormalities generally are not sufficiently severe to produce clinical symptoms of diabetes. Serum free fatty acids and various amino acids are increased and gluconeogenesis is decreased. The basal metabolic rate (BMR) is often elevated despite inanition. Cancer patients do not decrease their BMRs during semistarvation, unlike normal subjects (6). Energy expenditures for anaerobic glucose synthesis is excessive in patients with cancer. The multiple disruptions that result in decreased food intake and impaired control of metabolic regulation result in a profound catabolic state with progressive development of cachexia.

Direct anatomic and physiologic limitations caused by growth of tumors, as well as humoral mechanisms promoting malnutrition, may coexist in many patients. In addition, hormone production by endocrine tumors and the ectopic production of hormones or hormone-like materials, such as ADH, PTH, VIP, and ACTH, may produce profound fluid, electrolyte, and metabolic disorders that contribute to impairment of nutrition. Analgesics and other drugs used in symptomatic therapy, radiation therapy, surgery, and chemotherapy may all produce deleterious effects on host nutrition by a variety of mechanisms, such as anorexia, nausea, vomiting, stomatitis, gastroenteritis, and extensive bowel resection. However, since these therapies are not intrinsic to the natural history of cancer, they will not be discussed further.

Weight loss may not become evident to the patient who is becoming malnourished until it is of sufficient magnitude to cause looseness of clothing or thinning of the face. Occasionally, patients weigh themselves and note an inexplicable loss of weight. In some instances weight loss is masked by accumulation of fluid in the form of ascites, pleural effusion, or edema. In these cases abdominal swelling, dyspnea, or swelling of the feet may be the presenting symptoms. Anorexia is a common, but by no means universal, accompaniment of weight loss. There may be a general disinterest in eating or selective aversion for specific foods that previously were savored, such as sweets, meat, particularly beef, or fowl. Anxiety, depression, and withdrawal occur frequently in cancer patients who are aware of their disorder and contribute to loss of interest in food. As patients lose muscle mass, they first note diminished tolerance for strenuous activity. This progresses to general weakness and then to fatigue with even minimal activities. The act of eating, in itself, may require great effort, thereby leading to additional impairment of nutrient intake. Anemia related to nutritional deficiencies, impaired iron reutilization, and many other factors (Chapter 8) contributes to weakness and limited exercise tolerance. Dyspnea and palpitation may accompany slight exertion. As malnutrition progresses, patients often experience diminished taste sensation or a constant bad taste, dry mouth, soreness of the tongue and oral mucosa, cracked lips, and dryness of the skin. Menses may become irregular or may cease. With severe hypoalbuminemia the patient may develop an edematous state. Some patients have symptoms of hypermetabolism, including tachycardia, excessive perspiration, heat intolerance, and fever. With the development of cachexia the symptoms of asthenia become profound.

In some patients the apparent causes of malnutrition are reflected by symptoms relating either to impedence of the passage of ingested food or to excessive losses of nutrients, in addition to the general symptoms of malnutrition noted above. Such symptoms are the result of anatomic disturbances produced by the primary tumor or metastases and include odynophagia, dysphagia, easy satiety, nausea, vomiting, hematemesis, abdominal pain, abdominal swelling, obstipation, change in the stool caliber, melena, diarrhea, and steatorrhea. The symptoms consequent to cancer treatment that result in impaired nutrition will not be considered in this discussion.

Physical findings of malnutrition may not be evident in its early stages, particularly in the obese. If protein intake has been adequate and caloric intake inadequate, the major findings may relate to loss of fat. This is often evidenced by loss of the temporal fat pads; the temporal areas appear sunken. As more fat is lost, the malar areas become prominent. Skin thickness is diminished and the skin hangs loosely in areas such as the upper arms, breasts, and buttocks. The eyes may appear sunken. The skin is often dry and scaling. With combined protein and calorie malnutrition loss of muscle mass becomes evident. The circumference of the extremities is reduced. Muscle strength is significantly diminished, particularly notable in work against resistance. In cachectic patients the bones become very prominent, especially those of the face, the thoracic cage, and the pelvis; the ears and nose are accentuated. The patient takes on a skeletal appearance. The skin may appear hyperpigmented, particularly in the periorbital regions, and purpuric lesions may appear. The abdomen is often protuberant. There may be edema, ascites, or evidence of pleural effusion. The peripheral pulses and heartbeat are often accentuated, as are venous patterns over the face, neck, thorax, abdomen, and extremities, due to wasting of fat and muscle and thinning of the skin. The nail beds may be pale with alternating white and pink lines, and the nails may be ridged and brittle. Hair tends to be scanty, especially in the axillary and public areas and over the digits. There may be fissuring of the lips, angular stomatitis, and smoothing of the tongue due to loss of filiform papillae. The tongue may vary in color from pink to magenta. Recession of the gums and loosening of teeth may occur. White plaques due to candidiasis may be noted. Parotitis is occasionally present.

Laboratory findings in malnutrition are variable and nonspecific. Serum albumin and transferrin levels are often reduced in proportion to the degree of malnutrition (7). Low serum concentrations of iron, calcium, and glucose are common. Glucose tolerance is often impaired. Free fatty acids may be increased. In the presence of increased "third spaces" or if "sick cell syndrome" develops, there may be hyponatremia. Serum concentrations of folate, β-carotene, and ascorbate may be reduced. Excessive fluid and nutrient losses and malabsorption may markedly influence the type and severity of laboratory abnormalities. Some degree of impaired humoral and cellular immunity is frequently detected.

The treatment of malnutrition is accomplished through (1) replacement of deficient nutrients, correction of fluid and electrolyte disturbances, and provision of sufficient additional nutrients, including carbohydrate, protein or essential amino acids, lipid, vitamins, and trace elements to permit an anabolic milieu with rebuilding of body tissues, and (2) reversal of the causative factors through adequate cancer therapy. Oral alimentation alone is often unsuccessful in correcting severe malnutrition in cancer patients, since the development of malnutrition reflects the inability of these patients to meet their nutritional requirements by this route. While dietetic counseling, provision of appetizing menus and nutritious oral supplements, and efforts to stimulate appetite with drugs or aperitifs may be of benefit, severe anorexia, dysphagia, odynophagia, profound weakness, depression, and many other factors often limit the success of oral alimentation programs. Satisfactory enteral nutrition can occasionally be achieved with tube feedings when oral administration has been inadequate. However, intestinal obstruction, inability to accept or tolerate the tube, aspiration, diarrhea, and other problems may preclude the use of this method. Total parenteral nutrition (TPN) is an effective means of repairing nutritional deficits and of providing adequate nutrition to achieve an anabolic state and to improve immune competence (8). While TPN is primarily carried out in the hospital setting, it can be employed in selected out-patients. Such programs are expensive and must be monitored carefully to minimize infections and other catheter complications, as well as metabolic disorders inherent in such therapy. However, unless some degree of inhibition of tumor progression can be achieved, the benefit of TPN is limited. TPN can provide excellent preoperative nutritional support, particularly of value in debilitated cancer patients who require surgery. It can maintain adequate nutrition postoperatively in patients who may be unable to eat for many weeks and can also be used to support patients who have severe nutritional problems during radiation therapy or chemotherapy.

FLUID AND ELECTROLYTE DISORDERS

A multitude of paraneoplastic syndromes have been identified in recent years. Many of these produce derangements in metabolism, including fluid and electrolyte disorders. While the educational efforts that have created an awareness of these syndromes have certainly been justified, it should be emphasized that the majority of fluid, electrolyte, and other metabolic disorders in cancer patients occur for reasons other than paraneoplastic syndromes. For the most part, their causes are the same as those in patients who do not have cancer. The pathophysiology of these disturbances should be determined in each case by a careful analysis of history, physical findings, and laboratory data. Thus, hypokalemia is far more often due to vomiting, to nasogastric suction, to inadequate intake or replacement, or to diuretics than to ectopic production of ACTH. As in patients with disorders of fluid and electrolyte who do not have cancer, the presence or absence of symptoms, their nature, and their severity are functions not only of the magnitude of these abnormalities, but of the rapidity of their development. Disturbances that develop over weeks to months, although severe, may produce few symptoms; modest disturbances that occur within days may be very symptomatic. Similarly, symptoms, rather than serum concentrations of electrolytes per se, often dictate the urgency and form of treatment. This section will deal with some of the most common fluid and electrolyte problems that beset cancer patients, as well as those due to paraneoplastic syndromes.

Sodium Disorders

Hyponatremia
Hyponatremia and hypoosmolality evolve through two basic mechanisms: (1) deficits of salt in excess of water and (2) gains of water in excess of salt. In cancer

patients deficits of salt in excess of water often occur when these patients consume water freely after losing gastrointestinal secretions (vomiting, diarrhea) or after receiving diuretic therapy. These losses of sodium cause extracellular fluid volume contraction, which stimulates ADH (arginine vasopressin, AVP) secretion and water retention as well as thirst and water ingestion. The net result is the development of hyponatremia and serum hypotonicity. This may develop iatrogenically if patients with gastrointestinal losses (including nasogastric suction), blood loss, renal salt wasting, or adrenal insufficiency receive 5% glucose or hypotonic saline as replacement solutions. Gains of water in excess of salt are seen in a wide variety of disease conditions that may coexist with cancer, including chronic edematous states such as congestive heart failure, cirrhosis, nephrotic syndrome, and renal insufficiency. While the primary problem in these conditions is salt retention, reduction in "effective" plasma volume probably serves as the stimulus for both thirst and increased secretion of ADH with the subsequent establishment of chronic dilutional hyponatremia. Patients with advanced cancer often have significant pleural effusion, ascites, peripheral edema, and hypoalbuminemia and similarly develop chronic dilutional hyponatremia. Hypopituitarism, hypothyroidism, and adrenal insufficiency are also associated with hyponatremia.

The syndrome of hyponatremia and renal sodium loss probably resulting from inappropriate secretion of ADH was first identified by Schwartz et al. (9, 10). Subsequently, the syndrome of inappropriate antidiuretic hormone secretion (SIADH) was characterized by Bartter and Schwartz (11) in an extensive review of the subject in which they defined four groups of causes for the syndrome: (1) malignant tumors, (2) disorders involving the central nervous system, (3) diseases of lungs, and (4) idiopathic. In addition, many drugs can limit free water excretion either by stimulating secretion of AVP by the posterior pituitary or by action on the renal tubule, thereby producing the clinical characteristics of SIADH.

Small cell carcinoma of the lung is the tumor identified with SIADH in the majority of instances. Other tumors that have been associated with the syndrome are carcinomas of the duodenum, pancreas, esophagus, colon, prostate, adrenal, head and neck, nonsmall cell bronchogenic carcinomas, bronchial carcinoid, thymoma, Hodgkin's disease, and non-Hodgkin's lymphoma. SIADH with hyponatremia is thought to occur in about 10% of patients with small cell carcinoma, but may be somewhat more frequent. Elevated AVP levels have been found in a significant proportion of patients with small cell and other bronchogenic tumors and colon cancer without clinical evidence of SIADH. Up to two-thirds of patients with small cell carcinoma have been found to have impaired ability to excrete water when water-loaded (12).

The *central nervous system causes* of SIADH are diverse and include infections (meningitis, encephalitis, abscess), intracranial space occupying tumors, trauma (fractures, concussion, hemorrhage), Guillain-Barré syndrome, acute intermittent porphyria, pain, and emotional stress. *Pulmonary causes* (pneumonias, tuberculosis, aspergillosis, abscess) have also been associated with SIADH. Some of the drugs that produce the syndrome are Oncovin and cyclophosphamide, which are commonly used in cancer therapy, thiazide diuretics, opiates, and chlorpropamide.

The criteria for the establishment of the diagnosis of SIADH include (1) hyponatremia with corresponding hypo-osmolality of the serum and extracel-lular fluid, (2) continued renal excretion of sodium (>20 mEq-liter), (3) absence of clinical evidence of fluid volume depletion, (4) osmolality of the urine greater than that appropriate for the concomitant tonicity of the plasma (urine less than maximally dilute), (5) normal renal function, and (6) normal adrenal function.

The symptoms of hyponatremia and hypotonicity occur when the condition is either acute or profound. They include weakness, lethargy, headache, nausea, vomiting, painful muscle cramps and muscle twitching, personality changes, somnolence, convulsions, and coma. Focal neurologic findings may be present (as in other metabolic disorders, such as hypoglycemia) in the absence of cerebral metastases. In patients with cancer, of course, brain metastases may coexist with SIADH. Peripheral edema is generally absent in patients with SIADH.

Hyponatremia in a cancer patient is far more often due to causes other than tumor-related SIADH. These are often apparent upon consideration of the history and physical examination. Thus, a history of gastrointestinal losses and water replacement, of pulmonary infections, of CNS problems or therapy with drugs that inhibit water secretion, or the finding of an edematous state (heart failure, nephrosis, cirrhosis) or evidence of volume depletion, renal disease, or adrenal, thyroid, or pituitary insufficiency most often indicates the basis for hyponatremia. In a patient with no obvious explanation for hyponatremia, con-sideration must be given to an undiagnosed neoplasm, particularly small cell carcinoma of the lung. In patients with previously diagnosed small cell carci-noma, on the other hand, hyponatremia is quite likely to be due to SIADH. However, other causes should be considered, and the criteria for the diagnosis must be met. In these patients a CT scan of the brain should be obtained even if focal neurologic signs are absent. CNS metastases, secretion of ADH by small cell carcinoma, or both may be responsible for hyponatremia and focal neuro-logic findings, if present.

The management of hyponatremia depends upon its underlying cause. The treatment of chronic hyponatremic states, volume contraction, and chronic renal disease requires no discussion here. Treatment of SIADH should involve removal or amelioration of the underlying cause when possible (tumors, CNS problems, pulmonary problems, offending drugs) and the correction of hypotonicity. In patients with minimal symptomatology, restriction of water intake to insensible losses (500–800 mg/day) will result in elimination of excessive water and an increase in the serum sodium concentration over a period of one to two weeks. If the primary problem cannot be corrected, continued water restriction is dif-ficult to maintain, and daily treatment with demeclocycline in divided oral doses may permit liberalization of water intake (13). This drug blocks the effect of AVP on the renal tubule by blocking formation of cyclic AMP. Similar therapeutic results have been reported with ingestion of a concentrated solution of urea, which promotes an osmotic diuresis and net free water excretion (14).

Marked headache, lethargy, convulsions, or coma mandate urgent and ag-gressive therapy. Administration of 3% saline and furosemide intravenously can provide rapid improvement in these patients. Hypertonic saline acutely raises serum osmolality, and furosemide promotes a slightly hypotonic diuresis. This results in a net free water clearance (15). This program must be monitored carefully to avoid acute volume overload and other electrolyte disturbances. The mEq of sodium chloride required can be estimated by the formula: 140 − [Na]$_s$ × TBW (total body water). Half of this calculated amount should be administered with caution as 3% sodium chloride intravenously over a period of hours, the initial rate depending upon the urgency of the situation. Furosemide should also be administered intravenously as frequently as necessary to maintain a net hourly fluid loss. Vital signs, symptoms, cerebral and cardiovascular status, intake and output volumes, and serum and urine electrolytes must be checked repeatedly, and adjustments are made on the basis of these observations. In the first 12 hours, only a partial correction of serum osmolality should be attempted and is all that is needed to relieve acute symptomatology. Once severe symptoms and signs have been ameliorated, further adjustments in osmolality can be undertaken more gradually, as outlined previously. Patients with severe underlying cardiac or renal disease may require dialysis in preference to the above program, which might be particularly dangerous in such settings.

Hypernatremia

Hypernatremia results from a deficit of water in excess of salt and is relatively uncommon. This state of hypertonicity can occur in cancer patients who are obtunded or debilitated and who may be unable to maintain an adequate water intake. Hypernatremia may also develop in cancer patients who have uncontrolled diabetes mellitus or severe hyperglycemia and glycosuria secondary to adrenocorticosteroid therapy, or who have diabetes insipidus or renal insufficiency. Diabetes mellitus and diabetes insipidus may be coincidental disorders or a consequence of cancer. Reduced glucose tolerance is more common in bronchogenic carcinoma than in pancreatic cancer, though frank diabetes is more frequent with pancreatic cancer. Diabetes insipidus from metastasis to the posterior pituitary is most often due to breast cancer. Hypernatremia may also occur with intravenous hyperalimentation, if hyperglycemia and glycosuria are allowed to go unchecked, and may be observed in patients receiving tube feedings or protein-high carbohydrate supplements that are hyperosmolar. Severe hypernatremia is associated with thirst, weakness, irritability, delirium, and coma. The skin and mucous membranes are dry. The patient may have tachycardia. If dehydration is sufficiently severe, there may be vasomotor collapse. Primary treatment requires correction of the water deficit, which can be calculated as approximately equal to TBW − [(140/[Na]$_s$) × TBW]. Approximately half the calculated deficit should be given over 6–12 hours, most often as hypotonic (0.2–0.45%) saline, since there is often a deficit of salt as well as water. Subsequent adjustments are based on careful monitoring of vital signs, cerebral and cardiovascular status, intake and output volumes, and serial measurements of serum electrolytes, BUN, and creatinine. Diabetes mellitus and diabetes insipidus are treated conventionally.

Potassium Disorders

Hypokalemia

Excessive loss of potassium from the body either from the gastrointestinal tract or through the kidneys, without adequate replacement, results in hypokalemia. In cancer patients gastrointestinal losses are common. Bowel obstruction from intrinsic and extrinsic tumors may result in vomiting, and the patient often drinks low potassium-containing liquids for replacement. Vomiting may also be secondary to brain tumors that produce increased intracranial pressure, to analgesic drugs, and to cancer chemotherapeutic agents or radiation therapy. Nasogastric suction may result in hypokalemia consequent to losses of hydrogen ion and volume, primarily, and potassium, secondarily, if replacement of losses is inadequate. Diarrheal fluids are potassium-rich. In addition to the common causes of diarrhea, cancer patients may have diarrhea consequent to enteric fistulas, pancreatic insufficiency, bile salts, enteropathy due to invasion of the bowel and its lymphatics by lymphomas and other tumors, lymphatic congestion, mucosal ulceration, weeping of villous adenomas and the watery diarrhea hypokalemic alkalosis syndrome induced by "VIPomas" arising in non-beta islet cell tumors, lung tumors, pheochromocytomas, and ganglioneuroblastomas. Patients with VIPomas often have hypercalcemia and, less often, hyperglycemia in addition to hypokalemic alkalosis. As in patients who do not have cancer, the commonest cause of excessive renal potassium loss in cancer patients is the use of thiazide and loop diuretics. Hypercorticism due to ACTH production by small cell carcinoma of the lung and various other tumors, primary tumors of the adrenal cortex, pituitary tumors or dysfunction, and exogenous administration of adrenocorticosteroids may all produce hypokalemia by promoting renal potassium excretion. Primary aldosteronism due to an adrenal tumor can also cause excessive renal potassium loss, as may coincidental renal tubular disease in a cancer patient.

Hypokalemia is often asymptomatic. The major symptoms of hypokalemia are weakness that may progress to flaccid paralysis, polyuria due to nephropathy, polydypsia, and gastrointestinal symptoms (anorexia, nausea, vomiting, and abdominal distention due to ileus). Patients who have developed mechanical bowel obstruction and are hypokalemic may have a silent abdomen. The symptoms and signs of mechanical obstruction can reappear when the hypokalemia is corrected. Arrhythmias can occur in patients receiving digitalis preparations. The predominant physical findings of hypokalemia are reduced muscle strength, decreased deep tendon reflexes, and diminished bowel sounds. The EKG may demonstrate sagging of the ST segment, flattening and inversion of T waves, and prominent U waves. The magnitude of the potassium deficit cannot be calculated with precision from the serum value. A serum deficit of 1 mEq/liter often represents a body deficit of 150–200 mEq; a serum deficit of 2 mEq/liter may represent a body deficit of more than 450 mEq.

The treatment of hypokalemia should be accomplished by oral administration of potassium chloride whenever possible. Eighty to 120 mEq can be provided in four to six doses of various liquid potassium chloride preparations or in foods with the use of a salt substitute. Orally administered potassium preparations minimize the risks of dangerous increases in serum potassium levels. In urgent situations respiratory support may be required. Potassium chloride should be administered intravenously in a concentration of 20–40 mEq/liter. In the first hour up to 25 mEq may be given. The rate thereafter should probably not exceed 5–10 mEq/hour. Rapidly administered intravenous potassium chloride solutions may cause severe burning sensations at the injection site. The rapid injection of too much potassium may produce hyperkalemia and death. The serum electrolyte concentrations and pH should be checked with sufficient frequency to monitor changes during therapy and to make appropriate adjustments. It is generally considered advisable not to use potassium sparing diuretics in patients who are receiving exogenous potassium therapy because of the danger of inducing hyperkalemia. Alkalosis and acidosis, as well as dehydration, should be corrected in hypokalemic patients. It must be remembered that in acidosis the serum potassium is elevated by approximately 0.6 mEq/liter for each decrease in pH of 0.10 units and that potassium will move intracellularly as the pH is raised, with a subsequent reduction in serum potassium concentration.

Unexplained profound watery diarrhea with hypokalemia and alkalosis should suggest the possibility of a VIPoma. Symptomatic improvement of this syndrome often occurs with adrenocorticosteroid therapy. Continued renal loss of potassium in the absence of renal disease and diuretic therapy, with poor response to potassium therapy, should make one consider ectopic ACTH production or primary aldosteronism.

The syndrome of ectopic ACTH production (16) occurs most commonly in patients with small cell undifferentiated carcinoma of the lung. It is about one-fourth as common in these patients as SIADH. Both syndromes may coexist, and we have had several such patients. The syndromes may be present initially simultaneously or may develop sequentially. Ectopic ACTH syndrome has also been noted in a small group of patients with carcinoid tumors from various sites, islet cell tumors, pheochromocytomas, medullary carcinomas of the thyroid, and carcinomas of the gastrointestinal tract and other organs. Our own experience includes a patient with ovarian carcinoid and ectopic ACTH syndrome (17) and a patient with invasive lobular carcinoma of the breast with ectopic ACTH syndrome (18). ACTH produced ectopically appears to be identical with pituitary-derived ACTH. In patients with oat cell carcinomas, the physical characteristics usually seen with adrenal hypercorticism (moon facies, plethora, acne, buffalo hump, centripetal obesity, purple skin striae) are generally absent. Instead, the predominant findings are hypokalemia and metabolic alkalosis, proximal myopathy, hyperglycemia, edema and hypertension, and, less often, hyperpigmentation. The most frequent symptom is weakness. The diagnosis is often suspected when unexplained and persistent hypokalemia is detected in a patient with oat cell carcinoma of the lung, especially if the patient also has hyperglycemia and proximal muscle weakness. In patients with ectopic ACTH syndrome due to other tumors the clinical features of Cushing's syndrome may or may not be present. The ectopic ACTH syndrome is characterized by elevated serum cortisol and ACTH levels with loss of diurnal variation. In general, morning cortisol levels cannot be suppressed after 48 hours of treatment with 2 mg of dexamethasone every six hours. Regression of oat cell carcinoma due to chemotherapy or radiotherapy will cause remission of the syndrome, as will surgical removal of other tumors associated with ectopic ACTH production. Symptomatic control of the syndrome has been achieved with drugs such as metapyrone, aminoglutethimide, and o′,p′-DDD (mitotane), which produce adrenal insufficiency necessitating the administration of exogenous adrenal steroids, and with adrenalectomy.

It has been shown that all histologic variants of lung cancer contain a compound that is immunoreactive with ACTH (19). This compound has also been detected in the plasma of these patients, in the tissues and plasma of patients with nonpulmonary tumors, and in the lungs and plasma of patients with chronic obstructive pulmonary disease (20,21). The compound is a polypeptide precursor of ACTH, a prohormone that contains ACTH, MSH, and other biologically active peptides. The presence of so-called "big ACTH" in tissues and plasma is not associated with the clinical syndrome of ectopic ACTH.

Hyperkalemia

Hyperkalemia is most often due to impaired renal excretion of potassium. Hyperkalemia may result from severe volume contraction, intrinsic renal disorders, or obstructive uropathy. Excessive potassium administration, especially in patients with impaired renal function or volume depletion, may produce potassium intoxication. Hyperkalemia may also follow massive tissue destruction (rhabdomyolysis, tumor lysis due to therapy). Other causes include potassium sparing diuretics, metabolic acidosis, and adrenal cortical insufficiency. Manifestations may include weakness, paresthesias, flaccid paralysis, confusion, and lethargy. Cardiac manifestations are often the predominant evidences of hyperkalemia. The EKG demonstrates tall, peaked T waves and PR and QRS widening, which may progress to cardiac arrest. Hyperkalemia should be treated in the absence of symptoms if the serum potassium level exceeds 6 mEq/liter, because of the danger of cardiac arrest. Immediate treatment measures include the injection of 25–50 g of glucose as a 10% or 50% solution in the first half-hour with 10–20 U of insulin to move potassium intracellularly. Additional glucose can be given more slowly as a 10% infusion with 20 U of insulin per liter. Acidosis should be corrected with sodium bicarbonate infusion. Calcium gluconate should be given intravenously as a 10% solution, 10–25 cc, during the first few minutes of treatment to counteract the effects of potassium on the myocardium. Removal of potassium from the body can often be accomplished with Kayexalate, a polystyrene cation exchange resin in the sodium cycle. This may be administered orally, 20–30 g at 6–8 hour intervals, in a 100–150 ml solution of 20% sorbitol (to prevent resin-induced constipation), or as a sorbitol enema in patients who cannot be treated orally. Hemodialysis may be required in some patients, as in those with renal failure, for continuing therapy.

Calcium Disorders

Hypercalcemia

Cancer is by far the most common cause of hypercalcemia. In addition to being a frequent problem, hypercalcemia is often sufficiently serious to be considered a medical emergency that mandates prompt and vigorous treatment. Hypercalcemia occurs predominantly in patients with bone metastases, but in approximately 10–15% of cases metastases are not evident (22). The tumors that commonly metastasize to bone are cancers of the lung, breast, prostate, kidney, and thyroid and multiple myeloma. However, bone involvement may occur with tumors of almost any primary site and is not uncommon in cancers of the head and neck, esophagus, gastrointestinal tract, bladder, ovary and adrenal, in Hodgkin's disease, non-Hodgkin's lymphomas, and acute leukemia. The highest incidences of hypercalcemia have been noted in patients with myeloma, breast cancer, and epidermoid lung cancer. Since breast cancer and lung cancer are so common, they account for the majority of cases. However, hypercalcemia can occur with almost any tumor metastatic to bone, particularly when the metastases are osteolytic. There is no obvious correlation with the extent of bone metastases and the development of hypercalcemia. The rate of bone destruction and calcium release into the serum is probably a major determinant of hypercalcemia. Myeloma (23) and lymphoma (24) cells elaborate a peptide, first extracted from leukocytes, that stimulates osteoclast proliferation and bone resorption when these cells are incubated with bone in vitro. This peptide, called osteoclast-activating factor (OAF), may contribute to the bone destruction and hypercalcemia caused by these tumor cells as they lie in proximity to bone.

Hypercalcemia in patients without bone metastases is generally considered to be a paraneoplastic syndrome; there is ectopic production of a compound by the tumor that is released into the blood and increases the removal of calcium from bone. Ectopic parathyroid hormone (PTH) and ectopic prostaglandin (PG) are two substances that appear to account for some of these cases of hypercalcemia. Immunoreactive PTH has been demonstrated in the plasma of many patients with hypercalcemia and in tumor extracts (25,26). Many tumors have been shown to synthesize immunoreactive PTH. However, serum PTH and serum calcium concentrations in cancer patients often do not bear the same relationship as they do in primary hyperparathyroidism, in that PTH levels are usually much higher in primary hyperparathyroidism (22). There is some disagreement as to whether ectopic PTH is identical with pure bovine PTH. The percentage of hypercalcemic cancer patients with elevated serum PTH levels also varies with the type of immunoassay. If a patient with cancer has hypercalcemia and an elevated serum PTH level, this may be due to primary hyperparathyroidism rather than ectopic PTH. In fact, patients may have both conditions simultaneously. Ectopic PTH probably accounts for many cases of hypercalcemia without bone metastases. Several types of evidence (27) could help confirm ectopic PTH production as the basis for hypercalcemia in patients with elevated serum PTH concentrations, such as reduction in PTH and calcium levels with reduction of tumor burden and the converse, an increased concentration of PTH in the tumor venous effluent, a lack of an arteriovenous PTH gradient across the parathyroid glands, identification of high concentrations of PTH in tumor tissue, and synthesis of PTH by tumor cells. However, while such types of evidence have been obtained in a few carefully studied cases, most physicians have neither the facilities nor the expertise to conduct such investigations. In most clinical settings hypercalcemia in a cancer patient, coupled with a low or normal serum phosphate and an elevated serum PTH, in the absence of metastases, suggests ectopic PTH production. If reduction of tumor burden lowers the serum calcium and PTH, the diagnosis is probably correct.

There is evidence of ectopic PG synthesis by several animal tumors (22). These tumors produce large amounts of PGE_2 in association with osteolytic metastases and hypercalcemia. Treatment of animals with these tumors with aspirin or indomethacin, inhibitors of PG synthesis, prevents the development of bone metastases and hypercalcemia. Thus, PG production by these tumors appears to play a role not only in the development of hypercalcemia, but in the establishment of metastases. A related observation has been made in women with breast cancer. High in vitro osteolytic activity of primary breast cancers that could be blocked by PG synthesis inhibitors appears to correlate with the subsequent development of bone metastases. Increased secretion of PG in the urine has been found in breast cancer patients with bone metastases compared to those without bone metastases. Elevated plasma PG concentrations have been reported in some hypercalcemic cancer patients compared to cancer patients without hypercalcemia. The excretion of a PGE_2 metabolite was found to be greatly increased in the urine of patients with hypercalcemia and solid tumors compared to its excretion to normal subjects or in patients with hypercalcemia due to primary hyperparathyroidism or hematologic tumors (28). There are several reports of improvement in hypercalcemic patients treated with indomethacin, although this is a variably effective form of treatment. All of these observations suggest a role of PG in hypercalcemia and possibly in the establishment of bone metastases. However, as with ectopic PTH synthesis, ectopic PG production can only be implicated in some patients. Undoubtedly, other factors will be found to play a role in cancer-related hypercalcemia.

Hypercalcemia is related to the primary neoplasm in the vast majority of cancer patients. As mentioned earlier, primary hyperparathyroidism is an uncommon cause of hypercalcemia in these patients. Even less common are other causes of hypercalcemia that may be observed in the general population, for example, sarcoidosis, milk-alkali syndrome, thiazide use, thyrotoxicosis, and renal disease with secondary hyperparathyroidism. Immobilization resulting from fractures or paraplegia may occasionally result in hypercalcemia, especially in patients with extensive osteolytic disease, such as multiple myeloma.

As with other metabolic abnormalities, the clinical manifestations of hypercalcemia appear to depend upon the rate of its development as well as the level of the serum calcium. We have observed asymptomatic patients with serum calcium concentrations above 15 mg% and profoundly symptomatic patients with serum concentrations in the range of 12–13 mg%. In the former instances hypercalcemia developed slowly and represented a fairly chronic state, whereas it developed acutely in the other patients. Major manifestations of the syndrome are gastrointestinal, renal, neurologic, and cardiovascular dysfunction. Gastrointestinal symptoms include anorexia, nausea, vomiting, constipation, and abdominal discomfort. While this nonspecific constellation is common in cancer patients, it should trigger inquiry regarding other symptoms of hypercalcemia when the symptoms have no obvious basis, such as chemotherapy, radiation therapy, or bowel obstruction. Renal symptoms are initially due to hypercalcemia, which initiates polyuria, and, secondarily, polydypsia. This "calcinuric diabetes" results from a direct effect of calcium on the renal tubule, possibly through inhibition of formation of cAMP, which is manifested as an impairment of urine concentrating ability. Volume contraction from renal losses is potentiated by anorexia, decreased fluid intake, and vomiting and leads to azotemia and progressive renal insufficiency. Hypokalemia and alkalosis are often present.

Neurologic symptoms of weakness, lethargy, somnolence, personality change, and stupor that may proceed to coma often dominate the clinical picture. Such symptoms may develop insidiously or within a relatively few hours.

Cardiac symptoms are unusual, but electrocardiographic changes, such as shortening of the QT interval, prolongation of the PR interval, T-wave inversion, and arrhythmias, may occur. These problems are more common with high serum calcium concentrations. Digitalis toxicity may be precipitated in patients receiving this drug who become hypercalcemic. Digitalis administration in patients with hypercalcemia may produce cardiac arrest. In some patients hypercalcemia produces hypertension.

The treatment of hypercalcemia is directed at reduction of the serum calcium level, removal of precipitating and contributory causes, and reduction of tumor burden. In most instances, hypercalcemia is related primarily to tumor progression. Hormonal therapy in breast cancer is the precipitating cause in some patients, particularly in the first few weeks after treatment is instituted. Some reports indicate that in some patients it is possible to treat the hypercalcemia, continue hormone therapy, and eventually achieve a hormonally induced remission. We have had great difficulty in controlling the serum calcium levels in patients when this approach has been used and have only rarely achieved remission. Consequently, it is our practice to permanently discontinue the hormonal agent that precipitated hypercalcemia. Thiazide diuretic therapy should also be discontinued in hypercalcemic patients. It is unlikely that a low calcium diet has a role in therapy, since the symptomatic patient is not eating and the hypercalcemia primarily is due to calcium derived from bone. When the patient is able to eat, we do not restrict the diet (unlike the situation in milk-alkali syndrome). Our approach to the treatment of patients with symptomatic hypercalcemia or of asymptomatic patients with serum calcium levels above 15 mg% is basically that recommended by Suki et al. (29) at our institution. Sufficient isotonic saline is administered intravenously to restore vascular volume, and furosemide is then administered intravenously every one to two hours to effect a forced diuresis. This results in a significant outpouring of urinary calcium. It is critical to rehydrate the patient with saline before injection of furosemide or renal function and hypercalcemia may be worsened by diuretic-induced volume contraction. When a diuresis is established, the saline infusion rate is matched to the urinary output on an hourly basis. Serum calcium, sodium, potassium, and magnesium levels are monitored frequently, as are vital signs, neck veins, lung bases, and sensorial status. Potassium and magnesium are replaced as needed. Magnesium supplementation is usually not required during the first 24 hours of forced diuresis. It is essential to avoid either volume overload or volume contraction. Once the serum calcium has fallen below 12 mg%, which usually takes 24–48 hours, saline is used to maintain hydration and furosemide is administered only in the event of fluid overload or if the calcium begins to rise rapidly. Sensorial changes may persist for several days after correction of the serum calcium. In the event that the serum calcium again increases, other approaches are also used, since forced diuresis is designed primarily for emergency treatment and is a difficult program to maintain. Most often we administer mithramycin in this circumstance. In patients who have previously demonstrated this series of events, mithramycin may be administered when forced diuresis is initiated. Mithramycin is given as an intravenous infusion over one to two hours in a dose of 15–25 µg/kg of body weight (1–2 mg). If this causes undue nausea and vomiting, subsequent infusions are given more slowly. Treatment may require repetition if the serum calcium has not decreased appreciably after 48 hours. Occasionally, a single dose of the drug may normalize the calcium level for weeks (30). Some patients can develop marked hypocalcemia. If mithramycin therapy is required repeatedly for control of hypercalcemia, it is essential to monitor the blood counts, the serum calcium, liver and renal function, and coagulation factors frequently. Despite such monitoring, toxicity may occur precipitously and can be fatal, that is, myelosuppression, hepatic or renal damage, multiple clotting disorders, and hemorrhagic phenomena that may be due to vascular damage. These severe toxicities are unusual with the low doses of mithramycin used to treat hypercalcemia, particularly if only one to three doses are administered initially and subsequent doses are required no more often than once weekly.

Adrenal corticosteroids may be effective in hypercalcemia therapy, particularly in patients with breast or prostatic cancer, myeloma, lymphoma, or leukemia. Corticosteroids may be of benefit in these situations because of a direct antitumor activity, diminution of gastrointestinal calcium absorption, increased renal calcium excretion, or inhibition of OAF. The problems of chronic therapy with corticosteroids and the variability in their efficacy limit the usefulness of these drugs. Indomethacin therapy is also of unpredictable efficacy. We reserve its use for asymptomatic hypercalcemic patients with serum levels below 13 mg%, in whom a short trial can be undertaken without jeopardy.

In most instances, when the serum calcium has fallen below 11 mg% and the patient can retain oral fluids, maintenance treatment is begun with oral phosphate solutions and appropriate antitumor therapy is instituted. If the latter is effective, phosphate solutions may be discontinued. We do not use intravenous phosphate solutions because of the potential complications of intravascular and metastatic calcification and of sudden, severe hypocalcemia. Intravenous sodium sulfate therapy has no advantage over forced diuresis and decreases the serum calcium more slowly, in our experience. Administration of calcitonin may reduce the serum calcium within several hours, and this drug can be used as a supplement to forced diuresis in the initial treatment of severely hypercalcemic patients. However, its effects are not predictable, and its efficacy often is diminished with repeated injections.

Hypocalcemia

Asymptomatic hypocalcemia is frequently noted in patients with osteoblastic bone metastases. Spontaneous tetany or other symptomatology is rare. We have observed one patient who developed profound hypocalcemia and seizures following initiation of chemotherapy, presumably as a result of rapid uptake of calcium by lytic bone metastases responding to treatment. This patient had skin metastases that decreased in size rapidly at the same time. Large quantities of intravenous calcium gluconate were required for several days until the serum calcium concentration was stabilized in the normal range.

Acid–Base Disorders

Acidosis

The common causes of acidosis in the general population are also common in cancer patients. Diabetic ketoacidosis may occur not only in patients with preexisting diabetes mellitus, but in those with pancreatic replacement by tumor. In patients with diabetes ketoacidosis may be precipitated by ACTH or cortisol-producing tumors and adrenal corticosteroid therapy. In the nondiabetic, however, corticosteroid excesses from any of these causes generally result in hyperglycemia, hypokalemia, and alkalosis. Metabolic acidosis may also be a consequence of preexisting renal disease (chronic renal insufficiency, renal tubular acidosis, Fanconi syndrome), of renal insufficiency related to cancer (see Chapter 3), and of excessive losses of alkaline intestinal secretions (diarrhea, fistulas). Other causes of metabolic acidosis include lactic acidosis and intoxications with salicylates, ethanol, methanol, ethylene glycol, or paraldehyde.

Lactic acidosis is most often due to severe tissue hypoxia secondary to shock, but may also occur in the absence of hypoxemia or hypotension in diabetic ketoacidosis, hepatic insufficiency, renal insufficiency, after the ingestion of oral hypoglycemic agents or of toxins that produce anion gap acidosis (methyl alcohol, ethylene glycol), and in some forms of cancer. In the cancer patient dehydration, hemorrhage, and septicemia are probably the most frequent causes of shock, although cardiogenic shock is not rare. Severe tissue hypoxia results in a shift to anaerobic glycolysis with the generation of large amounts of lactate. The normal liver has the capacity to metabolize this lactate. The development of lactic acidosis in hypoxemia states reflects diminished hepatic blood flow, impaired hepatic function, or a combination of these deficits. A small increase in serum lactate concentration in diabetic ketoacidosis is generally of little importance. Severe lactic acidosis in the patient with ketoacidosis has a dire prognosis and often is due to concomitant hypovolemic shock, renal insufficiency, myocardial infarction, or extreme acidosis. Rarely, patients with leukemia, lymphomas, and solid tumors may have lactic acidosis due to increased lactate production by these neoplasms, generally in association with some impairment of liver function.

Respiratory acidosis in cancer patients most often is due to preexisting chronic obstructive pulmonary disease. Respiratory depression and acidosis from opiates and other drugs is not uncommon in this group of patients. It may also result from central nervous system tumors. Acute respiratory obstruction and acidosis due to tumors, secretions, and improperly placed airways are less common causes.

The symptoms and signs of metabolic acidosis vary with cause, severity, and duration. The most consistent finding is hyperventilation and even this may not be evident clinically. Weakness, thirst, polyuria, anorexia, nausea, vomiting, abdominal pain, somnolence, confusion, and coma are variable findings. The underlying problems (uremia, dehydration, hypotension, sepsis, hemorrhage, shock) may overshadow the clinical picture. Acute respiratory acidosis may be suspected in patients with depressed ventilation due to drugs or central nervous system disorders. Chronic respiratory acidosis often can be anticipated from the history and physical examination.

The diagnosis of acidosis and its etiology are established on the basis of history, physical examination, and laboratory studies that include arterial pH, Pa_{O_2}, Pa_{CO_2}, serum electrolytes, BUN, creatinine, glucose, and ketones. In patients with a wide anion gap, metabolic acidosis unaccounted for by diabetes, drug or other intoxications, or renal failure, lactic acidosis should be suspected and serum lactate should be determined.

The treatment of metabolic and respiratory acidosis is dependent upon the cause and is well described in many standard texts. Lactic acidosis in cancer patients, when due to tissue hypoxia, requires urgent efforts to restore circulatory volume, correct hypoxia, and reverse the underlying cause. In addition, the administration of sodium bicarbonate intravenously is often essential for partial correction of the severe acidosis and reduction of serum lactate concentration. Several hundred milliequivalents of bicarbonate may be required. The prognosis is primarily dependent on the rapidity with which the underlying disorders are recognized and treated. The overwhelming majority of patients in shock with lactic acidosis do not survive. Lactic acidosis due to tumor and anaerobic glycosis is a less urgent problem and may resolve with reduction of the tumor burden by appropriate antitumor therapy.

Alkalosis

The common causes of metabolic alkalosis in cancer patients are loss of hydrogen ions from the stomach due to vomiting or nasogastric suction, extracellular volume contraction from any cause, and diuretic therapy. Ectopic ATCH production, adrenal corticosteroid therapy, Cushing's syndrome, WDHA, and primary aldosteronism are far less frequent causes of alkalosis. Metabolic alkalosis is often asymptomatic or the symptoms and signs may primarily reflect hypokalemia. The finding of an elevated arterial pH and serum bicarbonate, often accompanied by hypokalemia, establishes the diagnosis.

Treatment consists of correction of dehydration, usually with isotonic saline, and the administration of potassium chloride to repair deficits of potassium. In severe alkalosis, intravenous administration of $0.15\ N$ hydrochloric acid or arginine hydrochloride may be required. Adrenal corticosteroids, indomethacin, or lithium carbonate may ameliorate WDHA.

Respiratory alkalosis is the result of a variety of processes that produce excessive ventilation and hypocapnia. Anxiety is a frequent cause in cancer patients. Other causes are hypoxemia (pulmonary embolus, lymphangitic pulmonary metastases), fever, central nervous system disease, salicylate poisoning, and hepatic coma. Symptoms may include circumoral paresthesias, numbness and paresthesias of the extremities, and faintness. Carpal pedal spasms and tetany may be observed. The diagnosis is established by documenting an elevated arterial pH and a low arterial Pa_{CO_2} Treatment is directed at the cause of hyperventilation.

HYPERURICEMIA

In the general population hyperuricemia is usually attributable to primary gout, psoriasis, starvation or reducing diets, impaired renal function, hemodialysis, or drugs such as aspirin in low doses and thiazide diuretics. Cancer patients may have hyperuricemia for the above reasons, but also as a consequence of increased nucleotide turnover related to the proliferation and spontaneous death of neoplastic cells, massive destruction of neoplastic cells by cancer chemotherapeutic agents or radiation therapy, or diminished renal function consequent to cancer. Hyperuricemia due to increased cell proliferation and cell death is common in patients with acute and chronic leukemia, Hodgkin's disease, non-Hodgkin's lymphomas, multiple myeloma, polycythemia vera, testicular neoplasms, and oat cell carcinoma, and it occurs occasionally with other solid tumors. The turnover of cells releases nuclear proteins that are degraded to nucleotides and to free bases. The purine basis hypoxanthine, xanthine, and adenine are partially reutilized by resynthesis to nucleotides (salvage pathway) and partially degraded to uric acid. The body pools of nucleotides, purines, and uric acid are increased in patients with rapidly growing neoplasms. Hyperuricemia occurs when the renal clearance of uric acid is exceeded. In chronic myelogenous leukemia, polycythemia vera, and myeloid metaplasia, hyperuricemia is often chronic. Patients with these disorders may experience acute gouty arthritis, tophaceous gout, uric acid ureteral stones, and gouty renal disease, thereby resembling patients with primary gout. The local factors that cause deposition of sodium urate in tissues are not known in secondary or primary gout. Unlike patients with myeloproliferative disorders, in the majority of cancer patients with hyperuricemia the condition is asymptomatic. Occasionally, it is the cause of renal insufficiency, usually of mild degree, but severe renal failure may occur. Dehydration may be a contributory factor in some cases. Hyperuricemia due to renal insufficiency from pre- and postrenal as well as direct renal causes (Chapter 3) is common in cancer patients. Such hyperuricemia is in keeping with the etiology and degree of renal insufficiency. The most serious uric acid problem in cancer patients is iatrogenic acute hyperuricemia that results in uric acid nephropathy, a consequence of massive destruction of tumor cells by chemotherapeutic drugs or radiation. This syndrome has been most frequently encountered in patients with leukemias, lymphomas, and myeloma, rapidly proliferating neoplasms that are highly responsive to the destructive effects of drugs and radiation. Prior hyperuricemia is not essential to the development of this problem, but should serve to caution the physician to observe prophylactic measures. Sudden elevation of the concentration of serum uric acid increases its concentration in urine to the point where its solubility is exceeded and it precipitates in the renal tubules and collecting ducts and even in the ureters. Crystallization of uric acid is enhanced by a low urine pH and low urine volume. The consequence of this process is acute renal failure. Its diagnosis is generally obvious, that is, acute renal failure in a cancer patient (usually with leukemia, lymphoma, or myeloma) who has recently received chemotherapy and whose serum uric acid level is disproportionately elevated.

The treatment of chronic hyperuricemia in cancer patients is to reduce the production of uric acid by administration of allopurinol (31,32). This drug inhibits the enzyme xanthine oxidase, which catalyzes the conversion of hypoxanthine to xanthine and of xanthine to uric acid. Serum and urine concentrations of these precursors rise as uric acid concentrations fall. Allopurinol and its metabolite, oxipurinol, also appear in the urine. Reutilization of hypoxanthine and xanthine for nucleotide and nucleic acid synthesis (salvage) is increased when their oxidation is blocked by allopurinol. Since xanthine and hypoxanthine are more soluble than uric acid, these bases do not crystallize in the urine and they pass through the kidney without difficulty. When the concentration of uric acid is markedly reduced, nephropathy is avoided. Nephropathy due to uric acid precursors is rare.

Acute uric acid nephropathy is essentially a preventable disorder. Patients at risk for its development should be treated prophylactically with allopurinol to reduce their serum uric acid concentrations before chemotherapy. In addition, adequate hydration to provide a urine output of two or more liters daily and urine alkalinization to increase the solubility of uric acid will minimize the likelihood of uric acid precipitation in the kidney. Allopurinol is generally given in daily doses of 300–600 mg orally. Alkalinization can be accomplished with the administration of sodium bicarbonate orally or intravenously. Allopurinol, diuresis, and alkalinization are also used in the treatment of uric acid nephropathy. Allopurinol dosage should be reduced in patients with renal insufficiency since the drug and its metabolite are excreted only by the kidney. Fluid challenge and alkalinization should be undertaken carefully to avoid acute volume overload. Hemodialysis may be necessary in patients who fail to respond to these measures. The dosage of thiopurines must be reduced in patients receiving allopurinol since these agents are catabolized by xanthine oxidase. Some of the adverse reactions to allopurinol include rashes that vary from mild maculopapular eruptions to severe exfoliative reactions and Stevens-Johnson syndrome, gastrointestinal reactions, hepatic injury, renal insufficiency, vasculitis, marrow suppression, peripheral neuritis, and drug idiosyncrasy.

GLUCOSE DISORDERS

Hyperglycemia

Hyperglycemia in cancer most frequently reflects preexisting diabetes mellitus; diabetes may also occur as an unrelated phenomenon at any time after a patient develops cancer. Relative insulin resistance and postprandial hyperglycemia may be noted in patients with anorexia-cachexia syndrome. Hyperglycemia may also be due to replacement of the pancreas by tumor, surgical resection of the pancreas, ectopic ACTH production, adrenal adenomas and carcinomas, pituitary Cushing's disease, exogenous steroid therapy, glucagonoma, pheochromocytoma, VIPoma, somatostatinoma, and diuretic therapy. Hyperglycemia may be asymptomatic or may be associated with the various syndromes of diabetes (thirst, polyuria, dehydration; nonketotic hyperosmolar coma; ketoacidosis).

The etiology of hyperglycemia can often be determined easily based upon the history (i.e., prior diabetes, obvious pancreatic exocrine cancer or pancreatic resection for cancer, exogenous steroid administration, diuretic therapy). Physical findings of typical cushingoid features and other components of Cushing's syndrome in patients who have not received corticosteroid therapy suggest the presence of pituitary Cushing's disease or an adrenal tumor. Hyperglycemia accompanied by hypokalemia and metabolic alkalosis without the usual cushingoid features (moon facies, fat redistribution) suggests ectopic ACTH production, as does proximal muscle weakness, edema, and hyperpigmentation. Sustained or intermittent hypertension, palpitation, tachycardia, and excessive sweating in a patient with hyperglycemia may denote the presence of a pheochromocytoma. Patients with glucagonoma often have a distinctive rash (necrolytic migratory erythema) and elevated serum glucagon levels (33). Hyperglycemia is an incidental finding in patients with VIPomas; the clinical picture is dominated by the syndrome of watery diarrhea (34). The diagnosis of somatostatinoma requires demonstration of a pancreatic tumor that has high levels of somatostatin on immunoassay and no evidence of glucagon production (35).

Insulin may be required for the treatment of symptomatic hyperglycemia. If hyperglycemia is due to a tumor, it will be ameliorated by effective tumor therapy. The management of ectopic ACTH syndrome has been discussed earlier in this chapter.

Hypoglycemia

Hypoglycemia in cancer patients, as in the general population, most commonly occurs in diabetics as a result of a relative excess of exogenously administered insulin. The regulated diabetic who develops cancer may become more difficult to control as a result of anorexia, easy satiety, gastrointestinal problems, infections, and other disorders related to cancer and cancer therapy. Loss of regulation may lead to both hyperglycemic and hypoglycemic episodes. The sulfonylureas may cause severe hypoglycemia in patients who are not eating. Alcoholism is another disorder that may induce hypoglycemia, and alcohol intoxication is not unusual in cancer patients. Hypoglycemia that is a specific consequence of cancer is most frequently due to functioning β-cell tumors of the pancreas, insulinomas. These may occur independently or as part of the MEA I syndrome. Malignant functioning islet cell tumors constitute approximately 10% of the total. Patients with insulinomas have fasting hypoglycemia with elevated levels of immunoreactive plasma insulin and, generally, of proinsulin (36). Since the β cells normally produce insulin, hypoglycemia due to tumors of these cells is not unanticipated. As yet unresolved is the cause of hypoglycemia associated with a variety of nonislet cell tumors. These are usually bulky neoplasms. More than half of them are of mesenchymal origin (fibrosarcomas, neurogenic sarcomas, fibromas, mesotheliomas, hemangiopericytomas, leiomyosarcomas), 21% are hepatocellular carcinomas, 6% are adrenal carcinomas, and the remainder include many tumor types (e.g., lymphomas, gastrointestinal cancers, pheochromocytomas) (37). These tumors do not produce immunoreactive insulin. Several studies suggest that hypoglycemia in patients with these tumors is due to their elaboration into the plasma of growth factors with insulin-like activity that is not suppressed by insulin antibodies. These factors have been collectively referred to as nonsuppressible insulin-like activity (NSILA). Purification of this material has led to the recognition and structural identification of two substances, insulin-like growth factors I and II (IGF I and IGF II) (38). A number of techniques have been employed to measure these substances in the plasma. The results of some investigators suggesting that hypoglycemia due to bulky nonpancreatic tumors can be related to high plasma levels of IGF-like materials (39) have not been confirmed by other investigators (40). Until the technological problems can be resolved, the relationship between these substances and tumor hypoglycemia remains uncertain. It may well be that the syndrome is due to heterogeneous causes. There is no convincing evidence that excessive utilization of glucose by these tumors causes hypoglycemia. Massive replacement of the liver by tumor and ectopic production of a glucagon inhibitor have also been proposed as etiologies in several cases of tumor hypoglycemia.

Hypoglycemia is generally manifested by behavioral changes, confusion, stupor, and loss of consciousness. Focal neurologic findings may dominate the clinical presentations; often these change repeatedly over a short time span. These symptoms and signs are usually reversed by glucose administration, but permanent neurologic damage may occur. The symptomatology of hypoglyce-mia due to insulin overdosage may be that of sympathetic discharge (tachycardia, anxiety, diaphoresis, tremulousness, hunger). This may also be observed post-prandially in patients who have had gastrectomies. Tumor hypoglycemia usually occurs during fasting or after physical activity, rather than postprandially.

If a patient is suspected of having a hypoglycemic episode, a blood sample is drawn for glucose determination and 50 cc of 50% glucose is usually injected intravenously over a few minutes time and followed by an infusion of 5% glucose. If the diagnosis of hypoglycemia is subsequently confirmed by the blood glucose determination, further treatment will depend upon the underlying cause. The chronic therapy of tumor hypoglycemia can prove difficult. Some patients may benefit from frequent small feedings. Multiple injections of long-acting glucagon can be of value. High doses of glucocorticosteroids may help sustain normal or elevated blood glucose concentrations, but may also inflict upon patients the problems of hypercorticism. Effective treatment of the underlying tumor re-solves the problem of hypoglycemia. This is often accomplished by surgical removal of benign islet cell tumors. Treatment of the bulky nonpancreatic neo-plasms usually associated with hypoglycemia is often ineffective. Partial resection of masses, radiation therapy, and chemotherapy may be beneficial temporarily.

FEVER

Fever is common in cancer patients. In most instances it is due to underlying infection, particularly if a thorough search is conducted for an infectious etiology. Cancer patients are often immunoincompetent, and the degree of impaired immune response often reflects the clinical stage of the cancer. Anergy is com-mon in advanced cancer, even in the absence of malnutrition. The latter may contribute to impaired immunocompetence, as discussed earlier in this chapter. The obstruction by tumors of structures with lumens such as bronchi, ureters, and bile ducts, thereby inhibiting their drainage, provides an excellent setting for infection. Ulcerations of the oral mucosa, gastrointestinal tract, and skin serve as portals of entry for microorganisms. Surgery, chemotherapy, radiation therapy, and administration of adrenocorticosteroids may further depress im-munologic reactivity. Granulocytopenia secondary to chemotherapy, radiation therapy, or myelophthisis also reduces the defenses against infectious diseases. In the compromised host bacterial infections with the usual aerobic and anaerobic bacteria are frequent, as are infections with viruses, parasites, and opportunistic organisms. Such infectious causes of fever may only be uncovered after extensive evaluations that may include tissue biopsies, viral serological and cultural tech-niques, special stains and electron microscopy, in addition to the commonly used cultural techniques and serological studies. Careful attention must be paid to areas such as the nasal sinuses, the central nervous system, the perirectal tissues, the subdiaphragmatic region, and the pelvis, in additon to the common sites of infection. In some patients fever cannot be related to infections, is not caused by drugs, and appears to be due solely to tumor.

Tumors that have a propensity for causing pyrexia are Hodgkin's disease, non-Hodgkin's lymphomas, acute leukemias, hypernephromas, hepatomas, carcinomas of the stomach and pancreas, osteogenic sarcomas, myxomas, and tumors that have metastasized to the liver. Many other types of tumors have on occasion been associated with fever. Marantic endocarditis may also cause fever and embolic phenomena and occasionally can be diagnosed by echocardiography. The etiologic relationship between a tumor and fever can be established if the fever subsides with removal or regression of the tumor and recurs with tumor progression, in the absence of evidences of infection.

Tumor fever may assume almost any course. It may be chronic, low grade and unremitting, high and spiking in association with sweats, chills, and leukocytosis, or it may be present for several days or weeks with interspersed afebrile periods, as in some patients with Hodgkin's disease (Pel-Epstein fever). The cause of tumor fever is unknown. A variety of mechanisms have been invoked. Many studies suggest that tumor fever is related in some way to release of endogenous pyrogen from leukocytes, tumor cells, and other tissues. Fever in Hodgkin's disease has been blocked by cycloheximide, an inhibitor of protein synthesis. This suggests that a tissue-synthesized molecule caused the fever, but does not indicate the tissue source of the pyrogenic molecule.

Antipyretics, such as aspirin and acetaminophen, may be used in the symptomatic treatment of tumor pyrexia. These drugs may cause diaphoresis and are variably effective. Adrenocorticosteroids have been beneficial in some patients. In our experience the most effective agent for control of tumor fever has been indomethacin. In a dose of 25 mg at six to eight hour intervals, this drug usually causes defervescence without diaphoresis within 24 hours. Tumor resection or effective tumor regression induced by drugs or radiation therapy generally results in subsidence of tumor fever.

REFERENCES

1. Davis JD, Levine W: A model for the control of ingestion. *Psychol Rev* 84:379, 1977.
2. Theologides A: Cancer cachexia. *Cancer* 43:2004, 1979.
3. Costa G, Donaldson SS: Current concepts in cancer: Effects of cancer and cancer treatment on the nutrition of the host. *N Engl J Med* 300:1471, 1979.
4. DeWys WD: Anorexia as a general effect of cancer. *Cancer* 43:2013, 1979.
5. Schein PS, Kisner D, Haller D, et al: Cachexia of malignancy: Potential role of insulin in nutritional management. *Cancer* 43:2070, 1979.
6. Waterhouse C: How tumors affect host metabolism. *Ann NY Acad Sci* 184:610, 1974.
7. Daly JM, Dudrick SJ, Copeland EM III: Evaluation of nutritional indices as prognostic indicators in the cancer patient. *Cancer* 43:925, 1979.
8. Copeland EM III, Daly JM, Oto DM, et al: Nutrition, cancer, and intravenous hyperalimentation. *Cancer* 43:2108, 1979.
9. Schwartz WB, Bennett W, Curelop S, et al: A syndrome of renal sodium loss and hyponatremia probably resulting from inappropriate secretion of antidiuretic hormone. *Am J Med* 23:529, 1957.
10. Schwartz WB, Tassel D, Bartter FC: Further observations on hyponatremia and renal sodium loss probably resulting from inappropriate secretion of antidiuretic hormone. *N Engl J Med* 262:743, 1960.

11. Bartter FC, Schwartz WB: The syndrome of inappropriate secretion of antidiuretic hormone. *Am J Med* 23:790, 1967.

12. Ginsberg S, Comis R, Miller M: Syndrome of inappropriate antidiuretic hormone secretion in oat cell carcinoma of the lung. *Am Fed Clin Res* 435A, 1978.

13. DeTroyer A: Demeclocyline treatment for syndrome of inappropriate antidiuretic hormone secretion. *JAMA* 237:2823, 1977.

14. Decaux G, Brimioulle S, Genette F, et al: Treatment of the syndrome of inappropriate secretion of antidiuretic hormone by urea. *Am J Med* 69:99, 1980.

15. Hautman D, Rossier B, Zohlman R, et al: Rapid correction of hyponatremia in the syndrome of inappropriate secretion of antidiuretic hormone. *Ann Intern Med* 78: 870, 1973.

16. Liddle GW, Givens JR, Nicholson WE, et al: The ectopic ACTH syndrome. *Cancer Res* 25:1057, 1965.

17. Brown H, Lane M: Cushing's and malignant carcinoid syndromes from ovarian neoplasm. *Arch Intern Med* 115:490, 1965.

18. Cohle SD, Tschen JA, Smith FE, et al: ACTH-secreting carcinoma of the breast. *Cancer* 43:2370, 1979.

19. Yalow RS, Eastridge CE, Higgins G Jr, et al: Plasma and tumor ACTH in carcinoma of the lung. *Cancer* 44:1789, 1979.

20. Ayvazian LF, Schneider B, Gewirtz G, et al: Ectopic production of big ACTH in carcinoma of the lung: Its clinical usefulness as a biologic marker. *Am Rev Respir Dis* 111:279, 1975.

21. Wolfsen AR, Odell WD: ProACTH: Use for early detection of lung cancer. Am J Med 66:765, 1979.

22. Trump DL: Abnormalities of bone and mineral metabolism, in Abeloff MD (ed): *Complications of Cancer*. Baltimore and London, The Johns Hopkins University Press, 1979, p 263.

23. Mundy GR, Raisz LG, Cooper RE, et al: Evidence for the secretion of an osteoclast stimulating factor in myeloma. *N Engl J Med* 291:1041, 1974.

24. Mundy GR, Rick ME, Turcotte R, et al: Pathogenesis of hypercalcemia in lymphosarcoma. *Am J Med* 65:600, 1978.

25. Benson RC Jr, Riggs BL, Pickard BM, et al: Radioimmunoassay of parathyroid hormone in hypercalcemic patients with malignant disease. *Am J Med* 56:821, 1974.

26. Sherwood LM, O'Riordan JLH, Aurback GD, et al: Production of parathyroid hormone by non-parathyroid tumor. *J Clin Endocrinol Metab* 27:140, 1967.

27. Fields ALA, Josse RG, Bergsagel DE: Metabolic emergencies, in DeVita VT Jr, Hellman S, Rosenberg SA (eds): *Cancer: Principles and Practice of Oncology*. Philadelphia, Lippincott, 1982, p 1594.

28. Seyberth HW, Segre GV, Morgan JL, et al: Prostaglandins as mediators of hypercalcemia associated with certain types of cancer. *N Engl J Med* 293:1278, 1975.

29. Suki WN, Yium JJ, Von Minden M, et al: Acute treatment of hypercalcemia with furosemide. *N Engl J Med* 283:836, 1970.

30. Perlia CP, Gubisch NJ, Wolter J, et al: Mithramycin treatment of hypercalcemia. *Cancer* 25:389, 1970.

31. Krakoff IH, Meyer RL: Prevention of hyperuricemia in leukemia and lymphoma: Use of allopurinol, a xanthine oxidase inhibitor. *JAMA* 193:1, 1965.

32. De Conti RC, Calabresi P: Use of allopurinol for prevention and control of hyperuricemia in patients with neoplastic diseases. *N Engl J Med* 274: 481, 1966.

33. Higgins GA, Recant L, Fischman AB: The glucagonoma syndrome: Surgically curable diabetes. *Am J Surg* 137:142, 1979.

34. Modlin IM: Endocrine tumors of the pancreas. *Surg Gynecol Obstet* 149:751, 1979.

35. Krejs GJ, Orei L, Conlon JM, et al: Somatostatinoma syndrome: Biochemical, morphologic and clinical features. *N Engl J Med* 301:285, 1979.

36. Rubenstein AH, Kuzuya H, Horwitz DL: Clinical signficance of circulating C-peptide in diabetes and hypoglycemic disorders. *Arch Intern Med* 137:625, 1977.

37. Odell WD: Humoral manifestations of nonendocrine neoplasms: Ectopic hormone production, in Williams RH (ed): *Textbook of Endocrinology*. Philadelphia, Saunders, 1974, p 1105.
38. Zapf J, Rinderknecht E, Humbel RE, et al: Nonsuppressible insulin-like activity (NSILA) from human serum: Recent accomplishments and their physiologic implications. *Metabolism* 27:1803, 1978.
39. Gorden P, Hendricks CM, Kahn CR, et al: Hypoglycemia associated with non-islet-cell tumor and insulin-like growth factors. *N Engl J Med* 305:1452, 1981.
40. Froesch ER, Zapf J, Widmer U: Hypoglycemia associated with non-islet-cell tumor and insulin-like growth factors. *N Engl J Med* 306: 1178, 1982.

Index